Primary Care Meets Mental Health

Tools for the 21st Century

Edited by:
Joel D. Haber, Ph.D.
Grant E. Mitchell, M.D.

Foreword by:
Michael A. Freeman, M.D.

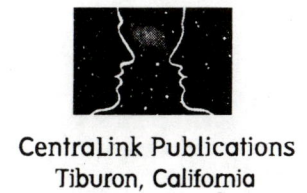

CentraLink Publications
Tiburon, California

©1997 by CentraLink Publications, 1110 Mar West Street, Suite E, Tiburon, California, 94920-1879. All rights reserved. No part of this work may be reproduced or utilized in any form by any means, electronic or mechanical, including photocopying, microfilm, and recording, or by any information storage and retrieval system, without permission in writing from the publisher.

Managing Editor: Ellen Tishman
Production: Ellen Tishman
Developmental Advisor: Marcia Byrnes
Editorial Advisor: Adam Richmond
Cover Design: Todd Crawshaw, Crawshaw Design
Interior Design: Todd Crawshaw, Crawshaw Design
Project Coordinator and Copy Editor: Cynthia Kahn
Copy Editor: Lynn Ferar
Composition: Archetype Book Composition

ISBN 1-887452-12-5

Printed in the United States of America.

This book is dedicated in loving memory to *Wilfred Haber*.

Many thanks to *Cynthia Kahn, Ellen Tishman, Marcia Byrnes, Shelley Byer,* and *CentraLink* for their time and dedication to this project. Thanks to *Paul* for support and direction in San Diego and *Bill* from MVH for guidance throughout the years.

Special appreciation to *Cindy, Scott, Alyssa, Evelyn, Rochelle,* and *Seymour* and *Mary Ellen, Michael, Alexandra, Joan, Arthur,* and *Meridith* for their unending support, patience, encouragement, and fun.

Contents

Foreword
Michael A. Freeman, M.D.   vii

Introduction
Marcia Byrnes, RN, M.P.A   x

Part I. Introduction

Chapter 1   From Fragmentation to Integration:
A History of Comprehensive Patient Care   3
Don R. Lipsitt, M.D.

Chapter 2   Integration of Primary Care and Behavioral Health:
The Driving Forces   13
David R. Selden, ACSW, LICSW

Chapter 3   The Roles of the Behavioral Health Professional in
Integrated Systems   27
Keith Dixon, Ph.D.

Part II. Barriers to Integration

Chapter 4   Overcoming Ecological Barriers to Integration   35
Carol L. Alter, M.D.
Steven Cole, M.D.
Mary Raju, RN, M.S.N.

Chapter 5   How to Structure the Financing of an Integrated
System/Medical Cost Offset Model   47
Stephen P. Melek, FSA, MAAA

Part III. Successful Models of Integration

Chapter 6   Building Partnerships of Lasting Value in Healthcare:
The Blue Cross and Blue Shield/Raytheon Collaboration   59
Nancy Langman-Dorwart, M.S., M.P.H.
Elizabeth Gatti, Psy.D.
Diane Duval

Chapter 7	The Integration Experience in a Group Model HMO: Northern California Kaiser-Permanente *Robin Dea, M.D.*	75
Chapter 8	Integrated Systems in the Workplace: The Delta/CIGNA/MCC Depression Initiative *David Whitehouse, M.D., M.B.A.*	87
Chapter 9	Depression and Its Management in Primary Care: The Harvard Pilgrim Health Care Experience *Steve Stelovich, M.D.*	93
Chapter 10	High Utilizers of Health Services: The Purchaser Perspective and Experience with the Personal Health Improvement Program (PHIP) *Paul B. Johnson, M.D.* *Lawrence B. Staubach, M.D., M.B.A.* *Anna P. Millar, M.B.A.*	99
Chapter 11	The Group Practice Model: Allina Health System *Michael Trangle, M.D.*	115
Chapter 12	The Quality Improvement Model of Behavioral Health Group Practices *Allen S. Daniels, Ed.D.*	121

Part IV. Working in Primary Care Settings: What You Need to Know

Chapter 13	The Primary Care Perspective: Culture and Reality *Michael D. Cirigliano, M.D.* *Mary F. Morrison, M.D.*	129
Chapter 14	Depression in Primary Care: Assessment and Management *Steven Cole, M.D.* *Mary Raju, RN, M.S.N.* *James Barrett, M.D.*	139
Chapter 15	Anxiety Disorders in Primary Care *Mack Lipkin, Jr., M.D.*	155
Chapter 16	Clinical Presentation, Screening, and Treatment of Substance Abuse in the Primary Care Setting *Thomas Horst, M.D., M.P.H.*	167
Chapter 17	Clinical Presentation, Screening, and Treatment of Somatization in Primary Care *Steven E. Locke, M.D.* *Katharine M. Larsson, RN, M.S., CS*	179

Chapter 18   The Mind-Body Connection:
             Outcomes Research in the Real World   193
             Marcie Parker, Ph.D., CFLE
             R. Edward Bergmark, Ph.D.
             Mark Attridge, Ph.D.

Part V. The Future of Behavioral Health and Primary Care Integration

Chapter 19   Training for Interdisciplinary Practice:
             Trends in Clinical Psychology and Family Medicine   213
             Thomas M. DiLorenzo, Ph.D.
             Harold A. Williamson, M.D., M.S.P.H.

Chapter 20   Computerized Technology: Integrative Treatment
             Outcome Technology in Primary Care Practice   229
             Len Sperry, M.D., Ph.D.
             Peter L. Brill, M.D.

Chapter 21   The Future of Primary Care/Behavioral Health
             Integration: Questions ... and Some Answers?   237
             Grant E. Mitchell, M.D.
             Joel D. Haber, Ph.D.

Annotated Bibliography   Treatment of Mental Disorders in Primary
             Care and Specialty Settings: Utilization, Recognition,
             Treatment Delivery, Outcome, and Quality of Care   247
             Marcia Kaplan, M.D.

Part VI. Appendices

Appendix 1   Mental Disorders in General Medical Practice: Adding Value
             to Healthcare Through Consultation-Liaison Psychiatry   255

Appendix 2   Levels of Systematic Collaboration Between Therapists
             and Other Health Professionals   293

Appendix 3   Symptom-Driven Diagnostic System—
             Primary Care (SDDS-PC)   297

Appendix 4   Prime-MD Patient Questionnaire   303

Appendix 5   Quick Guide to Patient Problem Questionnaire (PPQ)   305

Appendix 6   Teaching Medical Interviewing: The Lipkin Model   311

Contributors   323

Index   331

Foreword: Mind and Body— The Integration of Behavioral Healthcare and Medicine

Michael A. Freeman, M.D.

It is true that the mind is joined with the brain, and the brain with the body, and it is also true that the development of a healthcare system that fully integrates behavioral healthcare with general medicine is imperative. The failure to do so has had profound effects on the delivery, costs, and outcomes of health services. Current specialized substance abuse services and carve-out health plans are like a Band-Aid on a major injury because of their segregation from the rest of health and medicine, which limits their effectiveness. This critically important volume outlines the challenges that lie ahead in achieving integrated services and offers an industry-wide view of carefully laid out solutions to these challenges.

It is time to make the transition to different models of insurance and service delivery—models that respond to the healthcare needs of the whole person, rather than selected organs, and that meet the demands of the information and service economy of the future. As this book shows, dramatic restructuring of health insurance plans— from basic medical care to delivery systems and settings—must occur before behavioral and general medicine can be fully integrated. In order for change to occur, the deeply entrenched constraints that derive from the historical evolution of hospitals, health insurance, and medical education and training must be overcome.

It will be essential to develop incentives for individuals and groups to manage their own health behavior, lifestyle-related risks, and care models and systems in a person-oriented, collaborative infrastructure. Above all, mental health and addiction treatment services must be provided at parity with general medical coverage in a nondiscriminatory, comprehensive system.

Commercial health insurance plans were developed after World War II in response to the needs of a manufacturing and agricultural economy that relied on physical strength more than mental ingenuity. Most women held domestic roles, and families and communities were less mobile and more intact than today. Acute and catastrophic disabilities that interfered with the physical labor required to survive, such as fires and earthquakes, were viewed as unpredictable "acts of God" and were ameliorated by basic insurance mechanisms. Hospitals repaired the broken bodies that manned the machine-age economy, but the brain and the mind were neither addressed nor understood.

Now, agricultural and manufacturing production are largely mechanized or done overseas, and knowledge and service workers have replaced physical laborers. America's economic competitive edge relies more heavily on mental ingenuity and less on physical strength. Women have entered the workforce. The need for mobile and temporary labor has created transient communities and fragmented families. Now many health problems can be prevented or managed, and the fields of psychiatry, neurology, and behavioral neuroscience have produced a new understanding of the brain-mind-body connection. People with severe and persistent mental illnesses, who were once warehoused in vast, hopeless institutions, have a chance to function in the community, thanks to breakthrough medications and services.

However, the competitive edge our country thrives on and the economic security we know are imperiled. Purchasers who rely on health insurance plans and delivery systems to help maintain productivity and those with severe disabilities who seek a life in the community are relying on a system that is historically and systemically impaired.

In today's global, information-driven economy, Americans must continuously absorb new information. They must function efficiently in self-managing work teams, be resilient about ongoing change, and reconcile powerful and rapidly evolving computer technologies. Emotional stability, confidence, and interpersonal efficacy are needed to adjust to change, juggle the demands of job and family life, and handle the interpersonal challenges of work and community.

In this new and complex environment, innovative health plans and delivery systems are necessary to sustain individual productivity and health. This means integrated healthcare models, benefit plans, and services that fully respond to the needs of all the constituents of the American healthcare system, including children and the elderly. Plans and delivery systems must work to maximize our country's human potential, and must avoid discriminating against those with brain-based conditions and perpetuating the stigma associated with mental illness. And, while we improve behavioral health and effectiveness in the community, we must reduce disability costs in the workplace and in society.

The efficient prevention and management of chronic and acute conditions requires the participation of educated and responsible consumers, which means that education must be an integral part of treatment plans. Behavioral medicine must influence our lifestyles and health-risk behaviors, including our ways of thinking about health, dealing with emotions and stress, and making choices. In short, tomorrow's health plans and delivery systems must effectively reward individuals for the management of their own health.

In response to the cost-containment efforts of managed care, providers are consolidating as regionally integrated delivery systems that offer "one-stop shopping" to large healthcare customers. This trend has moved us closer to collaborative care, which integrates mental health services with primary care. We still have a long way to go, however. Truly integrated care with total health and cost management to improve functioning, enhance productivity, and to deinstitutionalize has not been the goal of twentieth century healthcare insurance plans and delivery systems. Current episode-based benefit plans are driven by financial incentives that cause health plans and delivery systems to see people as bodies, while ignoring their brains, their minds, and their emotions.

Coordinated care, collaborative care, integrated care, primary behavioral healthcare—these are just some of the innovative models now being implemented to unite behavioral healthcare and primary care settings. Those health plans and systems of care that are aligned with our healthcare goals for the next century must be rewarded, or implementation of these approaches will stall. We owe it to ourselves and to the next generation to see these experiments succeed. This volume, carefully designed to advance this agenda, brings us one step closer to achieving this goal.

This book takes us further down the road to a true integration of primary care and behavioral healthcare. Drs. Joel Haber and Grant Mitchell have collaborated with our outstanding authors to ensure the readers' understanding of the solutions and pragmatic tools presented here and to oversee the informed analysis and critical review expected in a volume of this nature.

After defining integration and reviewing its history, our authors articulate the business, clinical, and consumer rationales for integration. The authors know that professionals who read this book are likely to need support for favoring integration in their own organizations. They give specific suggestions for overcoming typical barriers to system integration, including financial barriers, and for assessing the new roles of health and behavioral health professionals that arise in integrated systems.

Perhaps the most useful aspect of this book is its presentation of a broad range of successful integration models. In order to best serve the various populations in the healthcare system, integration must come in different forms. This book describes integration methods that are currently working in large healthplans, corporations, HMOs, and primary care and behavioral group practices.

Clinicians who read this book will appreciate its spectrum of methods, tools, and models for specific clinical services. Issues are explored in detail regarding the culture of clinical service delivery, symptoms and patient presentation in primary care, screening and treatment methods for commonly encountered conditions, and clinical outcomes.

The road to collaborative care and health plan integration lies ahead of us. By identifying the main landmarks, getting our bearings, and testing our equipment, we are climbing the foothills that lie between us and the mountain we must ascend. The journey is progressing rapidly.

The book concludes by anticipating the future and its possibilities. Readers will examine the impact of technology in the workplace, particularly as it applies in the primary care setting, and explore issues related to the training of residents and primary care physicians. Also presented are treatment models, a discussion of key concepts, and assessments of our field.

While many important medical discoveries have been made, they have yet to be effectively applied. This book facilitates the process of upgrading antiquated health plans and delivery systems to meet present needs. It delineates a future where healthcare is truly integrated, treating the whole person and enabling him or her to achieve total well-being through health and fitness and to recover from acute, episodic illness. For the remainder of this century and into the beginning of the next, the work of the healthcare enterprise will take place, not in the laboratory, but in the naturalistic settings of continually evolving healthcare systems.

Introduction

Marcia Byrnes, RN, M.P.A.

We are all familiar with the statistics. Integration of behavioral health services can reduce the utilization of costly and inappropriate services up to an astonishing 50 percent for the elderly, according to some research documents. Integration also improves patient outcomes, with significant increases in satisfaction of care, patient competency, and improvement in the doctor/patient relationship. Lack of integration of behavioral healthcare services can result in significantly greater medical costs, and contributes to enormous costs in social and vocational disability.

It seems so simple. As a healthcare community, we are largely in agreement with the goal and principal benefits of integrating behavioral healthcare services within the general medical sector. Few would deny the growing mountain of research demonstrating the effectiveness, cost savings, and overwhelming satisfaction that patients, providers, administrators, and health plans experience within an integrated program.

If there is almost universal agreement that integration of behavioral healthcare services is a good thing, why should the issue pose such a conundrum to both primary care providers and behavioral health providers alike? The devil, as they say, is in the details. While stakeholders on all sides are motivated to create a system that has value and quality, the how-to questions vary, depending on the perspective. There are as many distinct answers to those how-to questions as there are stakeholders. There is no standard one-size-fits-all solution to the philosophical and operational problems in creating and implementing an integrated program that can be adopted by all health plans, purchasers, and providers.

Redesigning or reinventing anything requires a mutual assessment of the value of proposed changes. This assessment obviously depends on the perspective one holds. Patients, providers, health plan executives, and the purchasers all have their own views of what the questions are and what problems need to be solved. Recognizing that everyone wants improvement in quality, effectiveness, and in the control of healthcare costs, what is the unique question asked by each stakeholder?

For health plan executives, the question has always been, "How can costs be controlled while maintaining quality of service? How will I know it is worth the expense to redesign the system?" For purchasers the question is, "What is the best use of my healthcare dollar? What will improve the health and function of my employees at a cost I can afford?" Providers, facilities, and provider groups ask, "How can I best serve this patient population? What actions and resources will best meet the needs of the patient and improve patient outcomes?" Bearing in mind that at least 15 to 20 percent of patients who seek help from their primary care provider have clear anxiety and depressive disorders, behavioral health clinicians and program administrators are asking, "How do we become part of the system and improve services for these clients? How can we broaden the base of clients who we treat to capture the underdiagnosed and undertreated patients?" Primary care physicians, overwhelmed and beleaguered by the constraints of managed care, are desperate for resources to improve not only patient satisfaction, but their own job satisfaction as well. (Recent studies have documented the strong correlation between patient compliance and physician job satisfaction.) Perhaps for the patient the question is, "Who, how, and what will help me feel better without exceeding the amount I can pay out of pocket?" Sometimes it's hard to believe that we are all striving for the same goal.

As we have seen, a system in which behavioral and general medical healthcare work in separate systems begets many problems. Primary care physicians may underdiagnose or undertreat, leading to significant cost increases. Treatment is compromised when patient information cannot be accessed. Consultation between behavioral and physical healthcare systems can't occur until incentives, procedures, and outcomes are mutually developed and are a shared priority. And, as the quantity of mental disorders detected and treated in the primary care setting continues to rise, primary care clinicians—including physician assistants and nurse practitioners—need increasing support in their role as behavioral health service providers. As primary care practitioners become increasingly responsible for the double-edged sword of managing the resources through capitated contracts, the need to control costs while effectively meeting patient needs becomes one of the most complex issues in their medical practice.

What methods can be offered, and who should be responsible for instigating this design change—purchasers or health plans, providers or health systems? One of the most positive outcomes of addressing the issue of behavioral health integration is the shared investment in developing new approaches to health and medicine. For example, it is well researched and documented that a significant factor in the lowering of overall healthcare costs is prevention. Everyone operating within a capitated system has a genuine incentive to keep patients healthy. Purchasers have come to believe, and believe strongly, that improved quality and health status of their employees is the best and most important way to control costs and increase the value of the dollars they spend. The birth of improved and mutually developed screening measures, referrals to psychoeducational groups, and the development of guidelines and programs to engage the patient in the health improvement process, not only improves the overall caliber of medical care, but has clearly reduced the costs.

On a policy level, the Institute of Medicine has been more than explicit in its policy recommendations regarding primary care and mental health. Beginning with a fundamental definition of primary care as "the provision of integrated accessible healthcare services by clinicians who are accountable for addressing a large majority of healthcare needs," the committee also explicitly identifies "the reduction of financial and organizational disincentives for the expanded role of primary care in the provision of mental health services" as a critical initial step.[1] Additionally, they urge the development of evaluations for collaborative care models that effectively integrate primary care and mental health services. Clearly, neither of these recommendations are easily implemented, and can only be accomplished by the efforts of all stakeholders. The Institute of Medicine's recommendations underscore how critical, timely, and universal this goal is.

Building a new structure requires tools. A house cannot be remodeled without changes to a floor plan and at least some idea of how the finished house will look. Likewise, a new healthcare system cannot be built without a shared philosophy and vision. The authors of this book have brought to our attention some of the most critical and necessary philosophical shifts necessary to successfully integrate primary care with behavioral healthcare.

This volume is perhaps unique in its scope and practical applicability, hence its subtitle "Tools for the 21st Century." In this thoughtfully compiled text, complex issues are raised and addressed by the models that are proposed, and which are supported by a discussion of the history and the impetus behind the vision of integrated services. The editors' selection of contributing authors and their organization of chapters allow each of us to search out the models that work in the world in which we operate, and to find a representation that fits our individual stakeholder priorities. Operational questions are addressed in a philosophical context, and integrated services are presented with nuts-and-bolts models. In order to bridge the philosophical differences with real world concerns that naturally occur for primary care and behavioral healthcare clinicians, there must be a shared base of knowledge, ideas, and proposals. In answer to that need, these chapters offer all readers the opportunity to explore the clinical models, the administrative considerations, and the measurement and outcome methods—all the tools that are essential to build an integrated services system.

Reference

1. Donaldson MS, Yordy KD, Lohr KN, Vanselow NA (eds): Institute of Medicine. Committee on the Future of Primary Care: Primary care: America's health in a new era. National Academy Press, Washington DC, 1996.

Part 1.
INTRODUCTION

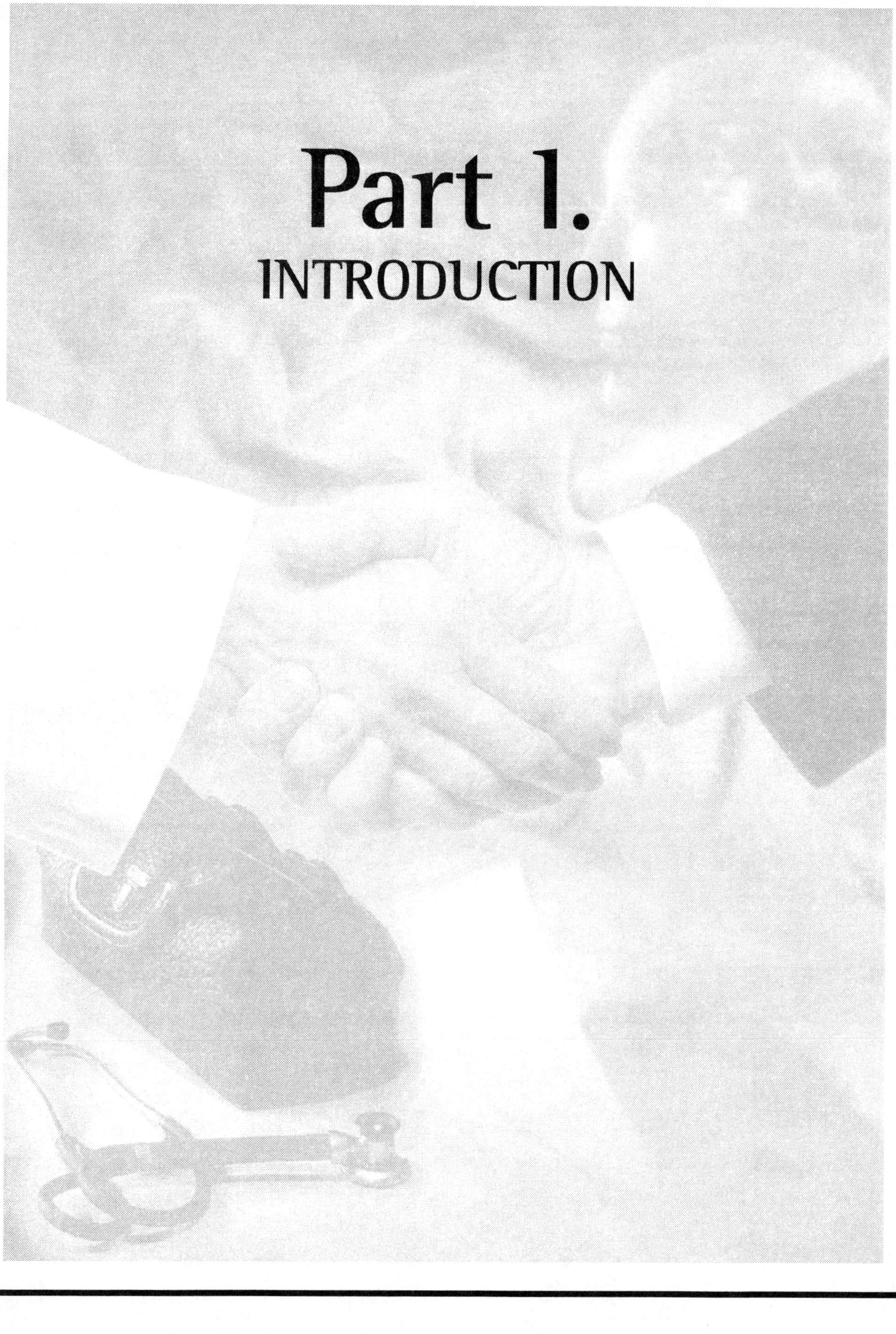

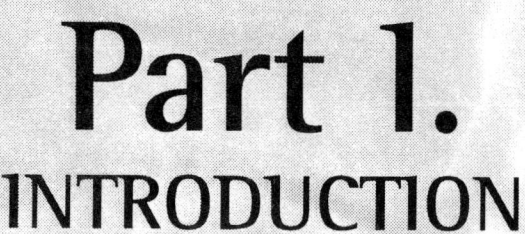

Chapter 1

From Fragmentation to Integration: A History of Comprehensive Patient Care

Don R. Lipsitt, M.D.

> We are not fighting for integration, nor are we fighting for separation. We are fighting for recognition as human beings. We are fighting for . . . human rights.
>
> MALCOLM X, SPEECH, BLACK REVOLUTION,
> NEW YORK, 1964

In the 1960s, the word *integration* conjured up essentially one idea: the racially oriented movement to open schools (and the buses that carried their students) equally to both blacks and whites. It was a time of turmoil, tragedy, and sadness, and a time that gripped the country in all its political, social, economic, and moral dimensions. In the years since then, integration–especially in healthcare–has eclipsed this connotation of a previous era. This chapter traces the evolution of the word and the concept from that time to the present.

Integration Clinic: "As Long as It Isn't Psychiatry, They'll Come"

It is no wonder that the May 1962 founding of a hospital-based clinic called Integration Clinic raised a few eyebrows in an institution that cared for both black and white patients.[1] Surprisingly though, it was the staff and not the patients who seemed uncomfortable about the name of the clinic. "The black patients will be upset," they said. It was the nurses who "forgot" to post the clinic sign on days that it met. In the more than eight years of the clinic's existence, not a single patient expressed concern about the clinic's name (except the paranoid man who wanted to know what this "Interrogation Clinic" was). The clinic had nothing to do with race relations or politics. It sprang from the recognition that many patients referred for psychiatric consultation from about 45 other clinics rarely seemed to make it to the Psychiatry Department at their appointed time or, if they did, they either dropped out after one visit or were considered "not suitable for psychotherapy" and returned to their referring physician. Patients who were previously "no-shows" when referred to psychiatry made their appearance with little hesitation when referred to the new clinic. For a particular population of patients, the "threat" of *integration* apparently carried less stigma than the implications of *psychiatry.*

The Dis-Integrated "Problem Patient"

Examination of the records of about 800 of these patients revealed a long history of clinic attendance (usually at many clinics), extensive "thick charts," multiple physical complaints often without concomitant physical findings (although established physical comorbidities were not rare), and hints of physician frustration in progress notes. Such patients were most at risk in the clinic setting of being labeled problem patients.[2] Their care was likely to be *dis-integrated* as a result of multiple referrals to clinics representing virtually every body part, disease, and symptom, and because of the lack of continuity and communication that accompanied these "rotating" patients.[3] Fragmented care was usually the result.

The most vivid of clinical experiences was reported by a 75-year-old diabetic, hypertensive man with a hiatal hernia and a wry sense of humor. He told of going to the gastrointestinal clinic for care of his hernia. There he was advised to buy two, three-inch wooden blocks from a lumber yard to place under the head of his bed, as part of his medical regimen. After instituting this treatment, his ankles began to swell. He reported this to the hypertension clinic, where he was advised to buy two, three-inch blocks to insert under the foot of his bed. In Integration Clinic, where he felt he had permission to complain, he jokingly told how everything was just the same, except "now it is three inches higher."

These high utilizers of medical resources are usually not "psychologically-minded" (now referred to as alexithymic), mostly women, and frequently complainers of somatic symptoms thought to be unfounded in physical etiologies (somatizers). Half-hour appointments, usually at monthly intervals, seemed ample for this population. The objective was to offer continuity of care, and to provide psychiatrically informed treatment that respected the defense of somatization. The caregivers were either psychiatrists or social workers who worked within the patient-therapist relationship to establish trust, a sense of connectedness, and an atmosphere of caring without caring too much. This meant walking the therapeutic line of allowing dependency while supporting and building defenses of independence or even counterdependence, to maximize use of strengths without awakening fears of abandonment. The modal patient could be managed for a year with an annual total of 6 hours (12 half-hour sessions) of face-to-face contact—a highly economic as well as therapeutic achievement.

In the pre-managed-care era, it was possible to accomplish these health promoting objectives with an open-door policy that said, in essence, "you will never be terminated from this clinic," and "you can decide when to extend intervals of time between appointments for more than one month" until many were secure and comfortable enough to use the clinic for only an occasional phone call or an annual visit. Over time, these patients learned (and believed) that it was not necessary to have a physical crisis or complaint to be accepted in the clinic.

The Many Meanings of Integration

It is virtually impossible now to read about healthcare reform and not encounter the word *integration*. Where does it come from and what does it mean? The dictionary offers us the etymological roots of the word: Latin gives us *integer*, not touched, not broken, intact, entire, whole; and Greek gives us *tekton* for architect, builder, or carpenter, one who assembles, constructs, or builds. The derivative *integrate* means to make complete, or to establish close cooperation among distinct entities, forming a whole by the addition or combination of parts or elements.

The word is broadly used. It applies not only at the level of single organisms, as small as an amoeba or larger than a human, as a way of referring to the biologic processes that function interdependently to sustain life, but also at the macro level to refer to the interaction of large nonhuman systems, as in industry, in reference to product development or collective operations. In between, one finds reference to integration in the application of mathematics to the measurement of volumes, using the odd symbols of *integral* calculus, first devised by Leibniz, a philosopher-mathematician who wrestled with the notion of the unconscious.

Sociology gives us the concept of integrated social classes or ethnic groups living and functioning in harmony. The superheterodyne radio, predecessor to the revolutionary electronic chip, would not have been possible without *integrated* electrical circuits. The biologic dynamic interplay of homeostasis attempts to maintain an *integrated* balance between catabolic and anabolic processes. Freud warned that an overzealous application of the techniques of psychoanalysis could risk regression and deterioration that might thwart the individual's inherent tendency toward developmental integration, synthesis, and health. Certainly, Freud's characterization of the psychosexual development of the child is an *integrative* psychology. Indeed, the concept of developmental integration of the human organism through many levels of function is exemplified in the psychobiologic realm by von Bertalanffy and in the psychosocial realm by Erik Erikson's description of the stages of the life cycle. More contemporaneously, pharmaceutical marketing now hawks the *"re-integration"* of the shattered individual through pharmacological intervention.

For our purposes, we will consider integration from three different vantage points: 1) the **individual**, as in the mind-body connection; 2) different **disciplines**, as in the relation of psychiatry to medicine, and of mental health disciplines to each other; and 3) **systems**, as in networks of care addressed by the continuum of services, both physical and behavioral (or emotional).

The Individual and the Mind-Body Connection

Integration is difficult business wherever it is attempted. Tension arises between the forces that drive the universe toward chaos, disorder, and death (entropy) and those countervailing forces attempting to resist or reverse this trend. From this general state of affairs, we have dualities of active and passive, good and evil, hot and cold, night and day, love and hate, life and death, and other opposing pairs. Every religion and philosophy has struggled with the tensions that arise between these forces. Even Descartes could not resist the temptation to accept the "Cartesian" notion that some interaction existed between the mind and the body. The robustness of this debate over the wholeness of man extends Descartes' philosophical treatise through a dialogue between a physician and his patient in de Mandeville's 1711 Treatise on the Hypochondriak and Hysterick Passions:

> The Metaphysical Principle of Monsieur Descartes, Cogito ergo sum, is a very good one, because it is the first truth, of which a Man can well be sure, and we all agree, some few Atheists excepted, that matter itself can never think, how elaborately fine soever it may be supposed . . . [I]t is a very just inference to say that we consist of a Body and a Soul. How they reciprocally work upon and affect one another, 'tis true, we cannot tell . . . [W]e can assert not only, that there must be an immediate Commerce between the Body and the Soul, but likewise that the action of thinking in which all, what we know of the latter, consists, is to our certain knowledge perform'd more in the Head than it is in the Elbow or

the Knee: From this we may further conclude, that as the Soul acts not immediately upon Bone, Flesh, Blood, etc. nor they upon that, so there must be some exquisitely small Particles, that are the Internuncii between them, by the help of which they manifest themselves to each other (p. 125).[4]

The Mysterious Leap: Too Big a Jump?

Philosophers have grappled with the effort of reuniting mind and body since at least the 17th century, when Descartes dualistically severed one from the other. And the challenge has been joined in the last hundred years by psychosomaticians trying to comprehend how mental events come to be represented in the body. What is this mysterious leap? asked Felix Deutsch and others, in their quest of understanding how emotional conflict translated into physical symptoms and illness.[5]

While it is a long jump from the "animal magnetism" of the 1700s to neuroendocrinologic transducers of the 1990s, the urge to find an *integrated* understanding of the workings of the mind and body is quite persistent. The same drive evident in religion's struggle to reconcile the sacred and the profane—or in the Chinese cosmological conception of yin and yang—gave rise to intriguing studies from the 1930s to 1950s that constituted the discipline of psychosomatic medicine. Conscientious efforts to address the wholeness of man, the expression of body and mind interacting together, enjoyed tremendous popularity. Adolf Meyer of Johns Hopkins University Medical School formulated a system of care referred to as "commonsense psychiatry" or "psychobiological medicine," designed to address the whole person rather than isolated parts. The spirit of psychosomatic medicine flourished until excessive promise and a few deflated theories diminished the influence of the field. The psychosomatic approach to illness has not been abandoned, but contemporary medicine holds that psychosomatic medicine is not distinct and separate.

Why is it so difficult to merge the dual dimensions of human distress? The striving toward and resistance to integration of mind and body is reflected by a mere hyphen in a paper by the psychoanalyst writer Donald Winnicott. In *Psycho-somatic Illness in its Positive and Negative Aspects* Winnicott states:

> The hyphen both joins and separates the two aspects of medical practice which are constantly under review in any discussion of this theme . . . . Psycho-somatics is in many ways a curious subject, for if one ascends into the sphere of intellectualization and loses contact with the actual patient, one soon finds that the term psycho-somatics loses its integrative function . . . . The split is certainly one that separates off physical care from intellectual understanding: more important, it separates psyche-care from soma-care (510–511).[6]

Winnicott postulates that a "psycho-somatic" illness constitutes a defense organization of the ego, which vigorously separates the somatic dysfunction from the conflict in the psyche; it is only the integrative forces in the patient that tend to make the patient abandon the defense. Further elaboration of the dilemma is expressed in the comment that some patients with psycho-somatic illness have to ". . . keep the doctors on two or more sides of a fence, because of an inner need; also that this inner need is part of a highly organized and powerfully mainstreamed defensive system, the defenses being against the dangers that arise out of integration and out of the achievement of a unified personality" (p. 514). "Our difficult job," Winnicott states, "is to take a unified view of the patient and the illness *without seeming to do so in a way that goes ahead of the patient's ability to achieve integration to a unit.*" In other words, it is the therapist's task to sensitively assist the patient's natural tendencies toward an integrative, holistic, homeostatic state and away from those internal forces that would pull the self toward more chaos and disorder.

Experiments in Comprehensive Care: Seeking the Elusive Ideal

It may be the very propensity of both patients and physicians to resist integration that has spawned the long struggle of psychiatry to rejoin the mainstream of medicine, from which it evolved. The pendulum has swung many times throughout psychiatry's history between the polarities of integration with and alienation from the broader field of medicine. The monotonous exhortations about the importance of combining physical and emotional healthcare seem not to have had much impact on the way medicine has been taught and practiced throughout medical history.

Nonetheless, the presumed benefits of a comprehensive approach to healthcare, in medical education and practice, have been idealistically extolled for centuries. The general practitioner and family physician have been the most vocal over the last four or five decades in their emphasis on the need for a comprehensive approach to healthcare.

Long before medical students were reminded that "it is as important to know the patient who has the disease as to know the disease the patient has," Cicero, in the first century BC remarked that "the competent physician before he attempts to give medicine to his patient, makes himself acquainted not only with the disease which he wishes to cure, but also with the habits and constitution of the sick man."[7] Some schools, as long ago as the 1950s, instituted "integration conferences" to put back together what the educational process had dissected into fragmented specialized disciplines. Any permanent advancement has been rare and transient. The battles of curriculum committees arise between the warring factions of basic scientists and clinicians, with every additional hour of time devoted to studying the "whole person" dearly won. This medical Humpty Dumpty is like a movie monotonously played first forward and then backward, displaying rapidly alternating states of intactness and fragmentation.

Experiments in comprehensive care were designed to demonstrate the validity of this orientation (before matters of cost-offset or cost-effectiveness were addressed). Perhaps the establishment of the General Medical Clinic at the University of Colorado School of Medicine in 1953 was the prototype of curricular changes acknowledging the deleterious impact of specialization on the teaching of comprehensive medical care. Teachers at Colorado School of Medicine were determined to tackle Humpty Dumpty's restoration. The study emerged from the conviction that "psychological and social factors are important influences on the well-being of the patient and that they may be the immediate and most important concern of the attending physician" (p. xv).[8]

The objectives of the project were "to create an environment that would not only foster thorough and deliberate teaching and learning, but also involve students, faculty, and patients in a clinic committed to the continuing, comprehensive care of the individual and the cultivation of a patient-student-teacher relationship in which the environmental, psychological, and cultural, as well as pathological, factors would play a very deliberate role in the formation of medical judgments" (pp. vii–viii). Students exposed to this experience in their senior year, compared to a control group, were found to develop a greater appreciation of the relevance of psychological factors in medical care, but disappointingly were no more inclined to deal with these problems in their face-to-face interactions with their patients than were students in the control group. One major finding of the study was that General Medical Clinic students considered learning traditional (organic) medicine to be much more important than learning principles and techniques of comprehensive care.

A similar program at Cornell Medical School in 1957 tried to foster a positive orientation toward social and emotional problems by exposing fourth-year medical students to community health programs in the hopes of altering their preference for the physically ill patients.[9] Here again, the disappointing finding was that, by the time these "experimental" students took their place with "non-experimental" classmates in clinical clerkships, they showed no difference in their continued preference for physically (as opposed to emotionally) ill patients. The outcomes of these experiments generated a less-than-optimistic prognosis for teaching the rudiments of psychosocial medicine in the years ahead. Indeed, contemporary studies have lent weight to the slim likelihood that graduating physicians will subscribe to or apply a comprehensive approach to patient care; the oft-replicated finding that physicians under-recognize and under-treat emotional problems in medical practice would seem to confirm this prediction.

The emphasis of medical curricula on the biomedical dimension of medicine, the tendency of colleagues and teachers to eschew affect and devalue the "touchy feely" side of medicine, and the influence of the specialty-oriented role models all conspire to deliver a lopsided education to the future physician. This unbalanced curriculum has been attributed, at least in part, to the sweeping reforms in medical education that evolved from the 1910 report of Abraham Flexner, a non-physician. He exposed the deplorable state of our country's medical schools, and by emphasizing the need for a more scientific rigor that relied on technologic advances, gave specialization a sizable boost. Indeed, Flexner is credited with the perpetuation of the dualistic approach to medical education, in which the whole is sacrificed for the particular. In a book called *The End of Medicine*, Carlson wrote that Flexner's report marked "... the period when medicine indisputably shifted its focus from the anthropological to the technical" (p. 208).[10]

Flexner's report also marked the beginning of a technological revolution in medicine. Although the Flexner Report is credited with dramatic improvement in the quality of the nation's medical schools and their curricula, it is also said to have contributed to the dehumanization of medical training, with disproportionately greater reliance placed on the tools of the profession, instead of on the skills of the practitioners.

In spite of the profoundly enhanced medical education obtained in post-Flexnerian medical institutions, physicians have often complained that they are

poorly prepared to recognize and treat the many patients who consult them with psychosocial or emotional complaints. For many years, psychiatry had been in the forefront in its endeavor to broaden the narrow biomedical training to include understanding and recognition of the role of emotional factors in general medicine. Following World War II, when psychiatrists worked closely with internists and surgeons, there was a flurry of interest in integrating psychiatry and general medical practice. The 1940s and 1950s saw a boom in psychiatric units in general hospital settings, in consultation-liaison services, and in psychosomatic research. It seemed that psychiatry was finally achieving the rapprochement it had sought since its severance from the mainstream of medicine in the early part of the century.

The 1960s witnessed the development of the community mental health movement and a high degree of collaboration among a variety of mental health specialists. Both the inpatient units and the community health clinics promoted the democratization of mental health treatment. Although this trend gave rise to identity and turf disputes, it established the foundation for later behavioral healthcare systems. In spite of these advances, most experiments that tried to achieve integration of the biomedical with the psychosocial produced the same discouraging results as the Colorado endeavor.

The challenge appears to be resurrected in 20-year cycles. In the 1970s, a pass at promoting primary care and family medicine was launched by the federal government. This was not so much to promote an integrated care model as it was a means to remedy the maldistribution of physicians. Guidelines suggested that primary care training should include at least 15 percent of curriculum time dedicated to "behavioral science." The discipline of the providers of this educational components was not specified; subsequent surveys revealed a paucity of psychiatrists, but a vast array of other "instructors in behavioral science," including sociologists, anthropologists, and the usual representation of psychologists and social workers. In 1977, an article in *Science* galvanized the mental health community with a plea for a new model in medicine. This essay, by respected internist-psychoanalyst George Engel, articulated what most students of the mind-body dichotomy had been feeling for decades, and the rallying cry for an integrated approach to healthcare was revived.[11]

The excitement gave way to frustration as new efforts at integrated models faded away. When grant money dried up, so did the thrust to train primary care physicians (PCPs). Now, in the 1990s, riding piggy-back on the economically driven managed care movement, primary care is resurrected with new enthusiasm. With the PCP now installed as "gatekeeper" to the entire healthcare system, former specialists are converting in droves to generalists, with no greater evidence of enhanced attention to the psychosocial aspects of medical practice. (See Chapter 19 for further discussion of these issues.)

Through it all, the subspecialty field of consultation-liaison psychiatry has carried the banner for an integrated, collaborative effort in patient care. Teaching by doing (consultation) and by formal and informal didactic pedagogy (liaison), consultation-liaison psychiatrists have been the foot soldiers of psychosomatic medicine in their efforts to dislodge the hyphen of Winnicott's model. But even these endeavors have been less than encouraging as a way to train physicians in the biopsychosocial model of medical practice described by Engel. Engel said "as long as physicians are imbued with the reductionism and dualism of Western science, there is no way in which the conflict between psychiatry and the rest of medicine can be resolved."[10,12] Furthermore, as the focus on money continues to drive healthcare reform, psychiatrists find themselves in competition with the less expensive psychologists, social workers, and psychiatric nurses as the providers of consultation and even psychiatric liaison—a state of affairs that has probably hastened a reassessment of the field and the benefits of collaboration.

The secret of integrated systems lies in the ability of the parts to function interdependently in a dynamically complete context that is different and most likely more than the sum of the individual parts. In the wake of the many failed attempts to merge psychiatry and medicine, the question has been asked whether the two are indeed compatible in a single system. From one vantage point, while both begin assessments with the patient's chief complaint, the internist seems to work centrifugally toward a narrower, parsimonious focus on "the cause" of the patient's complaint, while the psychiatrist begins at the same place but broadens the exploration centripetally to include "the multiple determinants" of the patient's plight in time. To expect both pursuits to occur simultaneously is to posit equal and opposite forces that may cancel each other out. Winnicott has colorfully portrayed "the rare physician who can ride the two horses (*psyche and soma*—italics added) simultaneously."[6] The result could well be a split up the middle!

But perhaps there is a silver lining to this multidisciplinary approach to patient care. Deriving as it does from the old community mental health model, there is increasing attention to the benefits of a "team" approach to patient care. To function as a system, the parts must be able to interact without slavish adherence to disciplinary boundaries. In other words, consensus building must displace turf battles; participants must work for the benefit of the whole, not of individual parts. To achieve such harmony among mental health disciplines is not always easy; to include internal medicine in the integrated enterprise is almost impossible. Nonetheless, there are renewed efforts to find ways to achieve the elusive ideal, including integrated training programs in family or internal medicine and psychiatry, as well as "seamless" systems of care, for which populations of patients are the magnet.

The Evolution of Systems Thinking: Modern Integration

What is the probability that integrated delivery systems are more likely to work now than in the past? There has been a change in the culture of the healthcare system and, with it, numerous paradigm shifts. The focus on the individual patient has broadened to encompass whole populations. There is a social move toward merger—motivated by economies and the need for survival, if not by the well-being of patients. With a relaxation of antitrust laws, industries, banks, and other corporate entities have responded to the marketplace by forming alliances that might have been prohibited years ago. Although many decry this corporate trend as lessening interest in the individual person, there may be opportunities not heretofore realized.

Hospitals (and even medical schools) have not been exempt from the urge to merge. Those who govern managed care companies and administer large industries have discovered that health plans that fragment delivery of services are more costly and less likely to be given high "satisfaction" ratings by patients than those that provide "one-stop shopping." But Descartes' ghost hovers over the efforts at horizontal and vertical integration in the form of "carved out" mental health and substance abuse services (behavioral healthcare). Mental health providers, and to some extent their patients, protest what appears to be discriminatory benefits for behavioral health services contrasted with those for physical illness. It is only recently that this force has been met with a counterforce that endeavors to carve back into medicine the psychosocial dimension of healthcare, fostered by the recognition that integrated care is not only better care but also probably more cost-effective in the long run.

Together Again by Popular Demand?

With the shift in focus from individuals to populations, and from separate disciplines to systems thinking and networks, there has come a softening of boundaries, less turf-oriented competitiveness, and a move toward collaboration and better integration. The ascendance of the PCP to the role of "gatekeeper" makes it imperative to find ways to serve the emotional as well as the physical needs of patients. The model of integrated multidisciplinary care exemplified by the Integration Clinic in the 1960s and 1970s reappears in the 1990s through innovative programs that bring behavioral healthcare to primary care. Recognizing that PCPs do not have the training or the time to attend properly to those patients requiring time-intensive care, efforts have been made to promote linkages that can offer the necessary services. Disciplines must work together for the benefit of the patient, and they must "inhabit a common neighborhood" without being threatened by one another.[13]

As we inhabit the brave new world of managed care, a dialogue ensues as to whether behavioral healthcare should be carved out (externalized) or integrated (internalized) into comprehensive healthcare systems. It is truly *deja vu* all over again, although on a much broader scale than we saw in the case of the individual or even different disciplines. Cogent arguments are made on both sides. Ludden of Harvard Pilgrim Healthcare makes the argument that carve-outs "undo the forward progress our healthcare system has made in the past few decades away from fragmented, un-coordinated, fee-for-service care toward well-managed, integrated, coordinated care."[14]

By contrast, Feldman points out the benefits of both carve-outs and carve-ins, in what he describes as "functional or patient-centered integration," in which the highest quality of care is most likely to come about when "a system of human services [is] composed of helping organizations that are freestanding but interdependent, specialized but with permeable boundaries, [having] a keen appreciation of how important it is for them to work together, and powerful incentives to do so."[15] Once again, we observe the uneasy tension in the integrative process as it strives for some dynamic balance.

Summary

The word *integration* has a long history; it has probably never been more exploited than in recent years, especially in the domain of clinical care and intervention. It is most especially applied to the broad and diverse field of what has become known as behavioral healthcare, an aggregate of mental health services. Generally it has positive connotations. But attempts to achieve it have been accompanied by angst, reaction, and resistance whether in the field of race relations or medicine. Nevertheless, we have evidence (outcomes) that demonstrate the benefits of integration, including less fragmented care, more economic delivery, and more efficacious treatment. If the result of integrated delivery systems of the future is to ameliorate the pitfalls of the dualistic healthcare of the past, a great advance will have been made. Hopefully, integration will not become mere shibboleth.

References

1. Lipsitt DR: Integration clinic: an approach to the teaching and practice of medical psychology in an outpatient setting. In Psychiatry and Medical Practice in a General Hospital. Edited by Zinberg NE. New York, International Universities Press, 1996, pp. 231–249.
2. Lipsitt DR: Medical and psychological characteristics of "crocks." Psychiatry Med 1:15–25, 1970.
3. Lipsitt DR: The "rotating" geriatric patient: challenge to psychiatrists. J Geriatr Psychiatry 2:51–61, 1968.
4. De Manderville B: Treatise of the Hypochondriak and Hysterick Passions (1711). Reprinted by Arno Press, New York, 1976.
5. Deutsch F: On the Mysterious Leap from the Mind to the Body: A Workshop Study on the Theory of Conversion. International Universities Press, New York, 1959.
6. Winnicott DW: Psycho-somatic illness in its positive and negative aspects. Int J Psychoanal 47:510–516, 1966.
7. Cicero: De oratore ii (55 BC): Quoted in The Complete Works of Montaigne, Stanford University Press, Stanford, CA, 1957.
8. Hammond KR, Kern Jr F: Teaching Comprehensive Medical Care: A Psychological Study of a Change in Medical Education. Harvard University Press, Cambridge, MA, 1959.
9. Merton RK, Reader G, Kendall, PL: The Student-Physician: Introductory Studies in the Sociology of Medical Education. Harvard University Press, Cambridge, MA, 1957.
10. Carlson RJ: The End of Medicine. J Wiley and Sons, New York, 1975.
11. Engle GL: The need for a new medical model: a challenge for biomedicine. Science 196:129–136, 1977.
12. Engle GL: Resolving the conflict between medicine and psychiatry. Res Staff Physician 26:73–79, 1979.
13. Paulsen RH: Psychiatry and primary care as neighbors from the promethean primary care physician to multidisciplinary clinic. Int J Psychiatry Med 26:113–125, 1996.
14. Ludden JM: Integrated care is the key to clinical quality and cost control. Behavioral Healthcare Tomorrow 3:40–43, 1996.
15. Feldman S: A marriage unconsummated. Behavioral Healthcare Tomorrow 3:47–48, 1996.

Chapter 2

Integration of Primary Care and Behavioral Health: The Driving Forces

David R. Selden, ACSW, LICSW

The Big Picture

Most health plans spend about four to six percent of their budget on behavioral healthcare. Because some view this as an inconsequential amount, behavioral healthcare has not received the proper attention when it comes to strategic planning or program development. The figure quoted above is misleading, resulting in the general undertreatment of behavioral health disorders and a failure to recognize and properly support the primary care setting, where a significant amount of treatment occurs for these disorders.

Why should we pay any attention to behavioral health services, since these disorders affect only a small proportion of the population? Aren't there more pervasive problems like cancer and AIDS that need more attention? The answer lies in the fact that the prevalence of behavioral health disorders is more widespread than many people assume. Undertreatment and nontreatment of behavioral health disorders—and the need for integrated efforts—is a larger problem than most people realize.

Prevalence in the American Population

Figure 1 illustrates the details of behavioral health disorder prevalence in the general U.S. population on an annual basis.[1] The overall occurrence of diagnosable behavioral disorders is estimated at 17 percent. Only half these patients ever seek any form of behavioral health treatment, with 50 percent of this group receiving treatment in the primary care setting.[2] Put another way, almost one-fifth of the U.S. population experiences some form of mental disorder in a given year. Only one-half of this group ever seek help. And of those seeking help, only half of them see a behavioral health specialist. This leaves a large percentage of the public in need of services and either untreated or undertreated.

For consumers with other medical disorders, behavioral health issues have a profound effect. The comorbidity of behavioral health disorders with physical disorders is strongly supported by recent data, as seen in Figure 2.[3] These behavioral health disorders are typically missed altogether or undertreated by primary care practitioners and other medical professionals not properly trained or supported to provide the needed care.

One result of this is the increased utilization of medical services by persons with these undiagnosed behavioral health conditions. In a 1990 study, 50 percent of high utilizers of medical care were found to be psychologically distressed. Figure 3 shows the specific nature of the psychological distress in this group.[4] This represents a

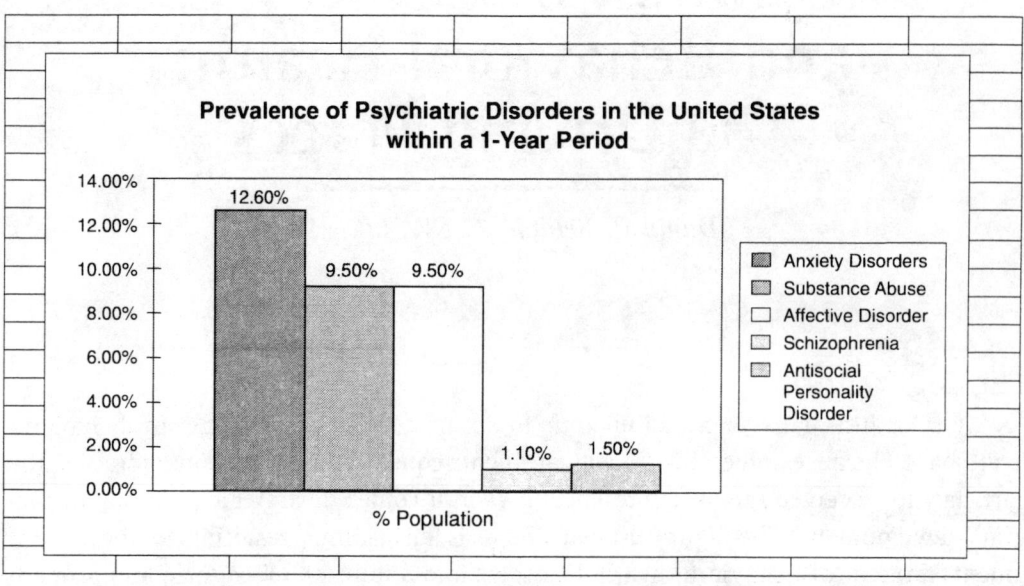

Figure 1

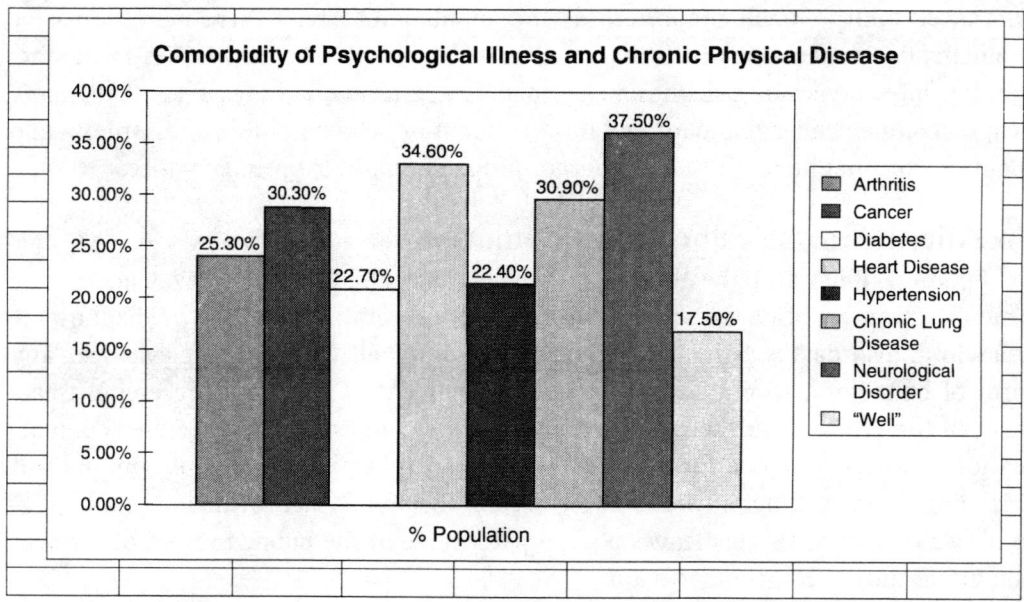

Figure 2

missed opportunity to improve patient well-being and decrease medical costs, since depressive and anxiety disorders can be effectively treated.

A study by Katon et al. at the University of Washington-Seattle provides additional information that reinforces the impact of behavioral health disorders in the general medical setting. Patients at a large health maintenance organization (HMO) who were identified as the top 10 percent of utilizers of healthcare were surveyed to

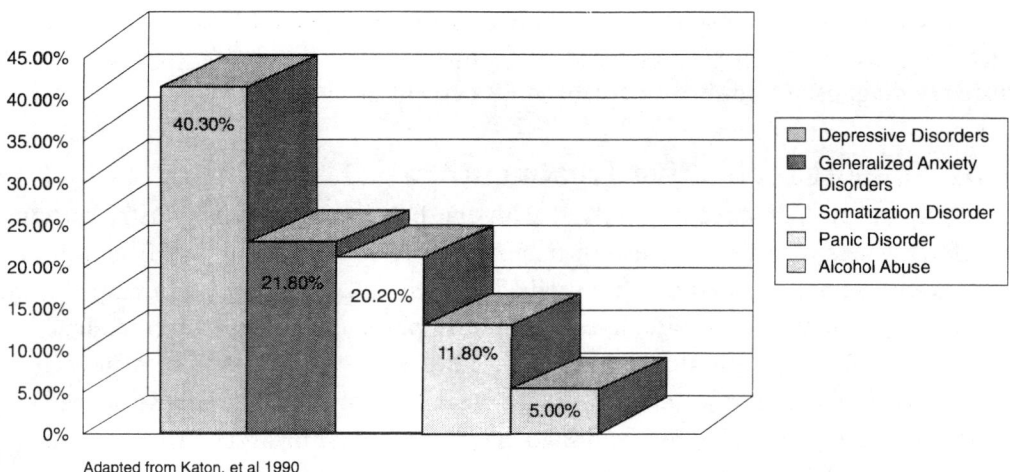

Figure 3

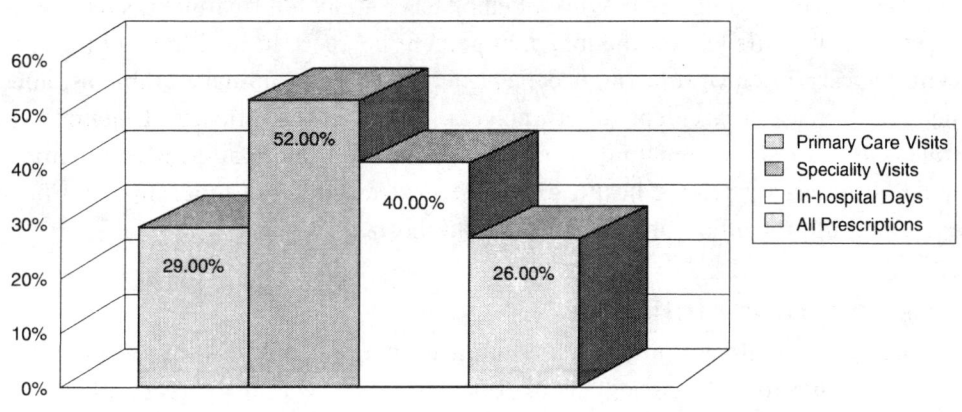

Figure 4

determine the degree to which this group utilizes healthcare services (Figure 4). The amounts signify the percentage of total healthcare services utilized by this group. If we combine the information from Figures 3 and 4, we can estimate the effect of the problem. Our lack of appropriate screening abilities and mechanisms, wellness and prevention initiatives, and funding incentives is driving a profound overutilization of inappropriate healthcare resources. The results are unnecessary expenses and poor quality treatment.

If We Ignore It, Will It Go Away?

A study sponsored by the World Health Organization predicts that by 2020 severe depression will be the second largest cause of death and disability.[5] The study also found depression currently accounts for 10 percent of productive years lost worldwide.

The National Depression Screening Day sponsored by the National Mental Health Association has seen 150,000 participants in previous screening days held over the past five years in 2,500 sites nationwide. In medical inpatient settings, depression is correctly diagnosed in only 14 percent to 50 percent of cases.[6,7]

Why Support Ineffective Treatment?

Many people not directly involved with the behavioral health industry question the effectiveness of behavioral health treatment. Questions arise in part from our lack of outcomes data. Recent studies are producing such data, however, and the results are compelling. Mental illnesses are more common in our society than cancer, diabetes, or heart disease. The success rate for treatment of heart disease ranges from 41 percent to 52 percent; in contrast, the success rate for treatment of schizophrenia is 60 percent, 65 percent for major depression, and 80 percent for bipolar disorder.[8] There is a growing awareness of these findings in the purchaser and health plan sectors.

Up to one-third of patients hospitalized for any medical condition have alcoholism, but in 5 to 50 percent of them the condition goes undetected.[9] The total healthcare cost for families with an alcoholic member is two times higher than for families without such a member.[10] A large automobile manufacturing plant, after implementing an employee assistance program (EAP) with an emphasis on alcohol treatment, saw a 49 percent decrease in hours lost on the job, a 29 percent decrease in health benefit use, a 56 percent decrease in leave time, a 64 percent decrease in disciplinary problems, and an 82 percent decrease in accidents after one year.[11] Data on the efficacy of mental health treatment grows more compelling every year. As a result, more aggressive attention to affective disorders by private health plans, integrated work-site programs, and further development of prevention programs are on the horizon.

Excessive Medical Inflation

On average, healthcare prices have outpaced general inflation by 50 percent for the past four decades. However, health price inflation was 60 percent higher than general price increases in 1995. Given historical and current trends, healthcare costs in 2030 could be 69 percent over current levels.[12]

For the first time during this period, in 1995, the increase in health insurance costs was below inflation. This could be viewed as a direct result of managed care and reflects the deep discounts and curtailment of intensive services experienced by providers in managed care penetrated areas. It would thus appear that we have the means to curtail costs, but this has not yet offset the expenses in other (e.g., uninsured) populations. The drawback for some people is that their care is now handled through a comprehensive, managed care approach. This approach typically takes the form of a well-managed HMO or a managed behavioral health "carve-out" company with an exclusive network and tight utilization controls.

The Aging of the American Population

An additional factor contributing to increased costs is the "baby bulge" that is just beginning to affect healthcare. In 1995, only 12 percent of the population was over 65. By the year 2020, this figure is predicted to rise to 16 percent and, by year 2040, 20 percent of the U.S. population.[13] Current annual per capita healthcare spending for men aged 30 to 34 is $1,528. The same figure for men aged 50 to 54 is $4,454.[12] There can be little question that costs will continue to rise.

The largest population group is the baby boomers, who are moving en masse into the over age-50 bracket. In addition, due to better medical treatment and increased attention to health, we are living longer. In 1960, there were 5,000 Americans 100 years old or older. Today, there are more than a million—and there will be 5 million by the year 2010.[14]

We can do little to change the costs of advanced medical technology. And there is nothing we can do to change the demographics of the aging baby boomer group. The one area we can control, and perhaps the biggest structural flaw driving the high costs and uneven quality seen in our current healthcare system, is fragmentation of the system. Numerous funding mechanisms are not well connected to each other or the services they support. Service systems are often a morass of uncoordinated specialties and redundant care providers. Consumers have been uninformed and distanced through lack of inclusionary programming and relevant information. A major example of this fragmentation is the relationship between primary care and behavioral health services.

Primary Care and Behavioral Health: A Dysfunctional Relationship

The current interface between primary care and behavioral health is dysfunctional (Figure 5). The dysfunction begins with the input to the system. Inadequate benefit structures, the stigma of behavioral health disorders, and poor consumer recognition of behavioral health disorders leads consumers to utilize the primary care setting rather than seek out appropriate behavioral health specialists. From another perspective, only 21 percent of behavioral health cases are actually receiving services from the area designed specifically to provide these services. There are three issues contributing to this dysfunctional relationship.[15]

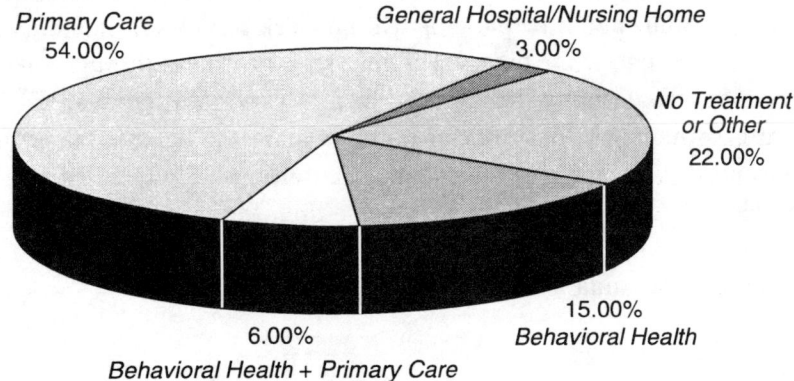

Figure 5

Benefit Structures

Benefit structures that only provide limited payments for outpatient services, sometimes with high deductibles for behavioral health rather than medical services, make it more economically sensible to access the primary care medical setting instead of the behavioral health counselor. In addition, if you exceed your outpatient annual maximum for behavioral health, you can always go to your primary care physician where no such cap exists.

Although risk sharing or capitation arrangements are prevalent throughout managed medical care, they are sparsely utilized in the behavioral health sector.[16] A capitation contract specifies a dollar amount to cover the annual cost of healthcare services for a person. If the person is healthy and does not utilize services, the provider receives the capitation amount as profit. If the person requires utilization of expensive services, the provider may provide more services than the capitation covers. The idea is to balance the "non-utilizers" with the "heavy utilizers" to meet expenses and, ultimately, make a profit.

A risk sharing arrangement between provider and payor can establish various amounts for which each of the providers is at risk for profit or loss. If a risk sharing arrangement does exist in a healthcare system, it is usually a dual system with the behavioral healthcare providers working from one risk pool and the medical providers working from another. This split fosters nonintegrated care and provides incentives to shift cases and costs from one sector to another. Behavioral health providers often are not familiar with medical issues, nor are medical providers always skilled in behavioral health problems. Hence, the issues are not addressed in an integrated manner.

Gatekeeper Systems

Gatekeeper systems usually require contact with the primary care physician (PCP) prior to any specialist referrals. This supports the dysfunction because many PCPs are inadequately prepared to assess behavioral health disorders. The purpose of a gatekeeper system is to establish a single point of accountability for the management of an individual's healthcare. When a PCP is the gatekeeper, there is an opportunity to integrate the PCP into all the healthcare issues of the patient. However, the gatekeeper can also serve as a barrier rather than a facilitator in behavioral health cases, due to confidentiality issues. Some potential patients will not seek services if they must communicate through a PCP first, while others will only seek treatment through their PCP.

The gatekeeper at many behavioral health carve-out companies (sometimes known as a case manager) does not always integrate the behavioral health services with the primary care and other medical care settings. Since so many behavioral health problems present in the primary care setting, the current structure supports a fragmented and redundant system that results in inefficient and inappropriate care, contributing to uneven quality and increased costs.

Consumers

The continued stigma of mental health and substance abuse contribute to consumers' reluctance to see a mental health professional. This leads to continued use of the primary care provider, necessitating improved training in behavioral health disorders and increased support from mental health professionals. Consumer education has long been neglected and results in most people being unaware of the basic signs and symptoms of easily treatable behavioral health disorders. Anxiety and depression are sometimes passed off as "fatigue" or "the blues" and are not addressed proactively. Similarly, early signs of substance abuse problems can be overlooked and the behavior "enabled," resulting in a visit to the PCP for gastrointestinal problems or other generalized complaints. One of the most significant examples of this is the accurate diagnosis and treatment of panic disorders (see Chapter 15).

Once in the system, the consumer depends on services from a professional who is often minimally trained to identify and treat behavioral health disorders. In addition, the health system usually provides weak incentives and sometimes even disincentives for the PCP to refer a case to a behavioral health specialist. In other cases, the physician is motivated to refer the patient out as quickly as possible, without any incentive to maintain contact with the case. As previously discussed, many behavioral health patients present as high utilizers of medical services. This type of patient may be quickly "turfed out" to another practitioner, sometimes a behavioral health specialist. This may bring positive results, but if there are concurrent medical disorders, the care can easily become fragmented and inefficient. In other circumstances, the PCP is unsure how to make a referral into the behavioral health sector. This may occur in a behavioral health carve-out plan, as well as in staff and group model health plans.

Results of the Dysfunctional Relationship

Many consumers are unaware of the effects of behavioral health disorders in their lives. An estimated 30 percent of family practice visits involve counseling for psychological stressors. A recent survey of patient visits to PCP offices revealed that 21 percent of the patients had clinically significant depression, yet only 1.2 percent cited depression as reason for their visit.[17] The result is a large untreated and undertreated population that contributes to reduced occupational functioning, compromised effectiveness in the home, and general dissatisfaction with the effects of health services rendered. Overall costs are higher for this population, as well.

In the corporate sector, effects of this dysfunction have been measured. A recent study at US West, a large "Baby Bell" communications company, noted that medical costs for families with behavioral health conditions were 32 to 36 percent higher when compared with families without behavioral health conditions.[17] These figures were for medical costs only; behavioral health costs were excluded.

In a large company (50,000 employees), the difference in costs can be substantial. Since 17 percent of the general population experiences a behavioral health disorder, 8,500 workers would be in need of behavioral health services in a given year. The average medical costs for the behavioral health service need group is $3,200 for the year, as compared with $2,100 for the non-behavioral health need group.[18] The additional cost to the company could be $9,350,000 (see Chapter 10).

In 1989 the McDonnell-Douglas corporation investigated the effectiveness of behavioral health interventions through their EAP. For a 4-year period (1985–1988), medical claims payments for employees treated for chemical dependency were $17,850 greater than payments for similar employees without a chemical dependency disorder. Excess medical claim costs for employees with a psychiatric condition were $7,500 for the same period. Although in part these figures were a result of the benefits plan and program management, it is clear that behavioral health disorders were driving considerable excess medical costs. Similar effects were seen in employee absenteeism and termination rates.[19]

Specialty Services

In another recent study, 5 to 18 percent of prenatal patients reported a significant problem with drug and alcohol abuse.[20] The direct result is newborns with complicated, sometimes lifelong difficulties requiring expensive healthcare services. This is directly and easily preventable through behavioral health intervention in the obstetrics/gynecology setting. Effective collaboration between primary care and behavioral health services produces powerful results, as seen in Table 1. Similar results of behavioral health interventions have been noted in breast cancer patients and patients presenting in emergency rooms with symptoms that indicated a possible cardiac disorder but were actually anxiety or panic disorders.

The Primary Care Setting

Patients with diagnosable mental disorders average twice as many visits to their PCPs as those without a mental disorder.[21] Nonpsychiatric physicians write approximately two-thirds of all prescriptions for psychotropic medications, and primary care patients are noncompliant with mental health referrals up to 74 percent of the time.[22]

A major problem in the primary care setting is the prescription of psychotropic medications.[23] Medications are sometimes not prescribed appropriately for patients in the primary care setting. This affects a large proportion of patients in need of behavioral health services. An example is the undertreatment of depressive disorders, the psychiatric disorder with the highest rate of treatment effectiveness.

The primary care setting is not prepared to manage behavioral health problems, although many of them emerge here. As discussed earlier, studies consistently demonstrate that 20 to 70 percent of cases seen in the primary care setting have some form of behavioral health disorder, which is missed in one-third to one-half of cases.[24-28]

None of this information is meant to blame the PCP for these problems. Their training has not given them sufficient skills to recognize some behavioral health disorders. There are structural and financial disincentives to diagnose and treat such

TABLE 1. KAISER-PERMANENTE OF NORTHERN CALIFORNIA'S EARLY START PROGRAM: OUTCOMES DATA 1995

Birth Outcome	Early Start women who quit using drugs/alcohol	Drug and alcohol users past 32 weeks of pregnancy
Premature births (<36 weeks)	4.6 percent	13.6 percent
Low birth weight (<2500 grams)	4.6 percent	13.6 percent
Average newborn length of stay	2.2 days	3.2 days
Neonatal intensive care unit admission	19.0 percent	27.0 percent
Average NICU stay	4.6 days	7.3 days

disorders appropriately. This can lead, in turn, to inappropriate use of more intensive and expensive medical services when behavioral health problems go untreated.

The Purchasers' Reaction

Although the wildly increasing costs of the late 1980s have moderated, healthcare costs continue to rise. The more progressive companies thus feel it is within their purview to continuously improve the quality of the healthcare system within a cost-conscious framework. They see this as a way to improve their competitive stance both locally and abroad. The use of Total Quality Management (TQM) or Continuous Quality Improvement (CQI) processes has been the most tangible implementation of these efforts. Other forms are employer purchaser coalitions, and development and implementation of employer/purchaser specific standards.

Integration of TQM/CQI process improvement programs and the use of sophisticated electronic technology to assess and manage performance are useful contributions to the medical field. Groups like the Employers Managed Healthcare Association and the Washington Business Group on Health commit significant resources to improving the current healthcare system.

In general, business purchasers adhere to principals of TQM/CQI. These processes are based on the idea that inefficiencies in a system drive down quality and increase cost. Leading edge purchasers increasingly recognize that separating or carving out behavioral health from other medical services may provide more immediate value, but can also create redundant and inefficient systems. The leading edge corporate purchasers are convening task forces, with their healthcare vendor partners, to address these issues.

Consumers, Providers, and Investors

In addition to corporate purchasers, there are other major constituencies with widely differing agendas. Consumers, providers, and investors can all achieve their goals through the better integration of healthcare services in general and, specifically, through the integration of primary care and behavioral health services.

Consumers want the best treatment and do not want to be shuffled from office to office in a fragmented system. Informed consumers will become empowered to recognize early symptoms of behavioral health disorders and push delivery systems to respond accordingly. In addition, electronic technologies hold great promise for the consumer. A number of health plans are now offering Web sites on the Internet where consumers may review the provider manual and other information about the health plan and their benefits. Other online information services under development may be able to provide consumers with real-time information about symptoms and basic healthcare management.

Benefits structures continue to hinder appropriate access to behavioral health services by providing primary care services for a lower out-of-pocket cost. The federal parity law scheduled to go into effect January 1, 1998, initially held some promise to address this issue, but the final structure may exacerbate the situation because it does not specifically address parity in co-payments or deductibles. As payors attempt to minimize the effect of parity on overall costs, one method of doing this will be to impede access to services through higher co-payments and deductibles.

Providers want to treat patients efficiently, but are hindered by fragmented training that emphasizes specialties. This occurs on both the primary care and the behavioral health side of the equation. Primary care physicians should be better trained to recognize the symptoms of anxiety, depressive disorders, and substance abuse problems (see Chapters 14, 15, and 16). They then need better information on how to access the behavioral health specialist system. Likewise, behavioral health specialists need to better recognize symptoms of biologically based disorders that can be better treated by a PCP. Behavioral health specialists also need to know how to work within the ecology of the primary care system. Again, electronic technology holds great promise to provide real-time linkage between the two systems. Although group and staff model health plans can co-locate professionals from either sector, thereby creating a real integrated team, independent practice associations and network model plans can link through computer and phone lines, creating a "virtual" team.

Current reimbursement structures also hinder integration. Many capitation arrangements provide payment to a PCP for the basic care of a defined population. However, payment for inpatient treatment is covered under a different financial model; thus referral to an inpatient unit does not financially affect the physician. This facilitates overuse of intensive psychiatric services in the inpatient setting and undertreatment of those patients who are too far from meeting the criteria for inpatient admission. Until financial mechanisms are better integrated (e.g., full capitation for all services in a system), integration of primary care and behavioral health will be difficult.

Investors must realize that long-term profits are not possible in an inefficient system. The volatility and short-term approach of stock market investors places emphasis on quick results that can be detrimental to healthcare delivery. Shareholders and investors need to understand that inappropriate and unintegrated clinical service delivery will ultimately erode their financial goals. There may be continued friction in this area, however, as the stock market often operates on "quick hits" that emphasize short-term activities without regard to long-term effects.

Recommendations

The question at this point should not be whether to integrate but rather how to integrate. As we implement our integration efforts, we should use a conceptual model to structure our efforts. There are currently three models that may be helpful in setting structure. The first model captures a specific aspect of an integration focus. The second and third are variations on the same theme that, if fully implemented, may result in an efficient, comprehensive healthcare system that provides high-quality services at the lowest possible costs.

Structural Models

1. *Managed Time Loss* is an integration model developed by consultants at William M. Mercer, Inc. This is an employer-focused model designed to integrate managed disability, workers compensation and related medical costs to facilitate employees' return to work and minimize risk liability. The model pre-

sents a process to evaluate all of the possible causes for decreased functioning, especially at the work site, and designs integrated programs (i.e., medical, behavioral, workers compensation, disability, EAP) to address these causes.

The Managed Time Loss model provides a single contact point for business, employees, and providers. Care is delivered through integrated clinical case management services. Integration with managed healthcare initiatives, employers' internal health programs, and return to work programs is included. Similarities with the following two models are inherent in the integrated case management approach and the emphasis on clinical program integration. The return to work emphasis is unique to this model.

2. The *Organized Systems of Care (OSC)* model, developed in 1993 by the Washington Business Group on Health (WBGH), calls for the integration of finance and delivery mechanisms with a coordinated focus on quality and cost management for a controlled panel of providers.[29] The result is a comprehensive healthcare service system driven by CQI processes and related incentives. Services are designed to meet the needs of a specific community and its residents, and include wellness and health promotion activities. The care provided is guided by clinical protocols that structure only appropriate and necessary services, and the overall system is accountable through data that detail cost, quality, and outcomes. Care delivery comes from care management teams that integrate physical, psychological, and administrative functions. The continuum of care ranges from prenatal to long-term care in settings ranging from the most highly technical to the home. The entire system and its processes are continuously informed through computerized information links (Figure 6). The result is a healthcare system that integrates delivery, administration, finance, and oversight in a continuous learning environment.

3. The *Organized Delivery Systems (ODS)* model was developed in 1996 by consultants at KPMG Peat Marwick's Strategic Health Solutions Practice.[13] This model is a variation of the WBGH OSC model described above, with added emphasis on

The Organized System of Care
Care Delivery

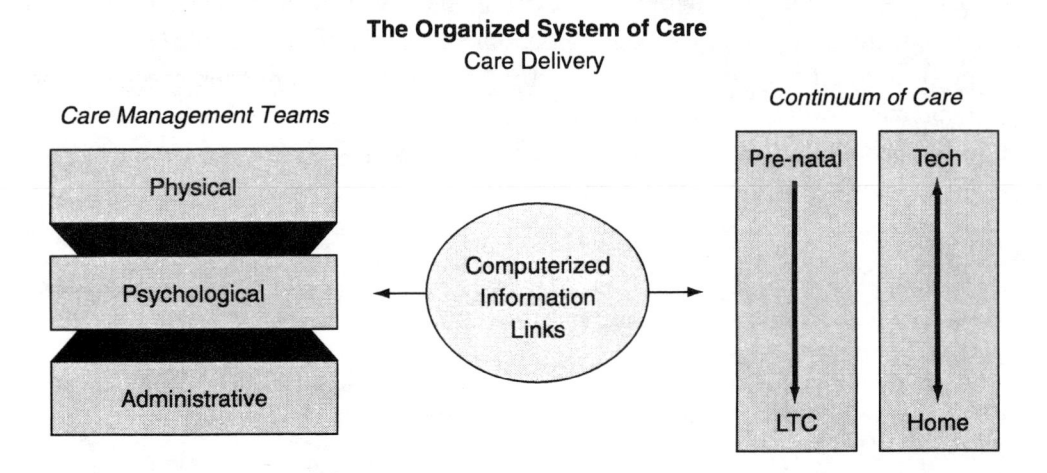

Figure 6

communication, information systems, and the need for providers to better prepare to manage capitated contracts. The ODS proposes a "systems" approach to the coordination and management of an individual's care throughout the entire spectrum of health services in a continuous, comprehensive, and systematic manner.

KPMG predicts that by the year 2010, integrated patient care will be defined by a focus on long-term value; increased interdependency of providers, suppliers, payors, and patients; a boundary-free culture (among all health system players); information empowered behavior; continuous outcomes improvement; and focus on the individual patient. The effective organized delivery system will consist of integrated information systems, an information infrastructure, aligned incentives, clinical guidelines, and public policy initiatives.[13]

Summary

The data demonstrate both the ineffectiveness of our current system and the effectiveness of focused behavioral health interventions on a number of psychiatric disorders in more integrated systems. We must become more efficient in the recognition and treatment of behavioral health disorders, or costs will continue to rise unnecessarily. Much of the need for behavioral health services remains in the primary care setting, and it is to this area that we must provide substantial resources.

Studies point consistently to the efficacy of behavioral health interventions in the primary care setting. Behavioral health services provided in the primary care setting have demonstrated up to 70 percent reduction in hospital costs and up to 30 percent reduction in outpatient medical costs, with the greatest effect on the elderly portion of the population studied.[30] With approximately one-quarter to one-third of the most common chronic disorders exacerbated by concurrent behavioral health disorders, a coordinated team effort—including at least one behavioral health professional—is needed to treat these chronic disorders. The Organized System of Care model provides one way to approach this challenge.

As we increasingly move toward capitated models and the use of the PCP as a general systems gatekeeper, the need is emphasized for a closer primary care/behavioral health integration. For patients that can be managed in the primary care setting we must ensure that primary care providers are properly trained and provided with appropriate support. For those requiring more intensive treatment from specialists, we must implement systems that appear seamless to the consumer and provide easy access to the behavioral health professionals. These specialists must then work in concert with primary care and other caregivers.

References

1. Regier D, Narrow W, Rae D, et al: The de facto US mental and addictive disorders service system: epidemiological catchment area prospective one year prevalence rates of disorders and services. Arch Gen Psychiatry 50:85–94, 1993.
2. Regier D, Narrow W, Rae D, et al: Use of services by persons with mental and addictive disorders: findings from the Institute of Health Epedemiolgic Catchment Area Program, Arch Gen Psychiatry 50:95–107, 1993.
3. Wells K, Stewart A, Hays R, et al: The functioning and well-being of depressed patients: results from the medical outcomes study. JAMA 262:914–919, 1989.

4. Katon W, VonKorff M, Lin E, et al: Distressed high utilizers of medical care: DSM III-R diagnoses and treatment needs. Gen Hosp Psychiatry 12:355-362, 1990.
5. Worldwide Study Predicts Severe Depression Will Become Second Largest Cause of Death. Via Internet PRNewswire, September 27, 1996.
6. Moffic HS, Paykel ES: Depression in medical inpatients. Br J Psychiatry 126:346-353, 1975.
7. Schubert DSP, Taylor C, Lee S, Mentari A, Tamaklo W: Physical consequences of depression in the stroke patient. Gen Hosp Psychiatry 14:69-76, 1992.
8. NAMI Heralds Historic Step Toward Ending Insurance Discrimination, via Internet by PRNewswire, September 19, 1996.
9. Moore RD, Bone LR, Geller G, et al: Prevalence, detection and treatment of alcoholism in hospitalized patients. JAMA 261:403-407, 1989.
10. Holder HD, Blose JO: Alcoholism treatment and total healthcare utilization and costs: a four year longitudinal analysis of federal employees. JAMA, 256:1456-1460, 1986.
11. Drugs and alcohol in the workplace: a guide for managers. New York: Facts on File Publications, 1988.
12. Watson Wyatt Worldwide Study. PRNewswire, April 30, 1996.
13. Integrated Patient Care: Managing Healthcare Costs, Maximizing Healthcare Value and Quality. A report prepared by KPMG Peat Marwick LLP, Strategic Health Solutions Practice, 1996.
14. Taylor W: What comes after your success? Fast Company No. 6:85, 1997.
15. Lipkin M: Can primary care physicians deliver quality mental healthcare? Behavioral Healthcare Tomorrow 5:52, 1996.
16. Melek S: Behavioral healthcare risk-sharing and medical cost offset. Behavioral Healthcare Tomorrow 5:39, 1996.
17. Zung WW, Broadhead WE, Roth ME: Prevalence of depressive symptoms in primary care. J Fam Pract 37:337-344, 1993.
18. Johnson P: The purchaser perspective on the need for primary care integration. The Primary Care Behavioral Healthcare Summit, San Diego, March 28, 1996.
19. Smith D, Mahoney J: McDonnell Douglas Corporation Employee Assistance Program Financial Offset Study, 1989 (unpublished).
20. Lieberman L: The Kaiser Permanente Early Start Program: how to integrate substance abuse services with perinatal care. The Primary Care Behavioral Health Summit, San Diego March 28, 1996.
21. Borus JF, Olendzki MC, et al: The 'offset effect' of mental health treatment on ambulatory medical care utilization and charges. A month-by-month and a grouped-month analysis of a five year study. Arch Gen Psychiatry 42:573-580, 1985.
22. Dea R: The Kaiser Permanente Northern California Model of Care. The Primary Care Behavioral Healthcare Summit, San Diego CA, March 28, 1996.
23. Wells KB, Katon W, Rogers B, et al: Use of minor tranquilizers and antidepressant medications by depressed outpatients: results from the Medical Outcomes Study. Am J Psychiatry, 151:694-700, 1994.
24. Rush AJ, Golden WE, Hall GW, et al: Depression in primary care: clinical practice guidelines, AHCPR. Behavioral Healthcare Tomorrow 5:61, 1996.
25. Katon W, Roy-Byrne PP: Panic disorder in the medically ill. J Clin Psychiatry 50:299-302, 1989.
26. Higgins ES: A review of unrecognized mental illness in primary care: prevelance, natural history and efforts to change the course. Arch Family Med 3:908-917, 1994.
27. Spitzer RL, Williams JBW, Kroenke K, et al: Utility of a new procedure for diagnosing mental disorders in primary care: the PRIME-MD 1000 study. JAMA 272:1749-1756, 1994.
28. US Department of Health and Human Services: Seventh Special Report to the U.S. Congress on Alcohol and Health. Alcohol, Drug Abuse and Mental Health Administration, Rockville, MD, 1990.
29. Cronin C, Milgate K: A Vision for the Future Healthcare Delivery System: Organized Systems of Care. Washington Business Group on Health, Washington DC, 1993.
30. Mumford E, Schlesinger H, Glass G, et al: A new look at evidence about reduced cost of medical utilization following mental health treatment. Am J Psychiatry 141:1145-1158, 1984.

Chapter 3

The Roles of the Behavioral Health Professional in Integrated Systems

Keith Dixon, Ph.D.

Several years ago John Kitzhaber, an emergency room physician (who went on to become the governor of Oregon) discussed Oregon's controversial approach to managing costs and quality of care, and the importance of the primary care physician (PCP) in our evolving system of health care.

Following his presentation to a group of physicians, a cardiologist remarked that we have dangerously raised our expectations of what a PCP can or should do, beyond the bounds of what is medically responsible. The cardiologist declared that PCPs will soon be expected by managed care companies to perform coronary bypass surgery on an outpatient basis following routine physical exams.

"Not to worry about that ever happening–it simply won't," Dr. Kitzhaber reassured him. "Coronary bypass surgery in tomorrow's managed systems will be done by the nurse practitioner!" Dr. Kitzhaber was obviously joking, but the laughs he received from the audience were nervous ones.

Specialists or Generalists?

Psychiatrists are experiencing the same worries as the cardiologist, because many in psychiatry have been accustomed to thinking of their roles as specialists–even as subspecialists–rather than as extensions of primary medicine. Dr. E. Fuller Torrey, a prominent U.S. psychiatrist and a very strong advocate for the mentally ill, recently stated that in medical schools, the department of psychiatry should be folded into the neurology department.[1] It should be noted that he does not suggest that the department of psychiatry be combined with the department of family practice or primary medicine.

Is psychiatry a specialty or a component of primary medicine? What is the role of this professional? In the disorienting environment in which we find ourselves, psychiatrists in the United States are now concerned about their role in the future healthcare arena. Some HMOs operate on the belief that many of the functions of the psychiatrist can be performed adequately by a PCP with a good team of social workers. They also argue that in this era of cost-consciousness, it can be done less expensively, with less administrative hassle, and with equivalent or better outcomes using this alternative model.

The roles of the clinical social worker, psychologist, and psychiatric nurse practitioner in the era of managed care are also in question. These professionals have PCPs available to them to prescribe medications. As we develop national guidelines and standardized approaches to illnesses like depression and anxiety, as medications become more efficacious, more readily available, and have fewer side effects, some believe that *any* doctor—regardless of specialty—could prescribe medication by adhering to treatment guidelines. In addition, a growing number of psychologists are training in the use of psychotropic medications and lobbying to obtain prescription privileges.

What is the future of psychotherapy? Can clinical social workers obtain equivalent outcomes delivering psychotherapy at a lower cost than other mental health "specialties"? Payors have also begun to question the value of psychological testing. For example, in one state the highest category of all Medicaid billings is for testing of children with attention-deficit hyperactivity disorder (ADHD). The state is facing the dilemma of cutting basic services in order to continue paying for the testing of these children. One managed care company is attempting to assess the value of the TOVA (a computerized diagnostic aid), popular with psychologists, but one that many pediatricians say is simply unnecessary. In an age of diminishing financial resources, difficult decisions will have to be made by determining the most effective and financially responsible treatments to be offered and deciding who should offer them. We do not have clear answers for this yet.

Changing Role Expectations

Given the diminishing role expectations for specialists across all areas of medicine, and the increasing role expectations for PCPs and their extenders, what boundaries should be placed on the PCP's responsibility for mental illness? Some of the practical implications of this question are revealed in the following example.

A primary care physician group with several thousand covered lives capitates professional fees for mental health treatment at $.50 per member per month (pmpm). Capitation rates for mental health treatment have been as low as $.20 or $.30 pmpm in some areas. These capitation levels may be acceptable if the PCP is trained to render psychiatric services and the psychotherapy is performed by social workers at lower cost. In this model, the role of the psychiatrist is perhaps to supervise and manage only the most severe forms of mental illness and/or the most chronic and difficult patients. Is this merely a reflection of harsh economic realities of healthcare today, or the result of more responsible, appropriate roles for practitioners and allocation of resources in our new systems of care? Obviously, one of the implications of this particular model is that we need far fewer psychiatrists than we currently have or who are now in training. This parallels the need for fewer specialists in many areas of medicine.

A second implication is that psychiatrists will increasingly become mere pill-pushers, seeing patients on short intervals that involve almost no "therapeutic bond." It remains to be determined whether such an arrangement is medically responsible or ethical. If patients improve and costs are reduced, what is wrong with this arrangement? The only people likely to object are those who may simply be mourning the diminution of a specialty and have a narrow interest in perpetuating a guild.

This kind of managed care arrangement, which has become commonplace today in areas of "mature" managed care evolution, raises important issues with respect to professional training. If we accept this role for the psychiatrist, we must teach psychiatric residents how to provide leadership and supervision to others—a unique aptitude involving a very challenging set of interpersonal skills. We must avoid preparing psychiatrists and others primarily for entry into solo private practice where the assumption is that the only performance they will ever have to worry about is their own. This is actually a corollary of a much larger structural issue. As Don Berwick observed recently in the *New England Journal of Medicine,* in the United States we still train doctors and nurses in separate schools, but expect them to function naturally as an interdependent team when they graduate.[2] In short, approaches to training, irrespective of the need to lower the number of licensed mental health professionals, have not kept up with the realities of managed care settings. Structure bears little relationship to function.

Integration: Image and Reality

When thinking about the integration of primary care with behavioral healthcare, two very different images emerge. My ideal image of integration is seeing my primary care physician for an annual physical exam and also being asked how I'm feeling. My family and work stressors are discussed. The doctor recommends some stress management techniques. She also refers me to a social worker just down the hall who offers an executive stress management program in the evening. When I return to the doctor six weeks later and have my cholesterol checked, she and I discuss the effects of the program.

However, this is not reality in most places in our healthcare system. First, physical examinations in many managed care settings are not done by physicians at all, but by physician assistants, who see patients on a rotating basis. There is no assurance that the patient will see the same practitioner on each visit. Typical physician encounters with patients in managed care primary care settings are short, and group practices often employ productivity measures to prevent a physician from becoming an "outlier" in this regard. In capitation, physician time is still money, but going in a different direction. Time available to discuss psychosocial issues is limited. If a patient is developing a depression, it is difficult to see how this would be diagnosed. The social worker down the hall (mentioned above) would probably be treating more serious mental illness than my executive stress. In addition, it is unlikely that my health plan would pay for mental health benefits for my stress (a V code), although I believe my physical and emotional well-being are clearly at risk and treatment would be cost-effective.

Moreover, emotional problems and mental illness frequently make medical doctors uncomfortable. This may be due in part to the nature of medical training, which can be isolating and authoritarian. It seems that behavioral healthcare, like other areas of healthcare, may expect too much now from PCPs when we require them to tease out the nuances of our emotional states.

The "Carve-out" Response

The so-called "carve-out market" for managed behavioral healthcare companies is a response to the shortcomings of integration. Carve-outs came into existence because employers did not like what general healthcare organizations—whether they are a health maintenance organization (HMO), PCP or multispecialty group practice, or hospital-based integrated delivery system—offered in terms of benefits and treatment for behavioral health disorders. Employers were not just obsessed with costs, because behavioral health benefits in HMOs were a very low percentage of a (relatively) low medical premium, yet employers still wanted this area of benefits carved out. So-called specialized carve-out companies now cover 120 million Americans and offer directly to employers a broad range of behavioral healthcare services that are still not generally available in HMOs or medical systems. These include employee assistance programs (EAPs), specialized workers compensation management, drug-free workplace screening and consultation, workplace crisis intervention, supervisor development, team building, and, yes, executive stress management. As long as medical practitioners and organizations are not thinking about the behavioral healthcare needs of the end customer, and ignore the compelling data and obvious common sense of the "offset" effects of mental healthcare, the carve-out market will thrive.

Many HMOs have not paid much attention to behavioral health until the marketplace pressure to receive National Committee for Quality Assurance (NCQA) accreditation forced them to pay attention. Now NCQA, with the help of American Managed Behavioral Healthcare Association (AMBHA) and others, is coming out with a distinct set of performance criteria for behavioral healthcare in HEDIS 3.0 (Health Employer Data Information Set). Recently many of the carve-out companies have been acquired by HMOs. This may help with NCQA accreditation for the parent HMO, but hardly ensures real integration at the service delivery level. For integration to occur, there has to be an operational and clinical interface between the mental health professionals in the carve-out company's networks and the PCPs contracted to the HMO or employed by the HMO in a staff-model configuration. And it is at this level that we face all the problems previously discussed. Few HMOs have been willing to grapple with these issues about professional roles and responsibilities in integrated systems of care.

Functional Integration

We should distinguish between *structural* integration as exemplified by the HMO that buys a carve-out company and turns it over to the management of its mental health benefit, and *functional* integration that requires a much more fundamental and more difficult effort to change clinical practices and processes throughout the organization. Functional integration obviously makes sense in terms of service, quality of care, and prevention. As of yet there is no single structural model for achieving this, just continuous experiments and innovations pushed by NCQA and the marketplace. Many carve-out companies have made strides toward integrating their networks and operations with PCPs who are not structurally aligned with them. In other systems, such as comprehensive medical group practices, there is often great teamwork between mental health clinicians and the medical staff of all specialties, but often little connection to the needs of the employer or the consumer with less serious mental illness.

All models have strengths and weaknesses. In carve-out companies, it is often a struggle to get close to medical providers and form collaborative relationships. In large group practices, it is often difficult to get close to the employer, who may be looking for something beyond what we customarily think of as behavioral healthcare—and carve-out companies are extremely nimble respondents to what employers need and want.

Summary

It is surprising that integration has only recently re-emerged as a major issue in healthcare. It has taken the economic pressures of managed care and the demands from employers for accountability to place integration in the spotlight. Without these pressures, we would most likely continue to focus our attention in behavioral health on the preservation of traditional professional roles and boundaries, instead of focusing on prevention and developing processes that produce the best outcome for the patient at the lowest possible cost. Integration challenges traditional roles and processes, forcing institutions in our field to change. In the sixteenth century Machiavelli said:

> It ought to be remembered that there is nothing more difficult to conduct, or more uncertain of its success, than to take the lead in the introduction of a new order of things. For the innovator has for enemies all those who have done well under the old conditions, and lukewarm defenders in those who may do well under the new.[3]

Role change, as sociologists know, can be profoundly disorienting to individuals and is often vehemently resisted by groups and institutions who have an investment in the status quo. That is where we are now in this field despite our current enthusiasm for this rather innocent-looking concept called integration. We should be confident that the innovators in healthcare will succeed. The economy and quality of care concerns demand it. I hope they receive something more than a lukewarm reception.

References

1. Torrey EF: Confronting America's Mental Illness Problems. Address to the National Alliance for the Mentally Ill. July 8, 1996, Nashville TN.
2. Berwick DM: Quality of health care. Part V: Payment by capitation and the quality of care. N Engl J Med 335: 1227-1231, 1996.
3. Machiavelli: The Prince. 1513 AD.

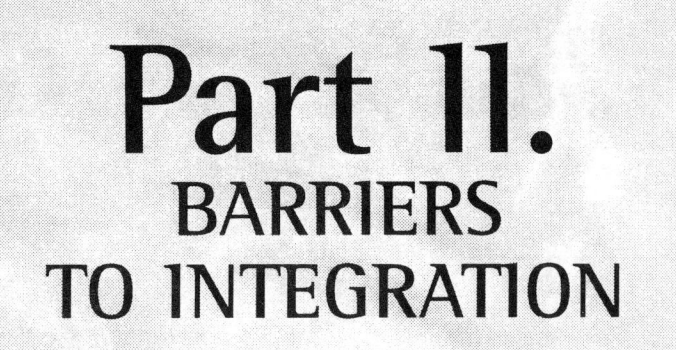

Part 11.
BARRIERS TO INTEGRATION

Chapter 4

Overcoming Ecological Barriers to Integration

Carol L. Alter, M.D., Steven Cole, M.D., and Mary Raju, RN, M.S.N.

Why don't patients with behavioral disorders receive appropriate care in the general medical sector, and what must be done to effect appropriate change? The answers to these questions involve not only the imperative to improve providers' knowledge and skills, but also the necessity to revolutionize the ecology of our current health systems, in the sense that *ecology* is the science of the relationship of an organism to its environment. We must examine the institutionalized relationships among the patient and the provider, and the health system in which they participate, in order to solve behavioral healthcare problems. As medical care is currently structured, an array of seemingly insurmountable obstacles block the development of a healthcare system that efficiently and effectively integrates behavioral and primary healthcare. Innovative paths to high-quality and cost-effective integration already exist, however, and more generalized solutions can be realized if health planners remain cognizant of and committed to program development that systematically integrates behavioral and general medical care on a day-to-day basis.

Overcoming Deficits in Providers' Knowledge and Skills

Western medicine based on Cartesian dualism, the separation of the mind and the body, historically has not been concerned with mental disorders. The thrust of general medical practice leads physicians toward a "biomedical reductionism," encouraging an approach to medical problems that focuses on ever smaller units of analysis, until, paradigmatically, a molecular explanation and solution can be found.[1] Given this conceptual approach to the practice of medicine, and the little education about the assessment and management of mental disorders in general medical practice that medical students receive, it is small wonder that physicians have inadequate knowledge and skills to deal with behavioral disorders.[2] Furthermore, in the current managed care environment, physicians often feel reluctant to investigate behavioral issues for fear of opening a Pandora's box that may lead them into an abyss of emotional chaos from which they may not be able to extricate themselves quickly or delicately.

Despite these problems, the need for a primary care physician (PCP) to begin addressing behavioral issues more systematically has now become imperative. Health services research clearly documents that undiagnosed mental disorders cost medical systems vast sums in unjustified, fruitless investigations, leading to unsatisfied patients, providers, and administrators.[3] Appropriate diagnosis and treatment of behavioral disorders in the medical setting, on the other hand, leads to more efficient and effective care and to more satisfied patients.[4] Contrary to concerns about opening a Pandora's box, physicians actually *increase* their efficiency as well as patient outcomes when they directly address behavioral issues. Avoiding emotional issues actually adds time and expense to patient care.

We have described elsewhere the concrete ways that health plans can begin addressing the knowledge and skills barriers presented by providers.[5] While overcoming these barriers is a complex task, new educational technologies can significantly improve physicians' communication behaviors with patients, leading to improved skills in the detection of mental disorders, more satisfied patients, and improved clinical outcomes. One study, for example, demonstrated that an eight-hour training program led to measurable improvements in physicians' communication skills, in detection rates of mental disorders, and in patient outcomes on measures of emotional distress six months after the training. These objectives were realized *without increasing overall interviewing time with patients*.[6] Another randomized, controlled study reported that physicians' knowledge of mental disorders was improved following two different focused training programs.[2] The MacArthur Foundation has recently developed an eight-hour training program for PCPs on the assessment and management of depression. The program has been piloted and is being tested in randomized, prospective clinical trials for efficacy. The educational monograph for this program is reproduced in Chapter 14 of this book.

By using validated educational strategies, training programs for primary care providers can be developed that have reliable, concrete, and expected outcomes. Objectives must be clear and understandable to both trainers and learners. They must be stated in behavioral—not general—terms. The objectives must align with the proposed teaching methods, and evaluation measures must assess the actual behaviors that are taught.[7] Teaching methods must be appropriate to the objectives selected. That is, programs focusing on increasing knowledge should differ from programs focusing on skills. While these educational "domains" (i.e., knowledge and skills) certainly overlap in practice, programs focusing on increasing knowledge can be best evaluated by testing what learners can report (or say) they *know*, while skills programs focus on what learners actually *do*. The best methods for imparting knowledge include learning approaches that communicate information in discrete, easily remembered "bundles." Skill development programs follow a time-tested approach that includes orientation, demonstration, practice, feedback, and repeated practice.[5]

While such programs will augment PCPs and assure that they can maximize their interaction with patients, the obstacles and their ultimate resolution lie beyond the individual relationship of physician and patient. Therefore, larger impediments must be considered, including economic and policy implications and mechanisms for addressing those concerns, in order to fully integrate medical and behavioral health systems.

Ecological Obstacles and System Solutions

The greatest impediment to patients receiving integrated care arises from the ecological and system variables that determine the nature of healthcare systems. Financial arrangements are often central to these outcomes. Whether a patient is receiving care through a plan with "carved in" behavioral health benefits, or whether benefits are "carved out," the ability to integrate that care in the medical setting is often limited. In the carve-out model, all requests for behavioral health input are outside the system. While most carve-out models of care develop "coordination of care" agreements between the medical and behavioral health providers, such agreements tend to focus on transfer of patient information and pharmacy concerns. Rarely do issues focus on how to obtain behavioral health treatment for patients within the medical setting, or concomitant with medical illness or treatment. Such issues are seldom addressed within these agreements. Because the behavioral health and general medical plans tend to use different panels of providers, significant problems of access can be created, especially when a healthcare institution/system has no contractual relationship with its affiliated or in-house behavioral health providers.

Carve-in or integrated plans should have seamless referral procedures for medical patients requiring behavioral health evaluation and treatment. However, these services tend to be focused on general psychiatric and emotional issues and are not aimed at resolving the special issues that might arise in the medical setting. Patients with complicated medical conditions—such as cancer, AIDS, chronic renal disorders, pediatric illness—that might put them at risk for developing psychiatric complaints, often need specialized behavioral healthcare. Rarely do these specialized services exist, even in an integrated setting.

In the current setting for a PCP or general medical plan that carves out behavioral health, what is the financial rationale to provide additional on-site behavioral health services? Similarly, why would the behavioral health provider invest resources in caring for a population that is not "his"? There is a significant disincentive, especially in the capitated environment, to increase costs. Unless there is compelling evidence that providing a greater number or intensity of services will lead to a short-term reduction in costs, extra outlays are often difficult to justify. There is a further disincentive for the behavioral health provider, because identifying additional cases within the medical setting can lead to increased demand for services and further expense.

Assuring Integration of Behavioral and Medical Care: Creating Workable Solutions

Psychiatrists and other behavioral health professionals have played active roles in medical settings, especially in those where patients have a high risk of developing psychological difficulties in conjunction with their medical conditions. Ideally, behavioral health providers will need to have increased involvement in both specialized and primary care medical settings and serve as team leaders to develop active, contributory behavioral health teams. On-site involvement of behavioral health providers can make ongoing education and consultation available to PCPs, and can reinforce and facilitate knowledge and skill training experiences. In addition, they can assist with preventive programs and provide important links to the behavioral healthcare system (including mental health providers with expertise in areas of high medical/psychiatric comorbidities) if patients require more intensive treatment.

The best approach to integrate medical and behavioral healthcare is to assure that mechanisms are put in place to reduce obstacles. Regardless of whether a plan is integrated or carved out, attention must be paid to the specific mechanisms established to assure integration. Administrators of health plans should ask themselves a series of questions to highlight where the system works and where it needs adjustment.

Several issues should be considered in order to ensure that care is maximally integrated: who provides services, how providers communicate with each other about medical and psychiatric care, and finally, who pays for services (see Table 1). These aspects of care are addressed in the following case study examples that show how components can be identified and included in the development and maintenance of an integrated care system.

Case 1: Psychiatric Consultation Performed in the Inpatient Setting

A patient with medical coverage from a medical plan, BestHealth, is admitted to the hospital for a myocardial infarction. His medical attending physician contacts an in-plan cardiologist to provide cardiology consultation. The patient is admitted to a cardiac care unit (CCU) for treatment and observation. On the second day of admission, the patient experiences confusion and agitation. Concerned about the management of his patient, the cardiologist contacts his colleague Dr. Smith, a psychiatrist, to do an evaluation of the patient. Dr. Smith discovers that the patient has a long history of alcohol abuse that was not revealed to the treatment team, and he is going through acute alcohol withdrawal. Recommendations for treatment are made, and Dr. Smith returns to visit the patient the next day to assure that he is receiving the appropriate medication and has shown clinical improvement. As the staff of the CCU is not particularly familiar with the detoxification of patients, they contact Dr. Smith on several occasions to review the recommendations, and Dr. Smith makes plans to return to the unit to educate the staff on alcohol intoxication and withdrawal syndromes and management.

TABLE 1. CREATING MECHANISMS TO ASSURE INTEGRATED CARE: A CHECKLIST

Who Provides
Clinical skills: which type of clinician for which setting?
Appropriate providers included in appropriate plan (behavioral health and/or medical)
Clinician should be privileged

Who Pays
Behavioral health plan
Medical health plan
Determined by primary diagnosis (medical versus behavioral health)
Risk-sharing agreements

How Paid
Established at time of contract negotiation
Establish and maintain adequate reimbursement rates
Eliminate onerous authorization procedures

Communication
Assure access to both behavioral health and medical records
Know your "gatekeeper"

When Dr. Smith returns to her office on Monday, she submits her fee slips to her billing manager. The manager submits the bills to BestHealth, who then informs the billing manager that they do not cover psychiatric services and suggests that the bill be submitted to the patient's behavioral health plan, BestMind. BestMind states that they don't have a contract with Dr. Smith, so they will not pay for the consult. They acknowledge, however, that they have responsibility for the patient, and if the patient's PCP had contacted the office before the consult (their hours are usual working hours), they would have been happy to send out a psychiatric nurse or psychologist to see the patient. Furthermore, the patient certainly could have seen a mental health professional in the outpatient center.

Who Provides the Care?

In this case, the patient's behavioral healthcare was carved out, and the plan did not provide service in the same institution as the patient's medical plan. The situation was further complicated by the fact that BestMind would have provided care, but of a different level of service (a nurse rather than a physician) to that patient in that hospital. One question Dr. Smith didn't ask was whether the nurse who could have done the consult was privileged at the institution. Because she sits on the privileging committee, she was surprised to hear of this offer: she knew of no mental health professionals outside of her department who held privileges to practice in her hospital.

Requirements for the Provider

In order to function in the system described above, the provider must:

— Have the appropriate skills;
— Be part of credentialed provider panels; and
— Have clinical privileges in the medical system in which the patient resides.

The provider must have appropriate levels of skill to meet the clinical circumstance. A psychiatrist will usually be needed to assess medical and psychiatric comorbidity, to make recommendations for further evaluation, and to make specific pharmacologic recommendations. While other professionals are often very important to the behavioral healthcare of medical inpatients, the role of each type of provider must be defined. Nurses and psychologists should not initiate medical or pharmacologic plans without physician support.

In addition to possessing the requisite skills, the provider must be part of the panel. Whether the provider is part of the medical panel or the behavioral health panel may depend on contract circumstances. If the provider is not part of the panel, obtaining reimbursement is either impossible or extremely difficult. In many cases approval may be granted, but only if pre-authorization is requested. In the example above, that would have been difficult to arrange.

Finally, the clinician must also be privileged in the medical system in which the patient receives care. In this example, it was discovered that BestMind's nurse was not privileged at the hospital, and that Dr. Smith was correct in assuming that her committee would have to review and approve any mental health professional for privileges. In areas where significant consolidation between hospitals and provider groups has occurred, assumptions are often made regarding the ubiquity of privileging across these new health systems; despite these changes, questions should be raised about who can do what and where.

The Need for Adequate Communication

This example illustrates two problems related to communication. Dr. Smith learned from the patient that he had a prior history of alcoholism, which had been addressed by BestMind. Neither the cardiologist nor the internist were aware of these issues, since neither participated in the ongoing care of this individual. Because records were shared on a case-by-case basis between the two plans, the patient did not volunteer his problem, consent was not obtained to query BestMind's data system, and the information was not revealed. Secondly, while it appears appropriate that the psychiatrist would communicate with the cardiologist in this case, both are consultants and neither had the right in this circumstance to provide or order services without the request of the internist.

Assuring Adequate Communication
In order to assure adequate communication:

– Records need to be shared readily and easily; and
– Lines of communication between physicians need to be solidified.

Legal mechanisms that respect local patient confidentiality statutes need to be established so that patient records of both psychiatric and medical treatment are readily accessible. Patients could sign release of information waivers on a routine basis, or whenever they have contact with either the medical or psychiatric system. In areas where such confidentiality statutes do not exist, a shared medical record or easy access to data between providers is critical.

In a gatekeeper system, consultants need to be educated regarding what can and cannot be done without permission. Systems that either carve out specialty care (e.g., oncology, chronic renal disease, etc.) or that allow a chronic illness provider to become a "PCP," obviate some of this confusion and diminish the need for referrals.

Who Will Pay?

In this example, it didn't appear that anyone would pay, but be assured that Dr. Smith would be less willing to volunteer to see the cardiologist's (or the internist's or the surgeon's) patients again without first guaranteeing that she was authorized to do so. Waiting for the mental health provider to obtain authorization, while the patient is standing on the ledge or threatening to assault another patient or staff member, will not ensure an appropriate or timely clinical response.

Creating a Financial Solution
Optimally, payment should:

– Be determined as part of the contract with either physicians or hospitals;
– Be easy to get; and
– Follow established rate structures.

Numerous models for payment are covered in more detail in Chapter 5. However, it is important to assure that someone is, in fact, paying. In some instances, agreements have been negotiated so that payment depends on whether the patient has primarily a psychiatric or medical diagnosis. In other instances the risk is shared based on an agreed-upon formula. In an integrated setting this may not be an issue, unless of course there is no appropriate provider privileged at the particular institution.

This scenario is not uncommon in the clinical setting. However, it has been the experience of many hospital-based departments of psychiatry that when their inpatient and outpatient mental health services are not included in a particular health plan or its affiliated behavioral health plan, mental health services for inpatients may be carved back in. In this way, psychiatrists who ordinarily provide psychiatric consultation and liaison services are included in the medical "panel" and can provide those services.[8]

In many settings, discussions with both the behavioral health and medical plans lead to solutions after contracts have been signed. An example described by Hails and colleagues involved the development of an agreement between a large behavioral health plan and several hospital-based departments of psychiatry.[9] In this plan, the behavioral health carve-out, which had not originally agreed to fund psychiatric consultations for the medically ill, agreed to do so but required pre-authorization for every consult or intervention. As the behavioral health carve-out plan had no experience handling medical problems, there were no clinically relevant forms to complete. The person giving authorization had little expertise in these areas and was often unwilling to provide authorization. Even when authorization was preliminarily granted, it was frequently rescinded, leading to further appeal and a lack of reimbursement for services performed.

Further, it has been found that psychiatrists seeing patients in this setting perform an average of two interventions. A behavioral health plan that allows for the initial consult and at least one follow-up visit without pre-authorization avoids significant oversight and authorization expense. Activity can be monitored over time to identify outliers, and overuse can then be addressed. If this is not possible, subcontracting with the medical provider may provide more efficient and appropriate utilization reviews, as they have greater capability to review the clinical needs in this setting.

While behavioral health specialists in the outpatient setting or inpatient psychiatric setting may negotiate reduced fees for service that may be appropriate or feasible for those settings, the work performed in the medical setting is in fact comparable to the kind of work performed by other consultants in the medical setting (e.g., cardiologists, endocrinologists). Fees should be predetermined based on market rates of other medical consultants.

The Outpatient Setting

Two characteristic issues occur in the outpatient setting. The first involves the availability of psychiatric and mental health input for the routine general medical patient. The second involves the special psychosocial needs of patients with chronic medical problems. Here too, issues of who provides, who pays, and how communication occurs predominate.

Case 2: Psychological Distress in the Primary Care Clinic

Mrs. Goodhealth has just switched medical plans. She is now enrolled in Best-Health's premier program, where she has been assured that she will have optimal physician choice and will benefit from numerous health-promoting activities. While generally healthy, she has had intermittent problems with insomnia that no one has definitively treated or diagnosed. In her first visit with Dr. Feelbetter, she reviews her medical history and discusses her chronic insomnia. He reviews her prior history and tests, then asks her to complete a brief questionnaire about her mood and other topics related to her emotional health. Dr. Feelbetter returns and lets Mrs. Goodhealth know that she has a minor case of depression and starts her on a course of Fluoxetine (10 mg/day).

Mrs. Goodhealth initially takes the medication but soon discontinues it. Six weeks later, when she sees Dr. Feelbetter again, she shares her experience with him, states she won't take pills anymore, and adds that in addition to not sleeping well, she now has headaches—and by the way, work has been very stressful for her. Dr. Feelbetter discusses further treatment for her symptoms and suggests that she can be referred to the mental health plan for follow-up if she is interested. She asks whether the clinic has any stress management courses available.

Who Provides the Care?

Both Mrs. Goodhealth and Dr. Feelbetter are representative of many typical patients and physicians. Mrs. Goodhealth's complaints appear to be vague, with little organic basis. Dr. Feelbetter, wanting to do the right thing but not having much time to do it, resorts to the best option he knows. The result was a lack of complete diagnostic accuracy and a practical attempt at management, with no improvement in outcome. One important question to ask is what other options were available to either the patient or the physician in this setting? What would have been the financial or clinical impact if on-site psychiatric input had been available? At what point, if any, would referral to the behavioral health team have been appropriate?

The Primary Care Provider:
Optimally, the provider:

— Must know how to provide behavioral healthcare services; and
— Have time to provide the services.

Or

— Must have the ability to collaborate with behavioral healthcare providers or make appropriate referrals to the behavioral health experts.

Studies that have examined the nature of psychiatric evaluation and treatment in the primary care setting by PCPs have found that the ability to accurately diagnose and treat psychiatric disorders is often limited.[10-12] However, studies have also shown that when there is ongoing and active psychiatric input, diagnosis and treatment are significantly improved.[13] This is true not only when the psychiatrist performs the assessment and implements treatment, but also if they have an active role in the teaching, supervising, and coaching of primary caregivers in the clinical setting.

As discussed earlier, there is a clear set of skills to be mastered in order to evaluate and treat psychiatric disorders. If the PCP is to provide these services, then training and ongoing education must be available and utilized. If the PCP is the mainstay of this care, attention must be paid to the amount of time necessary to provide these services. A seven-minute visit will not provide enough time to adequately determine the etiology or treatment of these complicated problems. Alternatively, the PCP can be supported/assisted by other mental health providers or can routinely obtain mental health services.

What is Provided?

In this instance, the PCP used a screening form to diagnose a psychiatric disorder. Is this an appropriate level of care? Would this be a sufficient way to diagnose diabetes or hypertension? Such screening instruments have been developed principally for use in the primary care setting. The two most widely used instruments, the PRIME-MD and SDDS-PC are patient self-report measures that are easily scored and that will arrive at a psychiatric diagnosis consistent with the *Diagnostic and Statistical Manual of Mental Disorders,* Fourth edition *(DSM-IV).*[14-16] However, studies have shown that these instruments are not foolproof and may, in fact, have a high degree of false positivity.[14,17] So while these instruments and other tools such as the AHCPR Depression in Primary Care Guidelines and the *DSM-IV PC* should help PCPs make appropriate diagnostic and treatment decisions, such decisions need to be supported by the availability of ongoing training and expert consultation.[18,19]

> *Quality of Care is Dependent on Provider Skills and Knowledge:*
> — Providers should be trained in clinical evaluations or in the use of standardized screening instruments. Training should be ongoing and reinforced over time; and
> — Treatment decisions should be consistent with acceptable guidelines for dose and duration of treatment. If psychosocial remedies are suggested, the provider should understand the implications and effectiveness expected.

Who Pays?

Mrs. Goodhealth's treatment, whether delivered by her PCP or by a mental health professional in the mental health setting, is certainly part of her benefit. She appears to have manageable psychiatric and psychosocial problems that can be readily treated with appropriate attention. The question is who should pay if mental health services are augmented in the primary care setting? Cost-effectiveness and cost-offset studies, as well as studies examining the indirect impact of anxiety and depression, show that costs of untreated mental illness are staggering, but adequate treatment can have a positive impact on reducing both direct and indirect costs.

> *Spend Money Wisely:*
> — Referring patients to the mental health setting will cost more than treating them early in the primary care setting;

— The absence of training or on-site support by mental health professionals can lead to poorly diagnosed and poorly treated patients, who may also be dissatisfied with their care; and

— The use of on-site behavioral health professionals can lead to decreased time spent by PCPs on psychiatric, somatoform, and other behavioral health problems.

Specialty Care: Ecological Care for the Future

Patients with chronic medical illness often have psychiatric and psychosocial difficulties related to their illness that are best addressed within the treatment context. This type of care has been provided in the setting of AIDS, cancer, chronic renal failure, and organ transplantation. Such care has been delivered by a host of individuals including nurses, social workers, psychologists, and psychiatrists. There is a large body of literature documenting the increased psychiatric morbidity for these patients and the benefit to both health-related and psychosocial outcomes with the presence of psychosocial assessment and support. This type of care is not only clinically important, but in some instances has been legislated, as in the case of the Designated AIDS Treatment Centers in New York. Each center must provide psychiatric, psychosocial, and case management services, and funding is provided to compensate these programs. The services have helped significantly in assuring that HIV patients can receive appropriate psychosocial and case management services without having to overcome significant cost and logistic barriers.

Another example of how psychiatric and psychosocial care can be integrated in a medical setting occurs within a nationwide network of outpatient cancer treatment facilities. Comprehensive Cancer Centers Inc. (CCC Inc.) owns and operates, in conjunction with partner hospitals, 11 cancer centers. Each center provides full-service medical and radiation oncology services, as well as comprehensive nutrition, psychosocial, and pain management services. In addition to a psychiatrist (who directs the program), the staff includes psychologists, social workers, a nutritionist, and a pain nurse who coordinates and delivers pain management treatment with a multidisciplinary pain management team.

Services are offered regardless of the ability to pay; however, some specialized services such as psychopharmacologic consultation, pain management, psychological and neuropsychiatric testing, and specific behavioral interventions are billed. Team members actively participate in medical and nursing team meetings and perform all of the functions described earlier.

This treatment style establishes clearly who will provide care and what care is to be provided. The question becomes: who pays? If patients are not held responsible for supporting the service, then how can the service be supported? Actually, the program costs only two percent of net revenues for each Cancer Center; this includes the support of a corporation-wide director and staff. These costs are seen as a non-negotiable component of care.

In settings where CCC Inc. has participated in full-risk capitated contracts, psychosocial services have been included. However, if the insurer with whom such contracts are being negotiated already provides mental health services for patients, will services provided by the Center be considered duplicative? The argument should be made that medically based psychiatric and psychosocial services can improve outcomes and are an essential component of case management functions of the treatment team. Furthermore, a risk/cost sharing agreement can be devised so that a small portion of the patient's ordinary mental health benefit can be diverted into the oncology benefit without significantly affecting the mental health program.

Political Issues

Health policy formulated on the national and local level heavily informs and determines how public sector healthcare is delivered. For providers and insurers alike, it is important to participate in the process of that policy development. The application of federal regulations and programs have led state and federal entities to develop Requests for Proposals (RFPs), which determine the specific characteristics of the medical and mental health plans offered. These RFPs are then used as the basis for managed care organizations to develop a proposal in order to provide services. All interested parties have the opportunity to participate in the development of RFPs. In addition, there is a review period during which interested parties may comment. Such comments can often lead to changes in the RFP and, hence, to changes in the standards that insurers must meet in order to receive contracts.

On the institutional level, participation in managed care committees and similar diligent review of all managed care contracts is critical to ensure that attention is paid to these issues. Such review, comment, and follow-through can have significant positive impact. Once policy decisions have been made and contracts signed, inclusion of services becomes more problematic.

Conclusion

There is clear evidence to suggest that a large proportion of patients receiving care for medical problems also have significant psychiatric symptomology. The cost—in terms of dollars and morbidity—of not treating these patients appropriately is staggering. Regardless of whether health plans attempt to integrate behavioral health and medical care, appropriate and specific behavioral healthcare for patients seen in the medical setting is often less than adequate. Financial and clinical solutions are available if policy, contractual, and clinical circumstances account for the need to include such services. With attention, diligence, and creativity, PCPs can become better behavioral health providers, mental health services that offer specific expertise in the medical setting can be provided, and patient care in general can be significantly improved, with little or no additional cost.

References

1. Engel G: The need for a new medical model: a challenge for biomedicine. Science 196:129-136, 1977.
2. Cohen-Cole SA, Boker J, Bird J, et al: Psychiatric education improves internists' knowledge: a three-year randomized, controlled evaluation. Psychosom Med 55:212-218, 1993.

3. Cole SA, Saravey S, Hall R, et al: Mental Disorders in General Medical Practice: Adding Value to Healthcare Through Consultation-Liaison Psychiatry. Kendall Hunt Publishing Company, Dubuque, Iowa, 1996.
4. Epstein Al, Budd MA, Cole SA: Behavioral disorders: an unrecognized epidemic with implications for providers. HMO Practice 9(2):53–56, 1995.
5. Cole S, Raju M: Overcoming barriers to integration of primary care and behavioral healthcare: focus on knowledge and skills. Behavioral Healthcare Tomorrow. 5:30–35, 1996.
6. Roter DL, Hall JA, Kern DE, et al: Improving physicians' interviewing skills and reducing patients' emotional distress. Arch Intern Med 155:1877–1884, 1995.
7. Bird J, Cohen-Cole SA, Boker J, Freeman A: Teaching psychiatry to non-psychiatrists: I. The application of educational methodology. Gen Hosp Psychiatry 5:247–253, 1983.
8. Gonzales JJ and Randel L: Consultation-liaison psychiatry in the managed care arena. Psychiatric Clin North Am 19:449–466, 1996.
9. Hails KC, Dichter H, Schindler BA, et al: A model for psychiatric care and the C-L service. Paper presented at the Academy of Psychosomatic Medicine Annual Meeting, Palm Springs, CA, November, 1995.
10. Brown C, Schulberg HC: The efficacy of psychosocial treatments in primary care: a review of randomized clinical trials. Gen Hosp Psychiatry 17:414–424, 1996
11. Katon W, Von Korff M, Lin E, et al: Collaborative management to achieve treatment guidelines. JAMA 273:1026–1081, 1995.
12. Katon W, Von Korff M, Lin E, Bush T, Orrel J: Adequacy and duration of antidepressant treatment in primary care. Med Care 30:67–76, 1992.
13. Katon W, Robinson P, Von Korff M, et al: A multifaceted intervention to improve treatment of depression in primary care. Arch Gen Psychiatry 53:924–932, 1996.
14. Spitzer RL, Williams JB, Kroenke K, et al: Utility of a new procedure for diagnostic aid for multiple mental disorders in primary care. The Prime-MD 1000 Study. JAMA 14:1749–1756, 1994
15. Olfson M, Leon AC, Broadhead WE, et al: The SDDS-PC: A diagnostic aid for multiple mental disorders in primary care. Psychopharm Bull 31:415–420, 1995.
16. Diagnostic and Statistical Manual of Mental Disorders, Fourth edition. American Psychiatric Association Press, Washington, DC, 1994.
17. Weissman MM, Olfson M, Leon AC, et al: Brief diagnostic interviews (SDDS-PC) for multiple mental disorders in primary care: a pilot study. Arch Fam Med 4:220–227, 1995.
18. Depression Guideline Panel: Depression in Primary Care, Volumes I and II. Clinical Practice Guideline No. 5. US Dept of Health and Human Services, Agency for Health Care Policy and Research. AHCPR Publication no. 93 0550, 1993.
19. Pincus HA, Vettorello NE, McQueen LE, et al: Bridging the gap between psychiatry and primary care: The DSM-IV-PC. Psychometrics 36:328–335, 1995.

Chapter 5

How to Structure the Financing of an Integrated System/Medical Cost Offset Model

Stephen P. Melek, FSA, MAAA

Financial Structure of an Integrated System

The successful integration of primary and behavioral healthcare depends on a successful financial structure that shares the risks and rewards appropriately among the various participants of the delivery system. The financial structure will likely need to include the development of a cost model, provider fee schedules, physician incentive programs and risk-sharing arrangements, and possibly subcapitation. Financial structures are put into place, and actual experience under the program is measured regularly, with changes made to the financial structure as part of a continual improvement process. The goal of such a process is to align the risks, incentives, and reimbursement arrangements so that there is fairness throughout the system, which fosters long-term success. This may include the design of medical cost offset models to recycle some of the medical cost savings generated from behavioral healthcare interventions, where such offsets exist, back into the behavioral healthcare programs.

Cost Model Development

The development of a cost model for healthcare delivery involves the establishment of expected utilization rates and average unit costs by type of healthcare service category (e.g., inpatient hospital medical days, outpatient hospital emergency room visits, primary care office visits, outpatient psychotherapy visits) for a given set of healthcare benefits to a given population of covered members. Typically, the benefit design details (copayments, limits of benefit coverage, etc.) and the demographics of the covered population (age, sex, geographic area, industry, etc.) are considered in the development of the utilization rates. The expected average unit costs would incorporate known levels of payment to providers (physician fee schedules, hospital per diems, discounts to usual and customary levels) as well as the expected mix of use of the various potential providers of healthcare, and the fixed versus variable cost pricing philosophy of the delivery system. The cost model may also include additional details by type of physician specialty.

The key is the development of a flexible model that will easily allow for changes in the underlying assumptions about expected utilization levels and average unit costs. It should also incorporate adjustments to the utilization and cost assumptions based on the expected impact of managed care. Increasing the degree of healthcare management generally reduces utilization rates and increases average unit costs due to severity. However, some services may have utilization increases if they are used as an alternative to more costly and restrictive forms of healthcare. Once this cost model is built, different categories of service can be combined or grouped together in the development of subcapitation rates, risk pools, or other types of financial incentive arrangements.

Fee Structures

Fee structures should be fair and reasonable to all of the various providers of healthcare services in the delivery system. This may involve scrapping old, ad hoc fee schedules paid to physicians, hospitals, or other providers in favor of schedules that are based on relative value to allow for better consistency between the time, cost, and value of services provided and the fees paid to the providers as reimbursement for the delivery of such services.

For physicians, fee scales are often based on either the McGraw-Hill or Resources Based Relative Value Scale schedules with various multipliers or conversion factors developed to obtain fair payments for delivery of medical, surgical, behavioral, maternity, radiology, and pathology services. For hospitals, per diems or diagnosis-related group-based (DRG) case rates are frequently used, with payments set at levels that also attempt to provide fair and reasonable reimbursement for the time, cost, and value of services provided. Other services, such as ambulance, home healthcare, or durable medical equipment, may be priced on a discounted fee-for-service basis (reductions from usual and customary charge levels), with the goal of achieving relative fairness to the physician fees and hospital reimbursement rates that have already been determined.

Provider Incentives

In managed care, outcomes are often dependent on provider behavior. Incentives are designed to facilitate behavior change in order to reach desired outcomes. Incentives can take the form of a financial or social reward (positive) or penalty (negative). The overall effect of a healthcare provider incentive system should be to encourage provider behavior that results in optimal delivery system performance—that is, high quality and cost-effective care with good outcomes. Successful implementation of an incentive system requires optimization of the healthcare management systems, reimbursement systems, and incentive systems together. In many cases, the reimbursement, incentive, and healthcare management systems have been developed haphazardly without considering the possibility that they might encourage conflicting provider behavior. The effectiveness of the provider incentive system can be maximized by recognizing and understanding the following key principles.

Natural Response versus Desired Objectives. The natural response to an incentive should be consistent with the desired performance objectives. This applies not only to the global incentive approach, but also to how risks and/or rewards are disbursed among individual providers. For example, an incentive pool based on utilization reduction may be counterproductive if the disbursement of surplus to individual providers is based on the provider's billed charges. This incentive will tend to reward high-use providers.

Provider Control. Incentives should be based on what the provider can and should control. For example, it is reasonable to vary primary care provider incentives based on specialist referral rates, but it is unreasonable to link them to the administration costs of a facility. A provider can choose one facility over another, but cannot dictate the operations of a single facility.

Equitable Risk Sharing. The incentive approach should be equitable in terms of provider risk and reward. To the extent that financial risk is transferred to a provider, the opportunity to share in any realized surplus should exist. Withhold arrangements common to many health maintenance organization (HMO) plans transfer utilization risk to the provider without any chance for reward. Such programs potentially destroy the plan's credibility with the providers, as well as any sense of partnership with the plan.

Clarity. The incentive approach should be simple. By keeping the number of goals and measures of success to a minimum, providers can more readily understand and focus on what is expected of them. Too many measures and goals dilute the provider's concentration on any one issue, and can create concern among providers that the results might be manipulated by the plan.

Provider Involvement. The providers should be involved in the process. Encouraging provider participation in establishing their performance goals and measures of success promotes a sense of ownership in the program. It is also likely that the providers are more aware of the areas that will produce the greatest yield. Goals should be periodically updated with provider input as conditions change.

Realistic Goals. Target utilization levels and other goals must be realistically and accurately set. Providers will quickly lose interest in a plan with unattainable goals.

Education and Support. It is usually insufficient to identify targets without a plan for achieving them. Providers often need educational resources and support to help them meet their goals.

Risk Sharing

Perhaps the most common form of provider risk-sharing involves the use of risk pools. A *risk pool* is a depository of revenues, usually paid on a per member per month basis, which is calculated to provide for a certain set of healthcare services. For example, using the cost model method, it may have been determined that the portion of the healthcare premiums (or other source of funding) available to provide hospital services is $40. Under a hospital risk pool concept, this $40 would be "deposited" into the hospital risk pool for each covered member in each month of the contract. Out of this risk pool fund, charges for covered hospital services are paid.

At the end of a predetermined period of time, the balance in the risk pool is determined (i.e., deposits less payouts to providers) and allocated to participating providers in the risk pool.

Risk pools are commonly set up for hospital and specialty physician services (usually separate pools), and sometimes for other services such as prescription drugs. Hospital risk pool participants usually include the hospital providers, specialty physicians, and primary care physicians (PCPs). Specialty risk pool participants usually include the specialists and PCPs. Participation rates are preset in the risk pool design. For example, hospital risk pool balances may be split 30%, 40%, 30% to the hospitals, specialists, and PCPs, respectively.

Risk pools have the advantage of including both positive and negative incentives. Surpluses and deficits are shared. Surpluses may be paid out entirely, or a reserve may be developed with some portion of the surplus to be used as an offset toward potential future deficits. Deficits may be carried forward for a period of time, or charged to the providers in the form of reductions in fee schedules or future withholds.

Financial Integration of Behavioral and Primary Care Providers

In integrated delivery systems, behavioral healthcare providers can be treated like other specialists. Behavioral healthcare inpatient facility costs can be reimbursed on a per diem or case rate basis comparable to the treatment of medical/surgical inpatient facility costs. Reasonable outpatient reimbursements can be scheduled for facility, program, and professional services—comparable on a relative value basis to other nonbehavioral reimbursements. And behavioral providers can be participants in risk pools just like other specialists.

A hospital pool could be established with per member per month revenue contributions made to the pool based on the expected costs of all facility services—behavioral and nonbehavioral. Outpatient services, per diems, DRG-based payments, and other services are preset, and reimbursements are made from this pool as services are provided. Balances are regularly allocated to facilities, specialists, and primary care physicians. These allocations can then be further divided among the individual providers based on various predetermined measurements, such as efficiency of treatment plans, quality measurements, and outcomes. Usually a minimum number of patients are required for a given provider in order to adequately measure their performance. Sometimes providers are grouped using pools of doctors for performance measurement purposes.

Efficiency of treatment plans can be based on the percentage of noncomplicated patients that conform to preset clinical pathways. Providers can also be "ranked" using quartiles where the highest 25% of those evaluated receive four "credits" from the risk pool surpluses, the next 25% receive two credits, the third highest 25% receive one credit, and the lowest 25% receive no credits. This evaluation can be reversed when deficits are achieved in the risk pool—where the lowest scoring groups are allocated the highest portion of the deficit and the highest scoring groups are not allocated any of the deficit.

The specialty risk pool can be handled similarly, but here the performance measurements may include actual costs versus target costs by specialty, percentages of primary care services actually performed by PCPs compared to specialists, quality indicators, efficiency of outpatient services, and so on.

The PCPs participate in the hospital and specialty risk pools. Their portion of the risk pool balances are predetermined. Allocations to individual PCPs or pools of PCPs are typically based on their efforts related to inpatient admits and lengths of stay, timeliness and appropriateness of specialty referrals, percentages of primary care services actually performed, and degree of efficiency of the specialists to whom they refer patients.

Even in integrated delivery systems, separate funds may be set aside exclusively for behavioral healthcare services. The same risk sharing and reimbursement concepts apply. However, the behavioral healthcare providers are sharing in gains or losses arising only from behavioral healthcare specific risk pools and not the larger pools that would be established in a combined behavioral and nonbehavioral approach. On the other hand, the behavioral providers are not sharing the results of their pools with any other nonbehavioral specialists.

Results Measurement and Continual Improvement Process

Fairness of the financial structures to all participants is very important as the system evolves and is evaluated. Initial risk pool targets may need to be modified. Fee schedules may need to be changed to better achieve consistent and relative reimbursement by type of service or type of specialist. Actual results should be regularly evaluated and fed back into the design and redesign process. This includes medical, surgical, and behavioral services across all types of providers and specialties.

Medical Cost Offsets

An additional structural area in the financing of integrated systems lies in the potential for medical cost offsets generated from the delivery of behavioral healthcare. The validity and credibility of such medical cost offsets have frequently been challenged, especially by medical care providers. Medical cost offset recognition is not common in the financial structures for various reasons, including the following:

- Desire to fix and isolate behavioral healthcare costs
- Difficulty in identifying and measuring any such medical offsets
- Subjective nature of some behavioral healthcare
- Natural cost savings being retained within behavioral healthcare organizations from their own carve-outs or risk pools when they are able to reduce their own costs

Several studies related to the existence and degree of such offsets have been conducted, including the influence of psychiatric group interventions on patients with malignant melanomas, the reduction of healthcare costs associated with alcoholism treatment, and psychological distress and cardiac rehabilitation.[1,2] Additionally, Milliman & Robertson, StayWell Health Management Systems, Chrysler Corporation, and the international union of United Automobile Workers jointly studied how an individual's health habits (including levels of mental health and stress) affect medical claims.[3] They all provide support, in different degrees, to the potential savings in medical costs as a result of behavioral healthcare services and interventions.

Integrated Risk Sharing Design Concepts Related to Medical Cost Offsets

In delivery systems that do not have separate, distinct budgets, capitation, or risk pools for behavioral healthcare services, medical cost offsets that are achieved may be shared with the behavioral providers naturally as a result of the risk pool structure. However, inequities could readily result in the distribution of these savings, since these favorable results are handled just like all other components of the risk pool. Additionally, medical cost offset savings could occur but not be shared if the pool still ended in a deficit position.

When it comes to medical cost offsets, separate structures may be necessary to handle the proper sharing of such savings between the medical and behavioral providers. The structures also readily apply where separate behavioral budgets or carve-outs are used.

Risk-sharing arrangements between medical and behavioral provider groups can be structured to encourage a joint effort between both provider communities to seek and achieve behavioral and medical wellness in their covered member groups. These approaches are distinct and separate from the risk-sharing approaches described earlier. Two different methods of structuring such risk-sharing programs are presented below—an *aggregate* approach and a *specific* approach.

Under either approach, a major task is to obtain agreement between the medical and behavioral groups on the amount of "risk overlap" between the groups. That is, how much medical cost influence do the groups agree is attributable to the behavioral healthcare providers. For example, if the expected medical costs are projected to be $100 per member per month, and the groups agree that $10 of these costs are highly correlated with behavioral healthcare delivery, then 10% can be established as the risk overlap rate. The higher the degree of behavioral healthcare delivery influence that is established, the higher the amount of risk overlap and risk-sharing (both for excess funds and fund shortfalls) structured into the arrangement.

Aggregate Approach

Under the aggregate approach, the financial results of medical healthcare delivery are directly shared with the behavioral healthcare providers by allocating proportions of the total medical healthcare "pie" via risk overlaps to the behavioral groups. No specific DRGs, CPTs, or individual services are identified. Instead, the medical group agrees to share its financial results on a proportional basis for *all* treated conditions. The medical group agrees that selected percentages of the profits/losses of its facilities, specialty physicians, PCPs, prescription drugs, and other costs will be allocated to the behavioral group via risk overlaps.

This approach can work well when the medical group has already established risk pools for its facilities, specialty professionals, and any other healthcare components. Percentages of each risk pool are attributed to the behavioral group using risk overlap rates. For example, if the risk overlap rate is set at 10%, then 10% of the results of any of or all the medical risk pools is identified as a medical-behavioral joint risk subpool. Then, a risk-sharing percentage is established to determine how to split the financial results of this medical-behavioral joint risk subpool (Table 1).

In this example, 10% of the financial results of the medical facility, specialist, and prescription drug pools are allocated to the medical-behavioral joint risk subpools, which are then split equally. The results of the medical facility risk pool yield a $.20 per member per month gain to the behavioral group ($4 × 10% × 50%), the results of the medical specialist risk pool yield a $.10 per member per month loss ($2 × 10% × 50%), and the results of the prescription drug risk pool yield a $.02 per member per month gain to the behavioral group ($.40 × 10% × 50%). This net gain of $.12 is relatively insignificant to the medical group, but represents a 3% increase to the revenues of the behavioral group ($.12 compared with its $4 cap rate) and turns a $.05 per member per month loss (costs of $4.05 compared with capitation revenue of $4.00) for the behavioral

TABLE 1. EXAMPLE OF AN AGGREGATE APPROACH TO RISK SHARING

Aggregate Approach Design Example Assumption*
Medical facility risk pool with $35 per member per month revenue
Medical specialist risk pool with $35 per member per month revenue
Medical prescription drug risk pool with $10 per member per month revenue
Behavioral healthcare capitation of $4 per member per month revenue
Medical-behavioral facility, specialist, and prescription drug joint risk subpools established using risk overlap rate of 10%
Financial results of joint risk subpools split 50% to medical group and 50% to behavioral group

Actual Results Assumed*
Medical facility risk pool costs of $31 per member per month
Medical specialist risk pool costs of $37 per member per month
Medical prescription drug risk pool costs of $9.60 per member per month
Behavioral healthcare costs of $4.05 per member per month

*Excludes maternity.

group into a $.07 per member per month profit. The medical group also profits significantly, obtaining a $2.28 total gain.

Specific Approach

Under the specific approach, specific DRGs, CPT codes, and other services that the medical group agrees to attribute to behavioral healthcare risk overlap are identified. This approach is more detailed and requires the establishment of utilization targets for each identified DRG, CPT, or service to be measured. The major steps in the specific approach include:

- Identification of all DRGs, CPTs, or services with behavioral healthcare risk overlaps, complete with expected unit costs for each service.
- Establishment of utilization targets for each such service to which actual results can be compared (days per thousand per year for each DRG, services per thousand per year for each other service or procedure, etc.).
- Establishment of behavioral risk overlap percentages attributable to each DRG, CPT, or service.
- Establishment of risk-sharing percentages of actual financial results for each DRG, CPT, or service.
- Measurement of actual utilization results for selected DRGs, CPTs, and services.
- Comparison of actual utilization results to targets and calculation of shared profits/losses.

The following examples illustrate how the specific approach would work for a few selected sets of services.

DRG 202–Cirrhosis and Alcoholic Hepatitis

Target annual days per 1,000 covered members = 0.43
Per diem cost = $1,800

Behavioral risk overlap percentage = 80% (indicating a high degree of cause-effect between behavioral and medical)
Risk share rate of 50% to medical and 50% to behavioral

DRG 140—Angina Pectoris

Target annual days per 1,000 covered members = 1.13
Per diem cost = $1,650
Behavioral risk overlap percentage = 25%
Risk share rate of 50% to medical and 50% to behavioral

CPT Codes 17260–17286—Destruction, Malignant Lesions

Target annual services per 1,000 covered members = 0.32
Per service cost = $145
Behavioral risk overlap percentage = 50%
Risk share rate of 50% to medical and 50% to behavioral

Actual Results Achieved

10,000 covered lives
DRG 202 had 0.29 days per 1,000 covered members
DRG 140 had 0.90 days per 1,000 covered members
CPT codes 17260–17286 had 0.16 services per 1,000 covered members

In this example, favorable results were obtained for the Cirrhosis and Alcoholic Hepatitis DRG, the Angina Pectoris DRG, and the Malignant Lesion Destruction procedures. The medical group realizes a $6,547 total gain from these favorable results before any behavioral group risk-sharing. The profits to be shared with the behavioral group are calculated below.

DRG 202: $(0.43 - 0.29) \times (1,800) \times (80\%) \times (50\%) \times (10) = \$1,008$
DRG 140: $(1.13 - 0.90) \times (1,650) \times (25\%) \times (50\%) \times (10) = \$474$
CPT 17260-17286: $(0.32 - 0.16) \times (145) \times (50\%) \times (50\%) \times (10) = \$58$

While this total risk-sharing profit amount of $1,540 may appear small compared with the $600,000 of annual revenue that the behavioral group would earn from 10,000 lives (at $5 per member per month), it represents the results of only a single DRG and a small group of professional services. When a full identification of all risk overlapping DRGs, CPTs, and other services is made, the potential for much greater risk-sharing profit is seen. Again, both the medical group and the behavioral group can benefit from savings generated from successful delivery of behavioral healthcare services.

Sample Programs Fitting the Specific Approach

Specific behavioral healthcare programs designed to result in medical cost offset savings can usually be mapped to specific DRGs, CPTs, or other services. Examples of these types of programs include the Early Start Program, certain emergency room case finding programs, and presurgery relaxation programs.

The Early Start Program is a model system for the early identification and management of substance abuse during pregnancy. The goal is to reduce neonatal abnormalities and medical costs associated with substance abuse. Drug and alcohol use can lead to pregnancy complications including prematurity, low birth weight, microcephaly, intra-uterine growth retardation, developmental delay, and birth defects. Targets for admit rates, lengths of stay, and costs per stay can be established by DRG for maternity deliveries, medical postpartum problems, complications of pregnancy, and newborn stays based on a healthcare delivery scenario that does not reflect the Early Start Program effort. Actual results with the impact of the program can then be compared to these targets to determine medical cost offset savings (see Chapter 7).

Emergency room case finding programs can be used to identify panic disorder cases that consume excess amounts of medical services in the emergency room before they receive appropriate behavioral treatments for their condition. Studies have shown that panic disorder patients can visit the emergency room many times before they are referred for appropriate treatment for their problem. Targets for specific services consumed in the emergency room related to these patients (EKGs, echocardiographs, observation without admit, etc.) can be established and compared to actual results after the case finding efforts to determine the level of medical cost offset savings.

Presurgery relaxation programs are intended to result in faster induction of anesthesia (with less required to maintain unconscious levels), lower rates of postoperative hypertension, fewer postoperative complications, shorter postoperative lengths of stay, and less pain and anxiety. Specific targets can be established for hospital costs by surgical DRG, anesthesia costs, pain medications, and so on; they can then be compared to actual results achieved with the program to determine medical cost offset savings.

Comparison of Approaches

Both approaches attempt to share the financial results arising from healthcare delivery between the medical and behavioral provider groups. The aggregate approach is simpler and easier to implement, if an agreement can be established between both groups that behavioral healthcare delivery can influence nearly the full gamut of medical costs. If the medical provider group is skeptical about the breadth of this risk overlap and is only willing to pursue selected areas of potential medical cost offsets, the specific approach can be developed and implemented.

One important fact should be reiterated—risk-sharing is a two-edged sword. It involves sharing of both profits *and* losses. Behavioral healthcare providers must be certain that they want to share in the results from their medical provider counterparts. Once the risk-sharing mechanism is in place, positive and negative results are shared, regardless of how they came about.

References

1. Fawzy I, et al: Malignant melanoma-effects of an early structured psychiatric intervention, coping, and affective state on recurrence and survival 6 years later. Arch Gen Psychiatry 50:681-689, 1993.
2. Holder HD, Blose JO: The reduction of healthcare costs associated with alcoholism treatment: a 14-year longitudinal study. J Stud Alcohol 53:293-302, 1992.
3. Milliman & Robertson, Inc. and Staywell Health Management Systems, Inc: Health Risks and their Impact on Medical Costs. Milliman & Robertson, Inc. 1995.

Part III.
SUCCESSFUL MODELS OF INTEGRATION

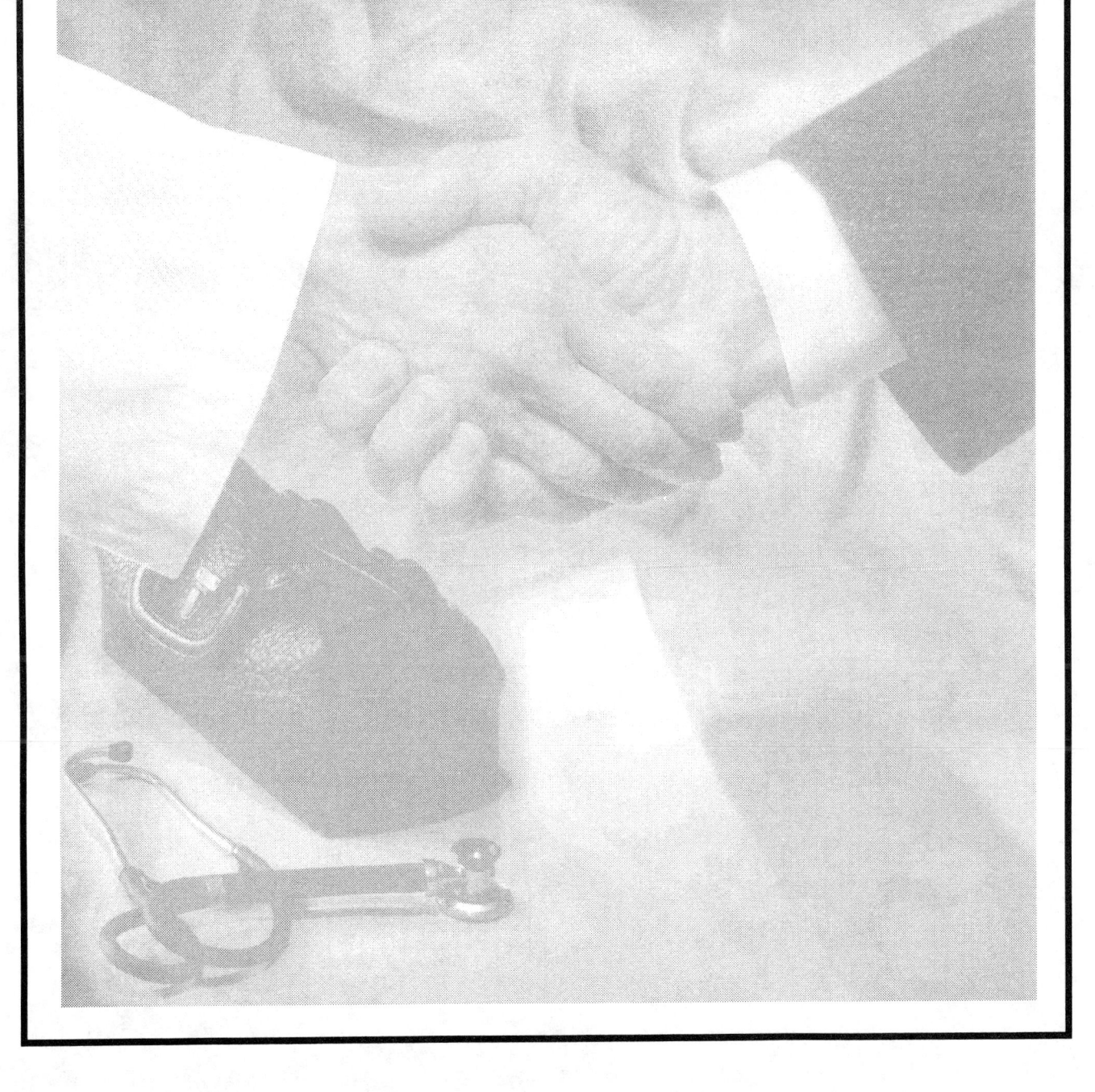

Chapter 6

Building Partnerships of Lasting Value in Healthcare: The Blue Cross and Blue Shield/Raytheon Collaboration

Nancy Langman-Dorwart, M.S., M.P.H., Elizabeth Gatti, Psy.D., and Diane Duval

Raytheon Company, the largest employer in Massachusetts, and Blue Cross and Blue Shield of Massachusetts (BCBSMA), the largest health insurer in Massachusetts, forged a unique strategic partnership in 1995 that challenged traditional relationships between corporations and insurers. As Raytheon explored a new model of healthcare partnership with BCBSMA, it recognized the potential to significantly change the delivery of healthcare to its more than 34,000 Massachusetts members. In addition, BCBSMA promised to save Raytheon millions of dollars in healthcare costs. Questions circulated as to whether or not two large organizations could really form a partnership that is aggressive and forward thinking in a time of consolidation and downsizing in both the healthcare and defense industries; and if it could be done, how would success be defined, delivered, and measured?

To meet this challenge, BCBSMA designed an integrated care management program. The model was designed with several guiding principles. First, primary care physicians (PCPs) are the core of all care decisions. Second, patients are active participants in their healthcare decisions. Third, behavioral and medical aspects of care are integrated. And finally, community supports are identified and utilized to maximize care. Key decisions included "carving in" mental healthcare into the general healthcare product and making prevention and wellness programs integral to the model. Prior to this contract, Raytheon's mental health program included traditional psychiatric and substance abuse services and was managed through a network of providers who did not typically coordinate with medical-surgical care.

The Corporate Partner

Raytheon Company, a Fortune 200 company, is an $11.7 billion international, high technology company that operates in four areas—commercial and defense electronics, engineering and construction, aviation, and major appliances. Between 1990 and 1995, the United States defense procurement budget was slashed from $96 billion to $46 billion. Raytheon was buffeted by these cuts and was forced to reduce its Massachusetts work force from 31,000 to 18,000. Originally dependent on defense funding, Raytheon diversified its business to include 65 percent commercial and 35 percent defense operations.

Concerned about remaining competitive with companies in states where the aggregate cost of doing business was much lower, Raytheon began to assess the high cost of healthcare within the corporation. The challenge was to balance the need to maintain a motivated and healthy work force, to control costs without compromising quality of care, and to assure the availability of affordable coverage for employees and their families. Raytheon developed an aggressive strategy to address these challenges, including a new partnership with a health insurer to both lower costs and raise the health status of employees and their families.

The Healthcare Purchaser

The increasing need for employers like Raytheon to develop a common strategy for healthcare is driven by globalization of business that increases administrative costs, liability issues, and employee intercompany transfer issues. A common benefit design that provides uniformity across a corporation, regardless of geographic location, can drive down administrative costs and ensure equitable benefit offerings. Raytheon's uniform strategy included a model for regional healthcare delivery with "best in marketplace" practice and enhanced preventive care benefits. The financial advantage of volume purchasing across subsidiaries was a key component. This strategy created a challenge for management to move their employees from a traditional indemnity product to a managed care product with the least amount of disruption and dissatisfaction.

To implement the new strategy, Raytheon issued a request for proposal (RFP) to local health services companies, seeking a new and innovative relationship. Raytheon wanted a partner interested in shared risk and responsibility who could deliver significant guaranteed reductions in healthcare costs without compromising quality of care. Raytheon's strategy was to select a plan that would deliver care as an integrated process, linking primary care and behavioral healthcare. The managed care product had to offer current technology in order to meet the expectations of Raytheon. Customer satisfaction was a key measure, and included not only member services but account and provider services as well.

The Healthcare Company

Blue Cross and Blue Shield of Massachusetts has 2.1 million members, 29 percent market share, and $3.5 billion in annual revenue. Originally known for its indemnity or traditional insurance coverage, BCBSMA had been reorganizing itself into a managed care company over the last several years and is gaining recognition for its creative use of technology. Despite its efforts to streamline and reorganize, BCBSMA faced a challenging environment with decreased membership, increased losses on regulated lines of business, escalating administrative costs, rapidly increasing medical claims costs (particularly in pharmacy, outpatient, and ancillary claims), and intense local market competition.

First, BCBSMA sought legislative changes from the state to be relieved of the burden of being the insurer of last resort, creating an economic disadvantage not currently shared by the other health maintenance organizations (HMOs) in Massachusetts. Also, BCBSMA had recently leveled the playing field in contracting and had been able to end a long era of the Rate Setting Commission controlling hospital contracts. In the new environment, BCBSMA was able to renegotiate all their professional contracts and receive competitive rates, allowing it to capture significant savings.

The response of BCBSMA to Raytheon's request for proposal was to offer a unique risk proposal that promised to deliver an innovative product including prevention and wellness, and to leverage technology to better serve customers. Their willingness to take on shared financial risk and work closely with Raytheon to evolve a customer-friendly and quality healthcare program won them the contract.

Strategy for the Future

One of the primary challenges was coming to an understanding of the culture and tasks of each organization and creatively designing "synergy points" to maximize each organization's strengths and minimize any weaknesses. The new product offering had to be driven by customer expectations, with *customer* defined broadly to include members, the account, providers, and internal customers of both companies. Faced with this challenge, BCBSMA encouraged Raytheon to integrate their behavioral healthcare with their medical care at BCBSMA rather than continue to carve out mental health benefits through a national behavioral healthcare company.

Raytheon's vision was to foster a synergy between the new partners that in and of itself would add value for both organizations. The parameters of the partnership evolved in early meetings between key BCBSMA and Raytheon staff, as they created a draft of the vision and values that would eventually become the guiding principles of the steering committee. The role of the steering committee was to provide leadership and direction for all activities between BCBSMA and Raytheon. Committee members included Raytheon benefits, medical, and human resources staff, and BCBSMA clinical, sales, and account management staff.

The first steering committee meeting included discussions of the mission of the committee and the expectations of all parties. The mission was to leverage the experience, expertise, and corporate resources of BCBSMA and Raytheon to continually improve the health status of and services delivered to Raytheon members. Further, the steering committee created a three-year strategy in which year one would involve stabilization and transition, year two would focus on continuous improvements, and year three would include innovation.

One of the first projects undertaken by the steering committee was selection and distribution of PCPs by Raytheon members. The data showed that 318 PCPs were taking care of 53 percent of Raytheon members. A further distillation showed 31 percent of the members were in care with 118 PCPs (Figure 1). The goal of the steering committee was to elevate the position of the PCP as the primary contact for all members needing medical attention, thereby decreasing the utilization of costly specialists for routine visits. If members failed to select a PCP, they would be assigned to a BCBSMA health center physician. Raytheon agreed to host several PCP focus group meetings to facilitate collaboration.

Between December 1995 and February 1996, the steering committee oversaw the transition of more than 1,000 members with complex healthcare needs from a non-managed care to a managed care model. More than 300 members who were receiving mental healthcare were transitioned into the BCBSMA network of providers. The medical management model was designed to support this innovative project, and BCBSMA analyzed the 1995 utilization data to better target specific programs. The goal of the

Members Choosing PCPs
Distribution Range

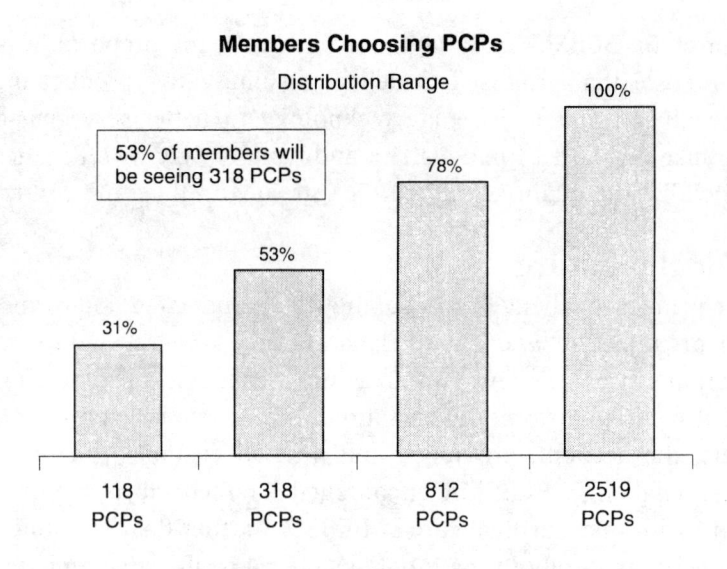

- 118 PCPs: 31%
- 318 PCPs: 53% (53% of members will be seeing 318 PCPs)
- 812 PCPs: 78%
- 2519 PCPs: 100%

Figure 1

BCBSMA medical management team was to maintain a focus on the family, which they believed added value to the more traditional patient-focused approach.

The initial entry of BCBSMA into the new managed care program offered opportunities to the customer. One such example is a member who was diagnosed with breast cancer and was concerned about her treatment coverage that had been ordered under her old medical plan. Exceptions were made for her treatment, and she was thereby assured that no disruption in treatment would occur. The message these decisions communicated to members was that BCBSMA would meet their needs with minimal disruption of care.

Today, the steering committee sets direction, monitors progress, and acknowledges success and challenges. Multiple working groups chartered by the committee develop key initiatives that support the broader vision. These include the Prevention Committee, the Members Communication Committee, and the Medical Staff Committee. These committees each have defined membership, with leadership provided by steering committee representatives. Committees meet regularly and report progress to the steering committee monthly. The steering committee sets aggressive goals each month that require significant effort on the part of these work groups.

Partnership with the Member

Establishing a partnership with Raytheon employees was perhaps the greatest challenge. Even though employees were familiar with BCBSMA and many had been long-term members, there were varying degrees of satisfaction with the health plan. The complexity of the relationship was due in part to escalating healthcare costs, which resulted in the loss of a traditional healthcare model. The point-of-service product required members to seek authorization from their PCP for all specialist care except mental health. Limited out-of-network benefits allowed members some flexibility, but deductibles and co-insurance added a financial burden. This change affected not only employees and family members, but also benefits counselors and the on-site healthcare staff whose role was to explain benefits, negotiate transition, and clarify expectations for employees. All members were required to select a PCP to coordinate care, and many had to give up the specialists they had accessed freely in the past.

While these changes were implemented, a plan was underway to add a national full-service employee assistance plan (EAP). The model Raytheon designed was for members to access all behavioral healthcare through an EAP toll-free number, along with an eight-session model of assistance for a broad range of problems, which was not applied to the mental health benefit. The selected national EAP vendor was Value Behavioral Health. Raytheon was instrumental in establishing the relationship between BCBSMA and Value Behavioral Health through its facilitation of ongoing working meetings involving key clinical and administrative staff.

Integrated Care Model

In response to Raytheon's healthcare delivery strategy and the rapidly changing healthcare environment, BCBSMA developed a proactive integrated approach to medical management. The concept of integration involved the co-location of medical and behavioral health professionals working together on the same team to coordinate and improve the quality of services Raytheon members receive. The goals of the co-management integrated team are to:

- Collaborate
- Strategize with patient and providers
- Hold joint physician/psychiatry consultations
- Ensure multidisciplinary team communication
- Coordinate services through joint case management

This model of integration was driven by research that has consistently demonstrated the profound effects of undiagnosed psychiatric comorbidities on employers' healthcare costs. It is estimated that more than one-half of chronic low back pain and carpal tunnel syndrome disability patients have psychiatric or personality disorders, and up to 80 percent of healthcare claims are at least indirectly driven by untreated mental health problems.

Comorbidity management is an area of opportunity in the managed healthcare environment to both improve quality and assure dollars are being allocated for the appropriate services. It was BCBSMA's expectation that the integration of medical and behavioral health services in the case management model would better influence the provider delivery system to improve efficiency and ensure appropriate care. This model of co-management of cases was designed because psychological issues often drive the utilization of primary healthcare services, and because PCPs often have limited training on the management of psychological aspects of illness. Training all staff on topics like hypothyroidism, growth hormone deficiency, and chronic pain, as well as on depression, anxiety, substance abuse, and panic disorders, would enhance case managers' skills in identifying comorbid conditions.

The integrated team at BCBSMA includes physicians, psychiatrists, psychologists, nurses, social workers, and case managers. In establishing and cross-training the team, BCBSMA hoped to influence care patterns as follows: 1) reduce visits to emergency rooms that result from psychological rather than physical causes; 2) improve the care delivered to seriously ill medical patients by offering psychological support services; and 3) find alternative treatments for patients with chronic pain before they either undergo unnecessary surgery or have addicting medications prescribed for them. As the program evolved, a disease management approach became the model of care for Raytheon members.

The integrated model of co-management allows BCBSMA to respond to members' needs. The team performs active case finding, collaboration, and education between the medical and behavioral health disciplines. Top priorities include assisting with identification of resources, discharge planning, and coordination of benefits to ensure that both medical and psychological needs are addressed. In the case of chronic illness or a catastrophic health event, the integrated team can answer questions and provide members with the resources they need. Case managers can actively refer members for psychological services such as support groups, psychopharmacology, or psychotherapy for problems like depression or chronic illness with a family member. The case managers foster a family-focused approach, recognizing the impact of illness on other family members and the need to acknowledge these issues and provide support. Currently, the integrated team is working with outcomes experts to define medical and behavioral health cost offsets and outcomes (Table 1).

Incentive Performance Standards

To encourage high performance, BCBSMA and Raytheon collaboratively developed performance standards and measures of results, along with financial incentives and penalties. A *standard* is commonly defined as the degree (or level) of excellence required for a particular purpose.[1] The performance standards developed for Raytheon included processing turnaround time for identification cards, average speed of answer and abandonment rate for both customer service and clinical services calls, and claims processing accuracy and turnaround times. In addition to developing a written survey for members, BCBSMA called every new member to welcome them to the plan and answer their questions about benefits and transition of care. This was the first of many communications with new members to encourage them to use the preventive and wellness services of their plan.

TABLE 1. MOST COMMON DIAGNOSES AMONG CO-MANAGED CASES

Asthma with adjustment disorder or attention deficit disorder

Cardiac conditions with obesity and/or phobia and/or substance abuse

Chest pain with depression

Chronic disease (Crohn's disease, multiple sclerosis, chronic obstructive pulmonary disease, chronic pain with depression)

Diabetes with depression and/or substance abuse and/or pain

Oncology with depression and family issues

Pediatrics with family issues

Other standards addressed completion of promised deliverables such as distribution of wellness surveys to members and an analysis of the results; distribution of *Living Healthy* magazine, a health journal for members; distribution of self-care guides; and a variety of other communication items. Other standards were based on HEDIS 2.5 (Health Employer Data Information Set), which included measures of mental health ambulatory follow-up rates, cervical cancer screening rates, mammography screening rates, and routine physicals. In addition to the minimum performance standards, BCBSMA could earn incentive payments for demonstrating improvements in overall member health status.

Disease Management: A Population-based Approach

Disease management addresses cost and quality concerns throughout the health care system, involving both patient and provider. Disease management programs seek to empower individuals to become more proactive in their health, while giving providers tools and systems to improve the consistency and quality of care delivery. The focus is not on an acute episode of a disease but on managing the long-term health of individuals. More specifically, disease management identifies and integrates all the components of care for a disease and uses outcomes analysis to determine the most effective care strategy.[2]

Investing in preventive programs for chronic ailments such as asthma and diabetes can dramatically reduce emergency room visits and expensive complications. For example, annual influenza vaccines, which average $10 each, reduce medical costs and sick days by $47 per patient. Disease management initiatives for the first year were based on reports of utilization of healthcare services, perception of need from surveyed employees, and recommendations from Raytheon health staff. First-year programs were selected based on an analysis of data gathered in 1995 and 1996 on the highest cost and highest utilization of services, as well as on results of the employee health survey.

In year one, asthma and diabetes programs were implemented. The plans for year two included implementation of programs addressing cardiac risk and musculoskeletal disorders. The goal of all disease management programs is the early identification of disorders, prevention of disease when possible, and maintenance or improvement of member health status through education, pharmaceutical intervention, and lifestyle change. Disease management is an evolving process that must continually reevaluate the health status and utilization patterns of members, as well as review current treatment technology.

Asthma Initiatives

About 10 million Americans are affected by the wheezing, chest tightness, and breathing difficulty that typifies asthma, according to the BCBSMA member self-help guide. Asthma is often considered an episodic disease, because acute attacks alternate with symptom-free periods. Our first disease management initiative for asthma included identification of high, moderate, and low risk members. We stratified risk by dollars spent on asthma-related healthcare claims such as visits to emergency rooms, physician offices, and hospital admissions. The risk data for asthma did not include pharmacy costs.

Risk was defined as a certain dollar amount of service used by members during an 18-month period that began one year prior to the Raytheon-BCBSMA partnership and included the first six months of claims in 1996. Our claims analysis identified 1,672 asthma-related claims (Table 2).

The lesson learned from our asthma initiative was one of timing. The program was developed in July, and members were called in August—a time when few asthmatics experience difficulties. Several members suggested we call them back in the winter. We responded by developing our winter initiative that included follow-up with members during early winter months by telephone. We also developed a newsletter, "Suggestions for Asthmatics: Tips to Make It Through the Winter," which was mailed to all asthmatic members. It was also made available in the medical offices at all Raytheon plants.

Diabetes Initiative

Diabetes is a multisystem disorder that often is not diagnosed or managed until serious health problems exist. As a result, diabetes is the fourth leading cause of death by disease in the United States. It has been estimated that diabetes costs the economy from $92 billion to $112 billion annually.[3,4] The prevalence and cost of diabetes were too high to ignore, and BCBSMA embarked on a case finding initiative for early identification. We identified 495 cases and, based on incidence and prevalence data, estimated that a significant number of undiagnosed diabetics existed among

TABLE 2. ASTHMA RISK MODEL AND INTERVENTIONS

Asthma Risk	Dollars Spent	Number of Members
High	1,000	37
Moderate	500–1,000	55
Low	500	1580

Interventions		
High Risk	**Moderate Risk**	**Low Risk**
Call PCP to discuss additional services for high risk patients.	Send letter to all moderate risk members offering home visit by an asthma educator.	No intervention; recheck claims at 6 months.
Call member to assess appropriateness for case management program.	Send "Asthma Tips" newsletter.	Send "Asthma Tips" newsletter.
Offer home visit by an asthma educator.		
Distribute peak flow meters.		
Send "Asthma Tips" newsletter.		

Raytheon members. The diabetes initiative was designed in collaboration with the medical staff at Raytheon and resulted in work-site placement of educational brochures and posters about the symptoms of diabetes.

A Raytheon steering committee member suggested reviewing the proposal with a Raytheon member who is a high-risk diabetic and is extremely knowledgeable about the disease. This led to development of a member-friendly, patient-oriented program that was well received. A second key event occurred when a BCBSMA case manager received a call from a Raytheon employee whose child is diabetic. The case manager carefully answered the employee's questions, listening for concerns and areas in which further assistance could be offered. Out of this interaction, the case manager developed a plan to call the school nurse and offer to provide an educational visit to the school. The parents' relief and appreciation caused us to add this to our protocol for childhood diabetics.

Cardiovascular Initiatives

Heart disease accounts for more than 40 percent of the nation's deaths.[5] Many heart disease deaths occur after long periods of disability and repeated hospitalizations, with costs nearing $100 billion for medical care alone. The indirect costs of lost productivity due to disability increase the costs of heart disease to almost $138 billion. In addition, 45 percent of heart attacks and 15 percent of heart disease deaths are in people under age 65.[6] This data prompted the steering committee to evaluate the prevalence of heart disease among the Raytheon population and formulate plans of intervention.

Case management staff at BCBSMA identified 445 employees and 307 spouses at high risk for cardiac disease based on claims data that highlighted the following criteria: high blood pressure, high cholesterol, excess weight, diabetes, smoking, heart attack, angina pectoris, and history of other vascular disease. Employees at several facilities were invited to undergo screening for participation in a work-site risk reduction program conducted by an organization called HealthMatters. Members whose blood pressure, cholesterol, and high density lipoprotein met HealthMatters criteria could enroll in a 12-week program focused on health education, behavior and lifestyle change, and stress management. The cost was shared between BCBSMA and Raytheon. For moderate to low risk individuals, information about cardiac health and lifestyle change was provided at work-site health fairs and health education displays attended by Raytheon nursing staff.

Breast Cancer Initiatives

Breast cancer is the most frequently occurring cancer among U.S. women, with an estimated 182,000 cases in 1993.[7] Among women, breast cancer accounts for 32 percent of all new cases of cancer. During this decade alone, 1.5 million women will be diagnosed with breast cancer, and 30 percent will die.[8] Significant nonadherence to treatment is common among breast cancer patients, often due to psychological difficulties such as depression. Data indicate that nonadherence to cancer treatment may have dramatic negative effects on patient survival.[9,10]

In planning disease management initiatives for breast cancer, Raytheon learned of BCBSMA's current research efforts in this area and realized that Raytheon members could benefit from participating in this research. BCBSMA, in conjunction with the American Psychological Association and the Linda Pollin Foundation of the Dana Farber Cancer Institute, is investigating the relationship between psychological adjustment and treatment compliance, psychosocial support, and treatment outcome. Newly diagnosed breast cancer patients are being recruited to participate in the study, which involves a group treatment design consisting of education, relaxation and stress management, and supportive/expressive group therapy. The steering committee decided to open the BCBSMA study to Raytheon members for their voluntary participation. Other initiatives included disseminating health information on screening and risk reduction at the work-site health fairs.

Prevention Committee

Raytheon and BCBSMA share the belief that prevention and wellness efforts will pay off in several ways, including improved customer satisfaction, prevention or reduction of disability and illness through early detection of preventable or treatable illness, and reduced sick time. For the first year of this partnership the prevention activities were designed by a central Prevention Committee. This committee was charged with setting a strategic framework for prevention and wellness programs that targeted quality, improved health function, and cost efficiencies for Raytheon. The Prevention Committee consisted of a prevention expert, a nurse coordina-tor with public health training, a physician with a background in occupational/corporate medicine, several high-level account staff representatives, and human resources staff.

The original Prevention Committee was to define a one-year prevention program aimed at both improving the health status of members and increasing their knowledge of health-related behaviors. The Prevention Committee reviewed many local and national disease management programs as well as best-practice guidelines for the treatment of disorders such as asthma and diabetes.

In the first year, wellness efforts included mailing Raytheon members a guide with basic information about common health problems such as sprains, strains, and earaches, presented in a decision tree format. A communication plan included refrigerator magnets and telephone stickers to remind members to use their guides before calling a doctor with routine questions or visiting the emergency room with a problem that could be treated effectively at home. Three on-site multi-topic health fairs that addressed safety for water sports, biking, and rollerblading, as well as wellness issues of exercise, stress management, cancer prevention, and healthy eating, were organized by BCBSMA and Raytheon staff collectively. All first-year programs avoided sensitive topics like acquired immunodeficiency syndrome (AIDS), and avoided invasive procedures such as cholesterol screening. The health fairs put BCBSMA at the work site with clinical and customer service staff.

After a successful first year of wellness programs that yielded participation levels above 30 percent, an even more aggressive strategy was planned. The focus for year two was on long-term prevention programs that targeted employees' and dependents' healthcare needs as identified by health status data. The goals of the program were to continue to improve health outcomes while reducing costs.

The Prevention Committee established long-term, focused goals and a budget. Staff were appointed to oversee the 1997 prevention initiatives, which were to be built on the foundation that was established in 1996 (Figure 2). The key strategy was to link knowledge of employee health status (from claims utilization data and the health status assessment) with data from the prevention field in order to contribute to improved health status and outcomes. This strategy included linking with national awareness programs and using multiple avenues of communication such as employee newsletters, posters at the work site, BCBSMA mailings to members, and work-site health screenings and fairs.

Partnership with Customer Service

Another effort to build a partnership focused on the customer service staff at BCBSMA, who often answered calls about medical benefits, and the case management staff, who also received customer service calls. Customer service for medical products is a mix of clinical and claims issues. Regular meetings were established to build relationships between the staff and to consider potential areas of collaboration. The first collaborative project resulted in a goal of improving referrals to the high-

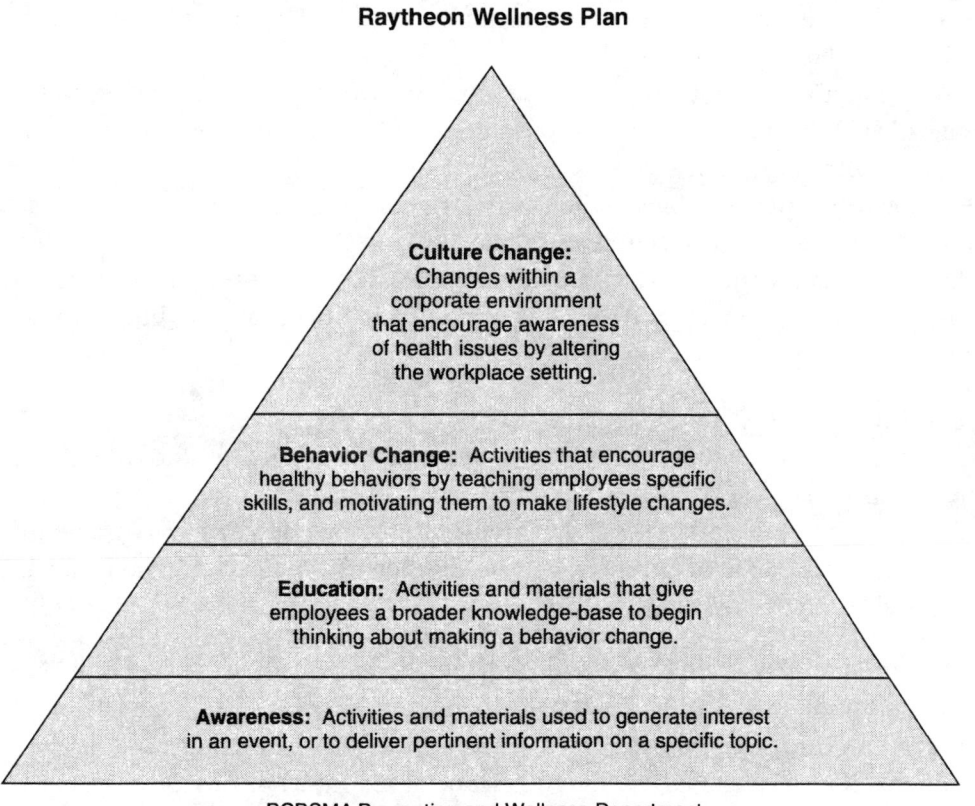

Raytheon Wellness Plan

Culture Change: Changes within a corporate environment that encourage awareness of health issues by altering the workplace setting.

Behavior Change: Activities that encourage healthy behaviors by teaching employees specific skills, and motivating them to make lifestyle changes.

Education: Activities and materials that give employees a broader knowledge-base to begin thinking about making a behavior change.

Awareness: Activities and materials used to generate interest in an event, or to deliver pertinent information on a specific topic.

BCBSMA Prevention and Wellness Department

Figure 2

risk maternity program. The goal of this program, called Lifestart, is to screen every newly pregnant woman so that high-risk pregnancies can be followed more closely by case management. The plan involved customer service staff seeking additional information from callers and providing education about Lifestart to anyone who asked about maternity benefits. The program also included the following strategies: 1) provide written procedures on Lifestart to the health centers at all Raytheon plants, 2) hang posters at the work site advertising the programs, 3) develop an educational approach for the health fairs, 4) review incentives currently used to encourage members to enroll in the Lifestart program, and 5) evaluate (through member satisfaction surveys) any impediments to enrollment in the program for pregnant women.

Member Services

Communicating with Members

Moving 33,000 members from an indemnity plan to a managed care product required the use of all available avenues of communication and education. We first communicated to members about transition of care issues prior to the implementation of the behavioral health change. Members currently receiving mental healthcare were encouraged to seek authorization for ongoing care to avoid misunderstandings. All Raytheon members received a welcoming letter at their homes, emphasizing the role of the PCP as the coordinator of their healthcare. In this letter, members were encouraged to schedule an appointment for a physical examination, a new preventive care benefit. Our goal was to get Raytheon members to their PCPs, in order to avert their seeking unauthorized specialist care.

A bimonthly corporate newsletter to employees featured a full page devoted to the new health plan and its focus on prevention of illnesses and coordination of care. Corporate communication channels were key to our ability to reach members. For 1997, the newsletter will have a health page with three sections. The health news contains information on current disease management initiatives such as Heart Month and our work-site Cardiac Risk Reduction program, a section on psychological issues such as post-holiday blues, and a safety section with articles on safe lifting and children and choking.

Infodial for Health

Another unique feature of the plan is our health information line, which allows members to access, via a toll-free number, basic health information on topics such as colds, flu, strains, and sprains. A recently added screen for depression uses a modified Zung 10-question tool to screen members confidentially for depression and offer them specific referral information.[11]

Blue Care Line: 24-hour Nurse Information

BCBSMA contracted with a national company to provide a 24-hour toll-free line that members can access to get healthcare questions answered rapidly and receive information about local resources, Internet services, and articles. Advice to members is based on protocols developed by national experts. The Blue Care Line encourages members to share their concerns about their healthcare with their PCP. Raytheon represents

2.8 percent of subscribers eligible to use the 24-hour Nurse Help Line. Due to aggressive marketing, Raytheon members currently represent 6.3 percent of all calls to the Blue Care Line. The Blue Care Line responds to general inquiries as shown in Figure 3.

Personal Health Assessment

A personal health assessment, administered confidentially by an independent firm, was conducted for Raytheon members. To gain steering committee support, the Prevention Committee proposed a pilot that allowed steering committee members and a limited number of human resource leaders to complete the assessment. After receiving their results, they offered input on how to promote this assessment to Raytheon members.

The steering committee decided that only employees would be offered the survey in the first year, and in the second year its use would be expanded to the full membership (i.e., eligible family members). The assessment mailings were preceded and followed by posters at work sites, along with reminder postcards. Health assessments identified patients' health risk factors in areas of nutrition, exercise, and cardiac-related symptomology. Participants received detailed personalized reports about their health status and how they might improve it.

The assessment revealed that tobacco use among Raytheon members was similar to the Massachusetts average. Nutritional education and intervention were clearly needed; therefore, we continued our collaboration with the dietitian at the work sites. Early efforts included menu changes in the work-site cafeterias, increasing healthy food offerings, and lowering the price of healthy foods. Additionally, brown-bag healthy eating seminars were offered at work sites during lunch breaks.

The health assessment aggregate data also showed that the most frequently reported stress conditions were insomnia and restless sleep; muscle tension in the neck, shoulders, and jaw; and lower back pain. These findings led to initiatives to address these concerns.

Blue Care Line Call Recommendation

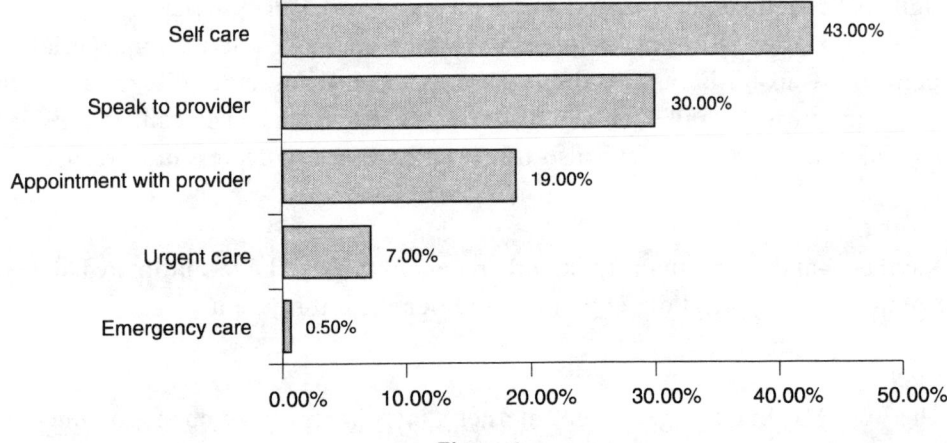

Recommendation	Percentage
Self care	43.00%
Speak to provider	30.00%
Appointment with provider	19.00%
Urgent care	7.00%
Emergency care	0.50%

Figure 3

Fitness was another key area identified in the survey. Results showed that 84 percent of respondents did not get enough aerobic exercise. This was especially true among women. The data was of concern to BCBSMA, given recent information showing that lack of exercise is correlated with increased mortality and morbidity to a greater degree than cigarette smoking. The health assessment findings led to a Prevention Committee discussion that produced the following recommendations:

- Develop walk paths and maps for each work site
- Facilitate walking clubs
- Encourage walking meetings
- Advertise discounts for memberships to health centers
- Explore link with an athletic shoe manufacturer for discounts
- Highlight different fitness alternatives at each health fair

Alcohol abuse was a new area to be addressed by the assessment questionnaire. The questions were modified from the CAGE questionnaire—a simple, easily administered, four-item instrument (see Chapter 16 for details on this questionnaire). Nine percent of respondents reported moderate risk, and 3 percent reported high risk alcohol use.

Technological Support

A fundamental part of the BCBSMA/Raytheon health plan is the use of leading edge technology. These technological innovations are described below.

Health Wire/Point-of-Service (POS) Devices

Point-of-service technology links BCBSMA with physicians' offices for referrals and authorization. A swipe of the BCBSMA card and a few keystrokes replace paper and phone processes. Health Wire allows electronic claims submission and easy access to claims status. Provider technology also notifies physicians of patients in need of routine screenings based on information from the claims database.

Kiosk

The kiosk is a virtual reality service center, with a video host to guide viewers through different menu features. Kiosks at each work site provide easily accessed member information, allowing members to change their PCP and look up specialists in the network. A health library on the kiosk provides articles about disease and illness, exercise and nutrition, and lifestyle and family issues. Each article can be viewed on-screen and printed. Members can also take a stress test or a depression screen.

Account Link

Raytheon and more than 1,000 other benefit offices have automated data exchange including application, eligibility, and benefit information.

Internet

The BCBSMA home page on the Internet allows access to company, product, benefit, and medical information.

Meditrax

Because every hospital emergency room in Massachusetts has Health Wire, a real-time information system, BCBSMA can respond to a PCP's request and notify him or her when a patient is seen in the emergency room or admitted to the hospital by another physician.

Medical Policy Fax on Demand

The medical policy area offers fax on demand policies so that providers can have easy access to medical policy as they practice. By calling a toll-free number, providers may access a policy as well as references to support the medical policy decision.

Physician Communication

Primary care physicians were mailed summaries about the general Raytheon population and utilization trends.

Team Building: Internal and External

What characterizes true integration is the development of cooperative behaviors that deliver optimum results. To achieve this ideal, BCBSMA selected staff who valued cooperation and team performance over individual success. The BCBSMA/Raytheon team spent a day together on a team-building event that fostered trust, cooperation, and maximization of individual skills to contribute to a group goal. Participants agreed that there was a better understanding of each others' strengths and styles, a respect for individuals, and an appreciation of the value of the team.

To promote integration, BCBSMA educated its own employees extensively about the goals and expectations for the Raytheon account. They sought to ensure that everyone understood the incentives for cooperation. Some incentives were financial, but others were relational and contributed to the longevity of the relationship with Raytheon. BCBSMA staff were taught negotiation skills and conflict resolution.

Most importantly, BCBSMA tried to "walk in Raytheon's shoes" to gain a deeper understanding of the perspective of the customer. BCBSMA visited Raytheon plants, pursued an understanding of their business and its challenges, read their annual report, and kept a notebook of press clippings from the media. Raytheon also made efforts to understand the unique problems and challenges facing BCBSMA. To understand and support each other was what the "commitment to partnership" meant in both words and action. The partnership continues to evolve, and the first year's success has built a firm foundation for the future.

Conclusion

In reviewing the first year of this unique partnership, we are pleased with the successes (Table 3). Bringing two such different and established organizations together in the midst of enormous industry change could have been problematic, but instead has been unmistakably positive. With an emphasis on integrated care, prevention, and disease management, great strides were made in delivering comprehensive services focusing on long-term improvement of health for Raytheon members. In the process, both organizations had the opportunity to collaborate, benefit from each other's

TABLE 3. YEAR ONE (1996) RESULTS

Health fairs were attended by more than 30 percent of members.
9 percent of employees completed health assessments.
51 percent of women between the ages of 21-64 had cervical cancer screening.
35 percent of members had a routine physical exam with their PCP.
56 percent of women over age 40 received mammography screening.
97 percent of members utilized In-Network providers.
Approximately 50 cases were co-managed with medical and behavioral health triage/assessment.

unique viewpoint and knowledge, and be challenged to provide the best healthcare delivery possible. The team approach to the integrated care model, demonstrated by relationships between behavioral and medical staff, PCPs and Raytheon members, and BCBSMA case managers and Raytheon members, has been the base upon which to build future successes. Staff involved in this partnership experienced pride and excitement in the programs they envisioned and implemented. The partnership model clearly supported both organizations to manage the challenges and foster the successes of quality healthcare delivery.

Acknowledgment

The authors thank Paul Hart, Blue Cross and Blue Shield of Massachusetts, for his contribution of important utilization and cost data.

References

1. Rosen A, Miller V, Parker G: Standards of care for area mental health services. Aust N Z J Psychiatry 23:379-395, 1989.
2. Hutcherson S: Disease management demystified: what can it do? Health Care Innovations Nov/Dec:25-27, 1995.
3. Direct and Indirect Costs of Diabetes in the United States in 1992. American Diabetes Association Inc, Alexandria VA, 1993.
4. Rubin RJ, Altman WM, Mendelson DN: Health care expenditures for people with diabetes mellitus. J Clin Endocrinol Metab 78:809A-809F, 1994.
5. American Heart Association: Heart and Stroke Facts: 1995 Statistical Supplement. American Heart Association National Center, Dallas TX, 1994.
6. Goodman RA: Medical care spending—United States. MMWR Morb Mortal Wkly Rep 43:581-586, 1994.
7. Boring CC, Squires TS, Tong T: Cancer statistics. Cancer for Clinicians 43:7-17, 1993.
8. Cancer Facts and Figures—1993. American Cancer Society, New York NY, 1994.
9. Ayres A, Hoon PW, Franzoni JB, et al: Influence of mood and adjustment to cancer on compliance with chemotherapy among breast cancer patients. J Psychosom Res 38:393-402, 1994.
10. Richardson JL, Marks G, Johnson CA, et al: Path model of multidimensional compliance with cancer therapy. Health Psychol 6:183-207, 1987.
11. Zung WWK: A self-rating depression scale. Arch Gen Psychiatry 12:63-70, 1965.

Chapter 7

The Integration Experience in a Group Model HMO: Northern California Kaiser-Permanente

Robin Dea, M.D.

Northern California Kaiser-Permanente is the joint collaboration between Kaiser Foundation Health Plan and Kaiser Foundation Hospitals, both nonprofit organizations, and The Permanente Medical Group, Inc., a for-profit professional corporation. The Permanente Medical Group contracts to provide professional medical care services within the medical centers and clinics operated by Kaiser Foundation Hospitals. Kaiser-Permanente functions as a group model health maintenance organization (HMO), having existed in the Northern California area since the mid-1940s. The organization services 2.6 million subscribers in the San Francisco Bay Area, Sacramento, and the Central Valley, utilizing 22 different medical centers or clinics.

A group model HMO system has inherent advantages for the integration of mental health and chemical dependency care with primary care. Northern California Kaiser-Permanente is a very comprehensive medical care delivery program. The system is almost totally self-contained, but does have the flexibility to allow some specialized services (radiation therapy and some cardiac surgery) to be contracted out. Most inpatient psychiatry is performed in community hospitals under contract to Kaiser Foundation Hospitals, and is closely managed by on-site teams of mental health clinicians from The Permanente Medical Group. In some areas Permanente Medical Group physicians are attending, and in others the clinical care is performed by a panel of community psychiatrists. The goal of the system is to offer high quality, integrated managed care to its members.

Unmanaged Integration

One of the key elements to integrated care is communication. Medical care is more fully integrated when all providers involved in a specific case are aware of the workings of other providers and collaborate in the clinical approach. Prior to 1993 most integration between primary care and behavioral healthcare was a result of the communication effort inherent in a group model system. Because all providers worked in the same general setting (even if separated by buildings), they still shared a common telephone system, interoffice mail system, facility meeting structure (including interdepartmental educational meetings), and a computerized appointment system. There was usually close communication between physicians and nurse practitioners in the medical area, and physicians, psychologists, and licensed clinical social workers in the behavioral health area. Although there were some joint clinical programs for specific problems, there was not much consistency from one facility to another.

While this system led to greater communication among practitioners, it was still generally unmanaged. Knowledge of the specifics of the overall care plan required the usual searching through often illegible outpatient medical records and required the thought and time to call a relevant provider. For example, it was frequently difficult to know which medications a patient was taking, and there were numerous duplications in laboratory studies in order to avoid time-intensive searches through the medical record.

Under this system, behavioral healthcare consisted primarily of outpatient psychotherapy and inpatient psychiatric hospitalization. For chemical dependency, medical detoxification was performed in the medical hospital and outpatient chemical dependency programs, but there was a lack of more intensive care for patients who required it. Numerous complaints were received from primary care practitioners about the poor communication with behavioral health providers. The primary care providers frequently felt that once a patient had been referred to behavioral heathcare services, they were unlikely to be contacted again regarding the clinical condition of the patient unless they specifically called and asked.

While primary care providers within the system had complaints with behavioral healthcare, the complaints from the purchasers of healthcare, primarily employers, were more significant. The system was simply not working. There were inadequate staffing levels in the behavioral health system to provide rapid access for anything other than acute emergencies. The result for many systems, including Kaiser-Permanente, was significant increases in inpatient hospitalizations, the most expensive form of behavioral healthcare.

The Psychiatry Model of Care

In early 1992 a committee of health plan, hospital, and medical group administrators, along with mental health and chemical dependency leadership, realized that unless important changes in the system were made, there was a significant risk of purchasers carving out behavioral healthcare. They organized a working group of behavioral healthcare providers, marketing and benefits specialists, and research analysts to write and develop a project called the Psychiatry Model of Care (PMOC). The PMOC has sections relating to benefits, access, practice guidelines, outcomes management, expanded levels of care, behavioral health education, and primary care integration. Although the latter is the focus of this chapter, it is important to understand the context in which these changes took place, as these elements all interrelate.

The starting point was access to care. The goals included improving access within specialty mental health and chemical dependency for self-referred patients (about 75 percent of the total) and for those referred from primary care departments and Employee Assistance Programs. At the same time that access was improving through specific redesign of the access process, practice guidelines were being developed for specific conditions. These included attention deficit hyperactivity disorder, panic disorder, major depression, behavioral health education, and outpatient chemical dependency services. Practice guidelines typically lead to an increase in specialty psychotherapy groups within mental health and chemical dependency. They also lead to the establishment of a wide variety of behavioral health education classes, available not only to patients within specific treatment programs, but also to all patients within the medical center.

Primary Care Integration

The effort to integrate mental health and chemical dependency services into primary care was seen within the overall model as a means to provide mental health/chemical dependency (MH/CD) services to a broader spectrum of the general population. Another goal was to achieve medical cost offsets and thus reduce overall medical cost. Integration revolves around communication and operations. All providers and support staff working with an individual patient have a need to know what the others are doing, and what their intent is. This must be organized operationally to create a planned treatment program for any individual patient, and carried out in such a way that all elements of the plan are implemented. In a group model HMO, as compared to other models, the ease of communication between providers is enhanced simply by the basic structure of the organization. Even having all provider phone numbers in a facility directory or on a computer mainframe increases the likelihood that communication will take place, but does not guarantee it. Operations must be designed in such a way that both written and verbal communication are enhanced.

In the Psychiatry Model of Care, five different elements were addressed in order to bring about integration. Due to the nature of rapid change both within Kaiser-Permanente and in the marketplace in general, this model is undergoing continuous analysis and improvement.

Case Finding

The first element of integration is *case finding,* which is the process of designing systems to enhance the detection of certain mental health or chemical dependency problems in the primary care or general medical center setting, so that treatment can be offered to the patient. One example of this involves chemical dependency services (CDS). Time is allotted on a daily basis for CDS providers to spend in the medical/surgical hospital, reviewing briefly the intake summary of all newly admitted patients, and searching for any signs in patients who may have chemical dependency or alcohol problems. When a problem is noticed, the provider discusses it with the attending physician and talks with the patient. The patient is offered treatment services within the CDS program. Over time this approach increases the likelihood that the attending physician will ask for a CDS consult when doing the initial work-up, and also builds close collegial relationships between attending physicians and CDS providers. The CDS staff also give grand rounds lectures to the medical staff to enhance the detection of chemical dependency problems in outpatient primary care.

Another example involves the practice guidelines for panic disorder. While these guidelines generally involve the treatment program for panic disorder within the department of psychiatry, there is also an educational and procedural element both for primary care and in the emergency department. An educational program is provided for the general hospital attending staff and is also given at specific departmental meetings. The program outlines the detection, diagnosis, and treatment of panic disorder and also outlines a mechanism for rapid referral. Although there has always been a written consultation process, sometimes (because of the slowness of interoffice mail) the system causes delays that prevent involving the patient in treatment immediately after detection of the problem. In the emergency department a postcard was developed on which the provider writes the name, medical record number, and phone number of the patient. The cards are simply dropped into a box and are collected on a daily basis by the MH/CD providers on their rounds. The card identifies whether the problem identified was panic disorder or chemical dependency.

Once the card is received, the patient is called and offered services in the appropriate treatment program. In order to make this system work, there must be periodic updates provided specifically to the departmental staff in order to remind them both of the existence of the program, and of the clinical signs and symptoms for which they are searching. As their awareness of these problems becomes heightened, patients are identified at a much earlier point, thus making treatment easier and avoiding further long-term medical consequences and costs. The programs have had a very positive response from primary care providers. They feel more supported in their efforts to avoid future medical complications, especially for the chemical dependency patients, and can avoid unnecessary utilization of procedures for people with panic disorder.

Specialized Programs

Another avenue for integration within primary care is specialized programs. These programs have a very specific procedure for detection and treatment of patients within the primary care setting, and they have designated personnel. One such example is the Kaiser-Permanente Early Start program in the obstetrics/gynecology department. This program places a CDS provider in the obstetrics clinic with the purpose of identifying newly pregnant women who are abusing alcohol or drugs. There is an initial short screening instrument to be filled out by all new patients. This questionnaire specifically asks about alcohol and drug use. If the answers indicate a potential problem, the CDS provider will then talk with the patient and request she fill out a more extensive questionnaire. A further conversation is held, and as a part of that discussion the patient may be invited to join the Early Start program if a clinically significant alcohol or drug problem is detected. The treatment program is done in a group, with all group members being pregnant women. This approach helps remove the stigma that would exist if these women were in a general chemical dependency program with nonpregnant patients (i.e., admitting alcohol or drug use during pregnancy).

As a result of the outcomes from the pilot program, it was implemented region-wide during 1994 and 1995. The Early Start program has led to a significant reduction of days in the newborn intensive care unit, and has been very successful in decreasing alcohol and drug use for the mother (Table 1). The providers in this program, while housed by and administratively reporting to the chief of the obstetrics/gynecology department, also have a supervisory and ongoing educational relationship with the CDS program within the department of psychiatry.

Another example of a specialized program is the pain management clinic. This program provides a multidisciplinary approach to dealing with patients with many different types of chronic pain problems. The program seeks to generate awareness

TABLE 1. EARLY START PROGRAM OUTCOMES DATA, 1995

Gestation	Early Start Women Who Quit Using n=150 (72%)	Users Past 32 Weeks n=58 (28%)
Birth Outcome:		
Premature births (<32 weeks)	4.6 %	13.6 %
Low birth weight (<2500 grams)	4.6 %	13.6 %
Average length of stay/newborn	2.2 days	3.2 days
NICU* admissions	19.0 %	27.0 %
Average NICU stay	4.6 days	7.3 days

* NICU = Neonatal intensive care unit

that cognitive-behavioral strategies and antidepressant therapy are effective for chronic pain. Response to neural blockade is unpredictable, and the use of certain medications (sedatives, anti-inflammatory agents, and narcotics) is frequently less effective and may even be counterproductive. The program goals include assisting patients in coping with chronic pain and removing pain medication that may have been abused. Primary care providers may either directly refer patients to the program or obtain phone consultation first.

The pain management clinic has a core group composed of a behavioral medicine specialist, a pain specialist (physician), and a care coordinator. Their functions include triage, diagnosis and evaluations, care coordination, and administration of the program. A care plan is created for each patient, and patients are tracked as they move through the program. There are associated professionals in primary care, physical therapy, health education, and anesthesiology as part of the clinic. They also have rapid access to other specialists as necessary. As patients move through the pain management clinic, their care is coordinated, they receive intensive interdisciplinary treatment, and there is ongoing communication with the primary care provider who made the referral.

A key element of the care plan addresses inappropriate medical utilization. The care coordinator performs intensive case management with high-utilizing or high-risk patients. The behavioral medicine component treats patients with significant psychobehavioral problems. Services include assessment, development of an exercise regimen, body mechanics, behavioral observation and management, relaxation training, cognitive/behavioral therapy, medication management, skill building, and education. There is also a very extensive behavioral health education component. The program is closely coordinated with physical therapy, anesthesia, and subspeciality clinics such as spine clinic, headache clinic, and CDS. There are also referrals for alternative treatments such as biofeedback and acupuncture.

As the implementation of these clinics spreads throughout the region, computerized tracking and analysis is being prepared to make it possible to measure medical cost offset data from patients attending the program. Although this has been available to evaluate a specific cohort of patients, newer programs will make evaluation possible for all patients.

General On-Site Integration

A third element of integration places a MH/CD provider in the primary care setting. These providers, usually psychologists or licensed clinical social workers, have joint appointment in the departments of psychiatry and primary care. There is psychiatrist back-up from the psychiatry clinic, but usually the psychiatrist is not on-site in the primary care clinic, although it can be arranged for a specific case.

The MH/CD provider in this setting is frequently called a behavioral medicine specialist. This is typically a clinician who has both a significant interest in and experience with the MH/CD aspects of primary medical care. The behavioral medicine specialists have several different functions. At the request of the primary care physician (PCP), they evaluate and do brief interventions with patients. While they may also evaluate the patient, they encourage and assist the PCP in providing ongoing care. Also, they may simply consult with the PCP and never see the patient, depending on the evaluation.

Both clinicians must decide which situations can be reasonably treated in the primary care setting and which require referral to the specialty mental health clinic. In situations regarding alcohol or drugs, there is usually a referral to the chemical dependency program as soon as the patient is willing to attend. In any case, the patient may also be referred to other resources within the medical center or within the community, including physical therapy, behavioral health education, and community programs. Behavioral medicine specialists are also available for more formal case staffing meetings with physician and support staff or for brief consultations. They need significant amounts of flexible time in their schedule, so that they may either do a quick hallway consultation with providers and staff or do a previously unplanned patient evaluation.

In addition to appropriately managing the psychosocial problems of patients, this approach allows a dual education function for both PCPs and the behavioral medicine specialists. Because the treatment approach by the behavioral medicine specialist is based on cognitive-behavioral therapy, the primary care providers over time become more sophisticated in their own use of these techniques. At the same time, the behavioral medicine specialists are exposed to a wide variety of medical problems. They increase their sophistication in the conceptualization of problems as a combination of biologic and psychosocial factors.

Behavioral Health Education

The fourth element of integration involves the design and implementation of an extensive behavioral health educational system. As this program has grown, its importance and effectiveness has exceeded the original expectations within the PMOC project. A practice guidelines team was established to set up the parameters of behavioral health education classes. There have traditionally been classes through each facility's health education department on general behavioral medicine themes, including stress management, weight management, parenting, and couples communication, in addition to a wide variety of classes that are more specific to particular medical diagnoses such as asthma or diabetes. The Health Education department managed these classes, having complete responsibility for their schedule, curriculum, teachers, and registration.

With the introduction of the PMOC, an integrated program was created between the health education department and the department of psychiatry. In the development of the Behavioral Health Education program, psychiatry departments hired at least a half-time behavioral health education coordinator. This person designs curriculum with a team, using the regionally developed guidelines. The coordinator also evaluates and hires instructors, coordinates the preparation of the materials, and is responsible for the internal marketing of all the courses. This includes frequent brief visits to staff meetings in primary and specialty care clinics, writing flyers, and sending voice mail reminders to providers and support staff about the specifics of upcoming classes. Advertising the number of people already signed up for an individual class spurs providers to make referrals so that the class will not be undersubscribed.

Classes are designed for the purpose of generally educating patients and family members about the problems they face, so that the time spent in a treatment provider's office is most efficiently utilized. Classes have been established in all areas listed in Table 2.

The mindfulness class is designed to teach the relationship between mind and body and, through workshop techniques, assist patients in increasing awareness of their own specific emotional triggers to certain behaviors or thoughts. With some classes (depression, ADHD) there is a free overview class of two hours to give attendees an idea of what a more extensive course will include. If a person then decides to attend the six- to eight-week course, he or she pays a nominal fee to cover the instructor's fee and materials. Instructors are usually hired from outside the Kaiser-Permanente organization, enabling providers to concentrate on the clinical treatment. People can attend these classes as part of a treatment program initiated in either primary care or the specialty mental health setting. They can also attend simply because they are interested in the topic or are deciding whether they wish to pursue a course of treatment. In the department of psychiatry, these classes are an integral part of the best practice guidelines for specific problems such as ADHD, depression, and panic.

The importance of ongoing, regular communication with providers in all settings about the existence and function of these classes cannot be overemphasized. Where communication has been diligently pursued, the class attendance has been excellent. When communication has faltered, so has attendance.

These classes have received very high patient satisfaction responses. Obviously some education still occurs during the treatment process, but the providers appreciate having patients come into the treatment setting with a good baseline knowledge of the condition.

TABLE 2. BEHAVIORAL HEALTH EDUCATION PROGRAM FOCUS AREAS

Depression	Panic disorder
Attention deficit hyperactivity disorder (ADHD)	Mindfulness
Anger management	Chronic pain and illness
Couples communication	Work stress
Parenting	Parenting through divorce

Data Systems

For integration, data systems must be developed to share knowledge between providers. This is an ongoing improvement process. In Northern California Kaiser-Permanente this is not yet fully achieved. However, the mainframe systems that exist have become sophisticated enough to enhance the treatment process and offer a competitive advantage over network model HMOs, where there is typically no clinical data repository to access.

All providers in the system have computer terminals on their desks with a program called the Clinical Information Presentation System. All laboratory results are available, which has decreased duplicate ordering by different physicians. It also makes it possible to easily scan results gathered over a long period of time, either for all results or by specific type (such as all thyroid tests, or all liver function tests).

The on-line system also shows all prescriptions that have been filled within the Kaiser-Permanente system, making it easy to see chronologically what medications a patient is taking, the doses, and even if the prescription has been picked up at the pharmacy. Because the system is pharmacy-based, however, it does not list all prescriptions written. If a patient has prescriptions filled in a pharmacy outside the system, it is not recorded on the computer. Some patients have used their knowledge of this fact to hide their usage of the same medication from two different physicians. Although this is rare, as the system improves it will provide information on all prescriptions written, not just the ones filled internally.

The Clinical Information Presentation System also displays patient demographic information, appointments, allergies, hospitalizations, immunizations, and provider schedules. This information makes it easier for all providers to share clinical information, to know who else is treating the patient, when they are being seen, and which appointments were kept. Since the regional phone directory is also on the same terminal (although not within system), it is easy for providers to access the phone numbers of others treating the patient.

Confidentiality is an important concern, and steps have been taken to safeguard information. These steps are frequently controversial because they attempt to balance the privacy of the patient with clinicians' need to be informed of specific data. In the primary care-MH/CD interface, there has been much discussion about how to accomplish this balance. All physicians are given access to the system, but nonphysician providers must be approved for access to the system by a department chief. An electronic trail is kept of all access to the system, and an alert to this fact appears when anyone first signs on to the system. In addition, a monthly report goes to department of psychiatry chiefs identifying non-mental health/CDS providers who have accessed mental health information. By calling up any clinical information on a patient, the provider acknowledges that they have a clinical need to know the information.

Some mental health information is handled differently from information generated in primary care. While laboratory and medication information generated within the department of psychiatry is available to all, drug toxicology screens and test results generated within CDS (a subdepartment of the department of psychiatry) as part of the treatment program are available only to the person ordering them. Drug screens ordered anywhere else in the system are available to all.

If a primary care provider wishes to access mental health information, there is first a warning screen specific to mental health. The provider is informed that continuing requires a re-entering of their password, and that an electronic trail is being kept. The information available is that a patient was seen, when, and by whom. After a lengthy committee process (including input from patients), it was decided not to include mental health diagnosis on this screen, because of the desire of patients to not have that diagnosis prejudice the judgment of providers concerning other medical problems.

However, there is a system whereby a provider can call and get the mental health diagnosis 24 hours a day if they need it to treat the patient. What most providers do is simply get the patient's permission to speak with each other. From a legal standpoint that is not technically necessary in the state of California in a system such as Kaiser-Permanente, but doing so leads to enhanced cooperation from the patient, and occasionally can be a tip-off to providers of a patient who doesn't want one physician to know what the other is doing. Chemical dependency visits are not viewable by primary care clinicians in the system due to restrictions imposed by federal law.

Redesigning Primary Care

In September 1996 the board of directors of the Permanente Medical Group, Inc. approved a plan to take a bold step in a new direction for primary care. According to Executive Director Harry Caulfield, M.D., this plan would be a "member-driven, physician-directed approach to provide the highest quality of care, service, and access at the lowest possible cost." The first component of this redesign would be the creation of a program called Adult Primary Care. A design group of 50 people from all specialties and primary care worked together for eight weeks to design a plan for a more member-focused care experience. The plan will be implemented throughout 1997 and early 1998.

Within each primary care setting, the Adult Primary Care program will develop teams of health professionals to serve about 20,000 adult members. The program will allow members great flexibility in choosing their healthcare professionals, rapid access to primary care and specialists, and convenient times for receiving care. It will provide a full scope of primary care services in one place, with the professionals working together in a managed, coordinated way, both in primary care and when specialists are involved. It requires the use of information services to track patients with chronic conditions and to manage clinical information and teleservice functions (electronic messaging via telephone and on-line).

The core of the program is the adult primary care team, a multidisciplinary group that can change its composition as it evolves. The initial plan is to have a combination of physicians, nurse practitioners, medical assistants, nurses, a manager, a behavioral health specialist, a health educator, and a physical therapist. These people will all work together in the same place and will function as a team, completely coordinating the medical care of their members. They also focus on prevention services with every patient contact. They work to provide the right kind of care the first time a patient comes in, with the right professional. Physician time is "leveraged" by utilizing the physician only when needed or upon patient request. Another leverage is that hospitalized patients will be cared for by hospital-based physicians, not members of the Adult Primary Care team, because physicians who specialize in inpatient care may be better able to manage the needs of hospitalization. Finally, this team gets to know the patients well over time, which makes interpretation of day-to-day problems far more accurate.

This program also requires some redesign in the specialty care clinics. Regional, specialist chiefs of service groups will develop service contracts with primary care to provide population-based disease management. This means utilizing regionally created practice guidelines and using both primary care and specialist services. Specialists will also provide rapid consultation on a situational basis and training for the primary care providers to enhance their knowledge and skills. The service agreements are reciprocal in the need for the Adult Primary Care team to provide primary care services for specialists.

The role of the behavioral health specialist (usually a psychologist or licensed clinical social worker) remains the same as in the previously discussed Psychiatry Model of Care plan. This provider focuses on detecting, triaging, and coordinating care for patients with psychosocial, behavioral, and treatment adherence issues. The behavioral medicine specialist may provide brief treatment (usually three to six visits of 30 minutes or less) or refer to psychiatry. Visits are offered for chronic conditions, consultation and referral for chemical dependency, and coordination of behavioral medicine services with psychiatry and behavioral health education. The consultation function within the team is important to help identify patients with behavioral problems and to train primary care providers to enhance their own skills of detection and treatment.

This overall plan builds on the already existing elements in the PMOC. Most case finding will shift into the primary care setting, and the previously mentioned providers in primary care will become the behavioral medicine specialists in Adult Primary Care (keeping in mind that some of them are also in pediatrics, not a part of the Adult Primary Care model). The department of psychiatry remains the center for specialty mental health and chemical dependency services. But the Adult Primary Care model significantly enhances the coordination of care for large numbers of patients, especially those with behavioral health problems who either would not have been referred to the psychiatry department or would not have come if they had been referred. While it takes personnel to make the management of cases actually work, the model guarantees that patients get the preventive and treatment services they need, without "falling through the cracks."

A cost structure has been proposed that will shift resources within medical centers to pay for the Adult Primary Care model. The model calls for slightly fewer physicians and more support staff than current standard care. It is assumed that there will be less overall utilization in this system because of a reduction in redundant visits that occurs due to not having all necessary providers in the same place and coordinating care. Patients will be able to have multiple services during a single encounter, and there will be more effective matching of resources to the patient's needs. The increased effectiveness of preventive services will also drive lower utilization in the long term.

The long-term effectiveness of the Adult Primary Care model on the department of psychiatry is unclear. One view is that the number of behavioral medicine specialists that are planned for now in the Adult Primary Care will increase case finding, so there will be many more referrals to specialty mental health. The opposing view is that many cases now referred to specialty mental health will be taken care of in the primary care setting. Either way, the emphasis on the behavioral aspects of medical care is viewed as a positive step for patients over the long haul.

Summary

The changes in the primary care/behavioral healthcare interface over the time period from 1992 to 1997 have been dramatic. Originally, the system was fragmented, with little programming consistency across a large geographical region. With the creation of the PMOC, a more coordinated effort was made to ease the communication between primary care and behavioral health systems. The programs developed as part of this model increased the level of integration with primary care. Those programs continue as a new overall structure for adult primary care is overlaid onto that system. The joining of the PMOC with Adult Primary Care (and the anticipated Child and Adolescent Primary Care) creates a powerful ability to have all the various aspects of day-to-day care truly working together in the interest of the patient.

As care is no longer based solely on what goes on when a patient is in the office with a physician, but instead is regarded as the whole spectrum of activities including prevention, behavioral health education classes, and computerized tracking of treatment in a disease management program, the experience of the patient becomes more seamless and more efficient. Patient input in the system assists in its continuing improvement. This approach to medical care allows the caregivers to continue to move toward the ideal of being very specific in the care of a particular problem, while still being able to view the patient as a whole person.

Chapter 8

Integrated Systems in the Workplace: The Delta/CIGNA/MCC Depression Initiative

David Whitehouse, M.D., M.B.A.

When medical costs were rising faster than inflation, and behavioral health costs faster even than medical costs, the idea of "carving out" mental health and substance abuse benefits and handing their management over to "experts" seemed like a great idea. For a time, costs did stabilize. Preferred practices, insistence on medical necessity, competitive contracting, and new approaches to treatment all played a part. The problem of "runaway costs rising faster than inflation" had been solved—or had it?

From the employer's point of view, the concern about medical insurance premiums decreasing the company's global competitiveness had been met and resolved successfully. Employer or healthcare vendors were now less likely to be interested in changing the healthcare system. After all, "if it ain't broke, don't fix it."

Part of the problem with carve-outs, however, may actually have been their success. Along with the desired results of decreased costs and a marked reduction in inappropriate utilization, an undesired but real result may also have been that those who could benefit from *appropriate* utilization may also have suffered. When utilization is the measure of success, the fact that the stigma of mental illness creates barriers to accessing help may be seen as a positive. Furthermore, because most carve-out companies need highly personal information to approve reimbursement for treatment, they too may compound the problem by their apparent intrusiveness. Success, therefore, seems to hide some unresolved issues. As the mist of this success cleared, outcomes data on the impact of depression on general medical costs, disability, depression-related workers' compensation costs, reduced productivity, and higher medical utilization revealed major problems in the system.

The degree of this "indirect" problem may have been accidentally compounded by the impact of the Americans with Disabilities Act, as well as by the possibly low level of sophistication among primary care practitioners who were managing depression-related disability. Now the *full* health cost equation is revealed, rather than just the part related to direct medical costs (Figure 1). Total healthcare costs related to a specific disease or process equal the sum of direct medical and behavioral health costs *plus* all indirect medical and work-related expenses that result from failures or delays in diagnosing or treating the illness (Total Health $ = Direct Medical $ + Direct Behavioral $ + Indirect Work-related $).

For any company, this equation impacts profitability. However, the equation contains the possibility that altering the weight of specific components might have a dramatic effect on the whole: the concepts, in fact, of *medical cost offset* and *work-related cost offset*. These concepts suggest that, if correctly managed, any increase in direct

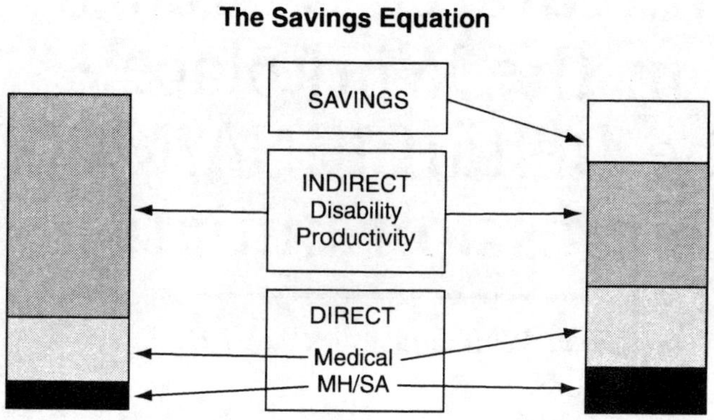

The Savings Equation

Figure 1. The health cost equation

behavioral health costs might well be more than offset by the impact of the interventions on general medical costs and indirect employer costs. These concepts give rise to the cost offset equation:

> Total medical and work-related cost offset equals the total healthcare costs during the time period studied minus the increase in direct behavioral care costs related to increased interventions during that time period minus the total healthcare costs for the same population at an earlier matched period.

Cost Offset

The impact of cost offset has already been well described in the literature (see Chapter 5). Approximately 70 percent of all healthcare visits are the result of psychosocial problems and not organically based physiological conditions.[1,2] Well-designed behavioral interventions can save anywhere from 20 percent to 40 percent of the previous total medical expenditure. A 1991 study shows that in elderly patients hospitalized for hip fracture, the direct cost of psychiatric interventions was $40,000, but the reduction in lengths of stay and other direct medical costs saved was $270,000—more than $1,300 per patient.[3] In another study, high-utilizing Medicaid outpatients who received behavioral health treatment achieved a 21 percent reduction in medical costs after 18 months, while those who received no behavioral services had a 22 percent increase in medical service utilization.[4]

Although the medical offsets achieved may show marked variability, they are clearly real. Among the elderly the largest effect comes from a decrease in patient costs, whereas among younger adults it is more commonly the result of decreased outpatient utilization. While the medical cost offset is clearly established, there are fewer studies in work-related cost offset. However, the evidence of its existence is compelling.

The Delta/CIGNA/MCC Initiative

Within this context, the Delta/CIGNA/MCC initiative was designed to increase our knowledge about work-related and medical cost offset by focusing on the current effect of depression on direct and indirect costs and then examining how increased availability and commitment to direct behavioral costs could result in happier and healthier employees. The medical director of Delta understood how a proactive, progressive approach could be extremely beneficial for individuals within the company who might suffer from depression. As a result, he initiated conversations between Delta, CIGNA, and MCC that led to a decision to study the impact of a proactive and intensified depression disease management program. Depression was selected because of its prevalence, its potential severity, its documented impact on psychiatric and medical costs, and finally, because of its well-established diagnostic criteria and treatment guidelines. For Delta, the concerns are safety, disability, and productivity. These concerns are vital because of economic and risk-related impact, and they combine to make a worthy focus for the study.

The aim is to establish an intervention that would benefit the patients, Delta, and CIGNA/MCC. An additional goal is to try to quantify the effects of the intervention. The gains for patients will come from a program of increased education, which will allow for better early detection and prevention; improved care due to the standardization of treatments and a more symptom-focused approach; as well as improved quality of life and functioning in the workplace. The gain for the health plan will be improved health for its members and a better understanding of the value of behavioral health services. The gain for the employer will be a healthier, happier workforce with improved productivity and decreased health costs.

The Intervention

From the beginning it was clear that this was not to be a minor adjustment to business as usual. Delta wanted to examine the potential effect of a comprehensive approach to the problem, namely, education of employees and supervisors for increased awareness, improved screening for early detection, best practices in standardization of treatment, and the analysis of individual, health-related, work-related, and economic outcomes. All of these were built into the final study design. If the scope was large, so were the potential problems. Certain elements were clear from the earliest planning stages. The fact that Delta had several concentrated locations of employees allowed one site to be chosen as the major intervention site, while other sites would serve as controls. Under the existing plan, detection of depression was limited to self-referrals and primary care referrals. Issues of stigma and logistical barriers following referral also added to the potential for missing patients, and resistance and lack of education about both the symptoms and the effectiveness of treatment for depression combined to complicate early detection.

To overcome these obstacles, there would have to be a focus on educational material (distributed through employee newsletters) to raise general awareness among employees and on health plan educational programs. At the same time, more formal training of supervisors would need to be undertaken to raise the level of education about the illness and its effects on the workplace. Primary care practitioners would need to receive training to increase their knowledge of the symptoms, comorbidities, and management of depression. While this might increase some referrals (self or on another's advice), more formal tools would have to be added to increase individual awareness of the risks and symptoms of depression.

Evaluations begin with the general health risk assessment (HRA) tool, since it contains some preliminary screening questions for emotional distress. Based on advice from others, the patient's personal concern, or the concern of a primary care physician (PCP), patients would then be advised to undergo a more formal screen for emotional illness (Figure 2). The SDDS-PC was chosen for its proven validity and reliability, as well as its ease of use. Computer-assisted telephone interview technology, for example, allows access to screening at any time or in any place that is convenient. The toll-free number would be available 24 hours a day, seven days a week. The results would be automatically faxed back to the primary care practitioner. If the patient screened positive for suicidal ideation, there would be an automatic transfer to a continuously operated crisis line for direct and immediate intervention.

The second part of the program would seek to enhance treatment by standardizing the specific clinical approaches based on the Agency for Health Care Policy and Research (AHCPR) guidelines. In addition, more PCP education, improved consultation capabilities for PCPs with toll-free consultation lines, and co-location of behavioral care teams in the PCP settings would be offered. Of the existing guidelines, the AHCPR guidelines were selected because they seemed to best meet the requirements of scientific validity, professional acceptance, and primary care setting compatibility. By looking at how to improve treatment in the primary care setting, one of the assumptions made was that, in the present system of carve-out care, many patients who are referred to

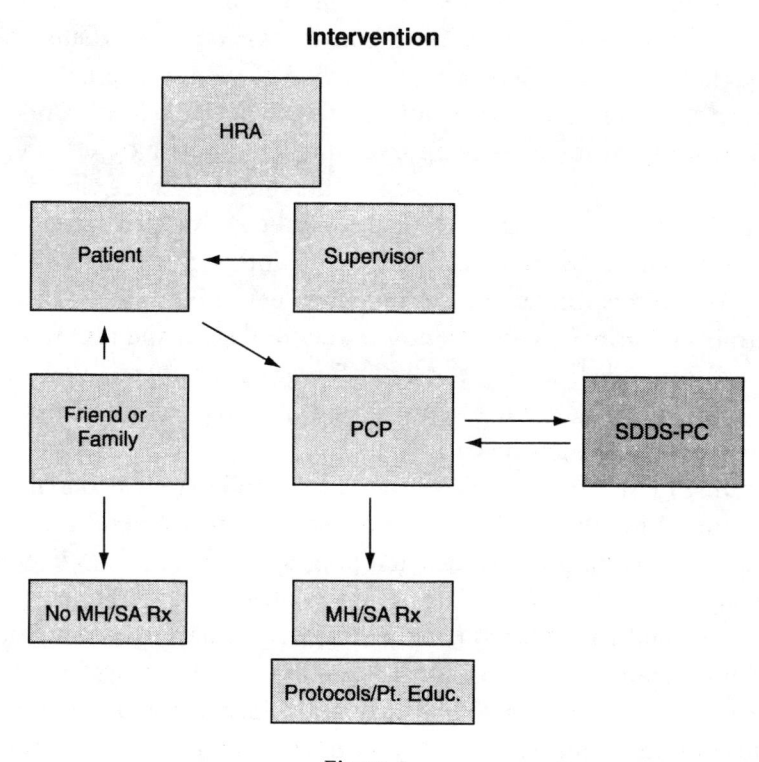

Figure 2

mental health specialists never make it to those referrals for a variety of reasons. To minimize this problem, it was strongly felt that the program must deliver most of its depression care in the PCP office, where the problem is often first detected.

Finally, detailed outcomes analyses would evaluate medical and work-related offsets, patient and provider satisfaction, levels of functioning, and quality of life for patients.

Preparation for the Study

The Employer

Two key issues that influence the acceptability of such a study are patients' concerns about stigma and confidentiality. The impact of these issues needed to be addressed within the whole framework of trust between employer and employees. It was important that there not only be a sense of genuine concern for the improved health of the employees, but that concern be evident and appreciated. Presentation of the goals of the study, reiteration of the sacredness of confidentiality, and honesty were clearly key ingredients. In a study like this, because of the obvious ramifications, the senior management team had to be fully behind the project. Barriers of corporate culture, current organizational structure, and openness to change were crucial elements to consider in the assessment. Supervisor training had to be evaluated for issues of receptivity and relative importance.

Even when these concerns are addressed, one of the greatest barriers to success relates to the data available to track the work-related effects of illness. Records kept on short-term disability, days lost from work, absenteeism, workers' compensation data, industrial accidents, and workplace violence were selected as variables to be examined and had to be researched as to their availability and integrity.

The Health Plan. The health plan similarly had issues to address. Key metrics required the availability of laboratory data, medical data, pharmacy data, medical utilization, and other health-related costs. In addition, work was needed to design the treatment protocol and also to select a screening tool while developing a training program for the use and interpretation of both. Primary care physician preparedness needed evaluation, and PCP educational material had to be developed and delivered. Finally, patient educational materials had to be prepared.

Lastly, both the employer and the health plan had to agree on the study design. Here issues centered on discussions of sample sizes, instrument identification, financial impact analyses, time lines, selection of comparison groups and variables, funding, expert partner identification, and advisory board choices. Information system issues were central. Data availability and integrity, and the absence or existence of metrics in areas such as work-related productivity and disability all presented significant barriers or major determinants to success.

Like every worthwhile project, preparation is the key to success. For Delta and CIGNA/MCC, joining forces with experts trained in this area has proven to be an integral part of the success of the project. Expertise in grant writing plus particular knowledge in the area of primary care integration have enhanced the final task of adding the details to the ultimate study design.

The final issue is having the patience to wait for the results. If this study succeeds in proving its point, as everyone believes it will, it has the potential to profoundly alter the way insurance is currently purchased. In winning the battle on direct medical costs, the employer may have lost the war on total healthcare costs. Reversing the situation could well prove to be the ultimate win—a win for the patient who gets better understanding, better education, earlier intervention, and better treatment; a win for the health plan that really provides better healthcare to its members and better value at the same time; and finally a win for the employer who has a happier, healthier, more productive workplace.

References

1. Fries J, Koop C, Beadle C, et al: Reducing healthcare costs by reducing the need and demand for medical services. N Engl J Med 329:321–325, 1993.
2. Shapiro S, Skinner E, Kessler L, et al: Utilization of health and mental health services: three epidemiologic catchment area sites. Arch Gen Psychiatry 41:971–978, 1994.
3. Strain JJ, Lyons JS, Hammer JS, et al: Cost offset from a psychiatric consultation liaison intervention with elderly hip fracture patients. Am J Psychiatry 148:1044–1049, 1991.
4. Pallak M, Cummings N, Dorken H, Hanke C: Effect of mental health treatment on medical costs. Mind Body Med 1:7–12, 1995.

Chapter 9

Depression and Its Management in Primary Care: The Harvard Pilgrim Health Care Experience

Steve Stelovich, M.D.

In the course of the last decade, four factors have emerged to exert tremendous pressure on the primary care/behavioral healthcare interface. First, studies have provided point prevalence rates for mental illness in the population at large.[1] With a more limited focus, and in respect to major depression in particular, high rates have been consistently demonstrated in primary care settings.[2] Second, improved understanding of costs, both direct and indirect, and of morbidity has been well documented. This too has been especially well illustrated with respect to depression.[3-5] Third, improved treatments appropriate for primary care settings have emerged. Here again, results in the field of depression are particularly robust.[6] And finally, the very nature of healthcare purchasing arrangements has evolved. Ever greater coalitions are overseeing the purchase, provision, and quality of service for larger and larger populations. The concatenation of these four factors increasingly pressures healthcare delivery systems to provide early detection and treatment for mental illness whenever appropriate in the primary care setting.

Appropriate Conditions for Primary Care Interventions

Traditionally, most psychiatric conditions have been treated in mental health settings. Though sporadic attempts have been made to provide some behavioral healthcare services in primary care, a comprehensive planning methodology has not been available. Several key factors shape any efforts to define appropriate conditions for treatment there. Such conditions must demonstrate 1) high point prevalence in such settings, 2) high morbidity and/or cost associated with lack of treatment, and 3) readily available first-line interventions appropriate for primary care delivery.

Using the above criteria, a "short list" of conditions becomes apparent. Most would agree that such a list would include major depression, substance abuse, anxiety disorder, and somatization.

Harvard Pilgrim Health Care (HPHC), a mixed model health maintenance organization (HMO) in New England with over one million members, used these criteria to initiate a program for the early detection and treatment of depression in primary care settings. The program was planned for and initiated within a capitated group of primary care physicians (PCPs), but many of the planning principles—as well as the program components—lend themselves to ready adaptation for other service delivery arrangements.

Principles and Practices in Program Planning

Four factors in planning were found to be of paramount importance: focus, simplification, minimization of practice interference, and starting small.

Focus

Major depression was ultimately chosen as the focus of work in the HPHC project. Significant pressure was exerted to broaden the endeavor. However, no natural endpoint for such expansion was evident. Further, each additional inclusion was understood to entail an increasing burden and complexity for PCPs to master. Ultimately, the goal became improving the quality of primary care practice rather than aiming for perfection. If improvements could be made through a focus on the detection and treatment of major depression alone as a first step, elaboration could follow.

In order to support such a focused endeavor, however, arrangements had to be made for dealing with related diagnoses and complex cases. A program of immediate consultation and/or referral was established to meet this need. Instruction was provided for the diagnosis of major depression using *Diagnostic and Statistical Manual of Mental Disorders IV (DSM-IV)* criteria.[7] Providers who encountered patients with any deviation from basic criteria were encouraged to call a psychiatric consultant, who was available by phone within five minutes of being paged. Such consultation was planned to support the primary care practitioner in furnishing treatment, if appropriate, to help determine whether referral was needed, and to provide a resource for obtaining emergency services when required. This ready availability was necessary to meet the needs of the busy primary care practice, to provide quality care, and to indicate the importance being attached to addressing such problems in the primary care setting.

Simplification

Throughout the planning process—which included input from expert panels, consultants, and primary care provider focus groups—the need for simplicity was reiterated. To achieve this goal, particular attention was paid to brevity, clarity, and responsiveness for each component of the program. Examples of such considerations included the following: 1) the use of a very simple three-item screen rather than a more elaborate option (such a screen was easy for patients to complete and could be scored with no more effort than a single glance at the page on the part of the physician), 2) *DSM-IV* diagnostic criteria for major depression were adopted, providing well-accepted standards as well as clarity, and 3) as mentioned, near immediate psychiatric consultation was available by phone to aid with any questions that might arise.

Minimization of Practice Interference

Considering the prevalence of major depression in primary care settings, one to two cases can be expected each day in an average practice. Because screening instruments are not totally reliable, additional "false positives" that will require further assessment can be anticipated. The diagnosis and initiation of treatment for appropriate cases of major depression will then inevitably have serious consequences for primary care practice.

In the HPHC program, it was anticipated that screening every six months and initiation of treatment for all appropriate cases in a practitioner's panel might require an additional 15 to 20 minutes from each physician each day. Such an addition to the existing work load was unacceptable. As an interim measure—and a fortuitous choice, as will be shown—the program was initiated on "well care" visits, i.e., those visits scheduled for routine check-ups and physical exams. Because these visits allowed slightly more time for the physician or physician's assistant to see the patient, the added burden of following through on a positive screen result was tolerable. In addition, on any one day, each physician had a limited number of "well visit" patients.

Start Small, Grow Large

The need to begin on a small scale, to allow for the working out of unexpected complications, and to build a foundation of success to assist in program expansion is clear. Of note, the success of the initial program at HPHC sites has led three additional capitated groups to request initiation of similar programs at their sites.

Program Components

The program for early detection and treatment of depression in primary care settings at HPHC was designed to consist of five components: 1) depression screening, 2) PCP education, 3) immediate psychiatric consultation back-up, 4) patient/physician supports, and 5) program evaluation.

Depression Screening

Several screening instruments were considered, but the three-item "yes or no" depression screen presented by Rost and associates was ultimately chosen.[8] This screen had a relatively high sensitivity and specificity, coupled with an ease of administration and scoring. The three questions are as follows:

1. In the past year, have you had two weeks or more during which you felt sad, blue, or depressed; or when you lost all interest or pleasure in things that you usually cared about or enjoyed?
2. Have you had two years or more in your life when you felt depressed or sad most days, even if you felt okay sometimes?
3. Have you felt depressed or sad much of the time in the past year?

At check-in for well visits, members are asked if they have filled out a screen within the past six months. If not, they are asked to do so prior to beginning their appointment with their doctor. The screening form becomes part of the patient's medical record (and in the HPHC depression project, a copy is retained for outcomes tracking). The PCP or physician's assistant is able to see at a glance whether any of the three questions have received a positive response, and whether further diagnostic exploration is warranted.

Education

Physician education, although critical to the success of the program, adds additional burdens to the physicians' work loads and had to be streamlined. A two-hour program was developed for a core presentation, with supplements planned via written materials and the psychiatric consultation back-up. Components of the basic module were as follows. The first hour included an overview of the problem of depression in primary care settings, an overview of the HPHC program, introduction to and administration of the screening tool, assessment techniques, basic rule-outs, and commonly missed cases. The second hour contained a presentation of treatment options in primary care, review of selective serotonin reuptake inhibitor (SSRI) and tricyclic antidepressant use, description of behavioral health program alternatives, presentation of the logistics of back-up, consultation and referral, and an evaluation of the overview program. Questions were encouraged.

In the basic education module, the lecture format was supplemented with written handouts, case presentations, and audiovisual aids that included both slides and video case examples for discussion.

Rule-outs included a basic presentation of suicide assessment, its associated documentation, and guidelines for consultation. Clinicians were encouraged to seek consultation if concomitant substance abuse or complicating psychiatric conditions were detected, and for any situation that deviated in any way from simple and uncomplicated major depression as they were being taught to diagnose it.

Particular attention was paid to the presentation of cases representing conditions in which major depression was most likely to be missed. These included cases in which a bona fide concurrent medical condition occupied center stage in the patient's presentation of chief complaint and reported symptoms, in which there was significant somatization that occupied the physician in extended medical evaluation, or in which the patient had a "reason" to be depressed (i.e., terminal medical illness, loss of body part). The latter category provided an opportunity to reinforce the difference between normal reactions of depression and major depressive illness, as well as to reinforce recognition of the fact that the two could coexist.

In the HPHC project, in-depth information was presented to make physicians comfortable with using at least one SSRI and one tricyclic agent. Practitioners were free to use any of the agents in the HPHC formulary, as well as to refer to a behavioral health program. Written materials, in addition to the psychiatric back-up system, were provided to supply additional education should the PCP wish to learn more about other alternatives.

Consult Back-up System

A psychiatrist with expertise in psychopharmacology was hired to be on call during working hours, with an expected response time of less than five minutes. Referrals to an associated mental health program were available, as were emergency mental health back-up programs. The logistics for these back-up components were reviewed during the teaching module.

Patient/Physician Supports

In addition to the consult back-up system, physicians were provided with treatment option summary cards for quick office reference. Additionally, the HPHC quality bonus program (wherein bonuses to the basic capitation for care could be enhanced through completion of quality improvement activities) was configured to encourage ongoing education in the early detection and treatment of depression in primary care settings. A continuing medical education program on depression in the elderly for home study using video or audio tapes was established. For patients, basic information for home review was available on depression as an illness and on medications prescribed.

Evaluation

Finally, physician participants were introduced to the major areas of outcomes evaluation that were important in the program. These included patient satisfaction, symptom reduction, general health status, medical costs, and indirect costs. A brief presentation was made as to how members who were willing to be followed would be contacted.

Initial Findings

The project was initiated October 15, 1996. As of January 22, 1997, 807 well visits had been screened. Of these, 243 (29 percent) gave a positive response to at least one screening question. Of the positive screens, 64 (27 percent of positive screens and 8 percent of all well visits) met *DSM-IV* criteria for major depression. Of the 64 persons determined to have major depression, 30 elected to begin a course of medication in primary care, 9 requested further discussion/counseling in primary care, 16 were referred to mental health, 2 received a one-time psychopharmacology consult (post-consult recommendations have not been reviewed in the program yet), 2 were referred to behavioral medicine, and 5 refused treatment. Of those who screened positive but were not found to meet *DSM-IV* criteria for uncomplicated major depression, 4 were determined to have alternative conditions for which medication was prescribed in primary care, 6 were receiving counseling in primary care, and 4 were referred to mental health.

An initial focus group among participating physicians revealed that the program was being well accepted and was not seen as a major imposition on practice routine. Parenthetically, one physician noted that an initial estimate of the 10 minutes necessary to complete an assessment and discuss treatment options following a positive screen was too optimistic for him as a "beginner"; however, he anticipated that with practice this goal might be reached. Several physicians have noted that positive screens in an otherwise well care visit gave them something other than just "one more physical" to do. In a significant number of cases, active depression was being uncovered, opening the door to helpful intervention. Finally, several physicians have made comments such as "I've had that patient in my panel for 10 years, and I had no idea he was depressed—it simply never came up before."

Summary and Discussion

Working with an expert panel, consultants, and primary care physicians, Harvard Pilgrim Health Care designed a program aimed at the early detection and treatment of depression in primary care settings. Guiding principles included focus, simplicity, minimization of practice interference, and starting small.

Initial results indicate that the program is able to uncover high rates of previously undetected depression, is accepted by physicians, and leads most patients to enter treatment in their primary care setting. At this early stage, other results have not been analyzed. Unexpectedly, it was found that very significant numbers of well care visits appear to be associated with active major depression. This observation raises the question of whether there is ever a true "well visit" to a physician's office. In addition, physicians experienced increased satisfaction by finding significant medical pathology that was readily treated.

References

1. Robins LN, Regier DA (eds): Psychiatric Disorders in America. Free Press, New York, 1991.
2. Agency for Health Care Policy and Research: Depression in Primary Care. Vol 1: Detection and Diagnosis. AHCPR Publication No. 93-0550. US Department of Health and Human Services, Washington DC, 1993, pp 24-25.
3. Katon W, von Korff M, Lin E, et al: Distressed high utilizers of medical care: DSM-III-R diagnoses and treatment needs. Gen Hosp Psychiatry 12:355-362, 1990.
4. Broadhead WE, Blazer DG, George LK, Tse CK: Depression, disability days, and days lost from work in a prospective epidemiologic survey. JAMA 264:2524-2528, 1990.
5. Simon GE, von Korff M, Barlow W: Health care costs of primary care patients with recognized depression. Arch Gen Psychiatry 52:850-856, 1995.
6. Agency for Health Care Policy and Research: Depression in Primary Care. Vol 2: Treatment of Major Depression. AHCPR Publication No. 93-0551. US Department of Health and Human Services, Washington DC, 1993, pp 1-6.
7. Diagnostic and Statistical Manual of Mental Disorders, Fourth Edition. American Psychiatric Association, 1994.
8. Rost K, Burman MA, Smith GR: Development of screeners for depressive disorders and substance disorder history. Med Care 31:189-200, 1993.

Chapter 10

High Utilizers of Health Services: The Purchaser Perspective and Experience with the Personal Health Improvement Program (PHIP)

Paul B. Johnson, M.D. (Part 1)
Lawrence B. Staubach, M.D., M.B.A. and Anna P. Millar, M.B.A. (Part 2)

The first part of this chapter describes findings on some of the limitations in our current health plan delivery systems from the perspective of a large, stable employer. Suggestions are offered for the design of new models of healthcare delivery that will better address current problems. The second half of the chapter describes an example of a successful new model, the Personal Health Improvement Program—a patient education program targeted to high utilizers of the healthcare system.

Part I: The Employer/Purchaser Perspective

US West is a regional telecommunications company operating in 14 states from the upper Midwest through the Rocky Mountain region to the Pacific Northwest. The average length of service among its employees is 16 years; the average employee age is 42 years.

US West offers health plan benefit coverage to all active employees and their dependents, as well as to a large retiree population. Active employees are enrolled in managed care plans throughout the region. Currently, 63 percent are enrolled in point-of-service (POS) plans, and 37 percent are enrolled in health maintenance organizations (HMOs).

Like most companies, US West pays wage replacement to employees who are absent from work. For record keeping purposes absences are coded by categories, which are individually defined by companies. The following categories are used by US West:

- Incidental absence—brief, acute illnesses or injuries
- Short-term disability (STD)—longer, more severe illnesses or injuries that, by US West's definition, begin on the eighth calendar day of absence from work
- Workers' compensation (WC)—any absences due to a work-related injury or illness

Management of absence from work for an illness or injury episode varies widely in U.S. business and industry from essentially no management to aggressive absence management. Where absence management occurs, a spectrum of approaches is seen. Generally, companies manage this function internally, outsource the function to an external administrator, or use a combination of these methods. Absence management is becoming more prevalent as businesses appreciate the significance of this additional cost and the necessity of having people at work to perform their tasks.

At US West, incidental absence is not medically managed. Rather, it is managed by attendance rules. All STD and WC absences, however, are medically case-managed by an internal professional medical or mental health case manager who is part of the health organization. In broad terms, the role of the case manager is to ensure that the absence is appropriate or that the person is, in fact, disabled from work. In addition, case managers make sure that care is appropriate and that the person returns to the right job at the appropriate time. We want absences to be *appropriate*—neither too long nor too short—as governed by the objective medical evidence of the case. Case management is an interactive process between the employee, their caregiver, the US West case manager, and a supervisor. Appropriate release-of-information forms are utilized, and strict confidentiality is maintained.

The Problem

An analysis of our absence data reveals that a small proportion of our workforce consumes a disproportionate share of our absence days and costs. This fact can be illustrated using the three previously defined absence categories.

Incidental Absence

In a calendar year, approximately 55 percent of the total workforce had an incidental absence. Approximately 25 percent of that group had more than one incidental absence episode. These "repeaters" were responsible for approximately 80 percent of the total incidental absence episodes.

Short-term Disability

In a calendar year, 85 percent of those employees who had an STD absence had only one absence episode. However, 15 percent of those employees who were absent on STD had more than one STD case. These repeaters, who represented 2 percent of the total workforce, consumed 30 percent of the total STD days lost.

Workers' Compensation

In a calendar year, approximately 75 percent of all workers' compensation claims had no associated time lost from work. Of that 25 percent who lost time due to a WC case, 12 employees had more than one WC absence claim in the year. These repeaters, representing only 0.02 percent of the total workforce, consumed 4 percent of the total days lost to workers' compensation.

Employer's Outlook

Overall, the absence rates and costs at US West compare very favorably with available industry data. Incidental absence rates and costs have remained essentially stable. Our actual absence rates and costs have decreased in each of the last three years in the STD and WC categories. This decrease is due, in part, to our case management efforts. Regarding the data on high utilizers, our current internal information systems do not permit us to easily recognize whether these separate small cohorts of absent employees actually represent the same individuals. However, our anecdotal experience is that they often are the same workers. To summarize, a small percentage of our employees are disproportionately absent from work, thus incurring disproportionately higher healthcare costs.

In addition, experience has shown that this population exerts other influences on the company. These employees and the problems they pose result in increased time spent by their managers, as well as by representatives from the health organization, labor, legal, and human resources who often must meet to attempt management of these individuals in a fair and equitable way. Other influences that have been noted include worker morale/frustration, replacement worker costs, and lost productivity. These factors (and others) exert a multiplier effect on the actual absence wage replacement costs.

The Repeater Population

This small population of employees who consume a disproportionate amount of absence time, costs, and management attention can be divided into two subsets. The first group consists of persons with well-defined disease states that are symptomatic, serious, chronic, and often progressive. The outcome in these cases is variable. Their absences are easy to understand based on the medical facts of the case. These people may often be legitimately absent from work—a situation we have to accept as a condition of their disease state. Alternately, we can define their abilities within their medical condition and adjust or accommodate their jobs to match their work capabilities. Finally, their disease may progress until they are no longer able to work. At US West, they can then leave the payroll and become eligible for long-term disability payments.

The second group is more problematic. These employees seem to have common characteristics. First, they are absent far more frequently than the average employee. Their absences variably occur under our three classifications of absences. Second, their employment records often document poor work performance or workplace behavior problems. Third, unlike the individuals mentioned above, these employees generally have no documented or easily understood disease state. Their absences are for multiple medical and behavioral health reasons. Too often, absences are for vague, subjective symptoms rather than well-documented diseases. Common examples include headache, fatigue, stress, and incapacitating pain syndromes. Their absences seem inappropriate or, at the very least, longer than normal for the diagnosed problem.

Finally, we have determined that these employees, as patients, see multiple physicians in multiple specialties. They frequently change primary care physicians (PCPs) and health plans, and seldom have a good mental health evaluation as part of their multiple diagnostic evaluations. From the health plan perspective, these are high utilizers of healthcare. As employers, the absence-related costs of these employees are a concern. Additionally, as purchasers of their healthcare, we bear the costs of their high utilization.

Analysis of Current Situation

Too often in this situation, the scenario is predictable. An employee is in trouble with attendance issues; the supervisor may advise the employee (with or without input from an internal medical case manager) to "go see your doctor." The employee then sees his or her doctor or doctors, who often pursue the evaluation and treatment of multiple presenting symptom complaints. As a consequence of the doctor-patient relationship occurring in isolation—and perhaps because too few physicians really understand the concept of disability—the employee receives a recommendation for time off from work.

Thus, the problem is perpetuated. The employee feels justified about lost time and about the severity of symptoms because their doctor recommended absence from work. In essence, the employee thinks, "I must be sick because my doctor said not to go to work until I feel better."

Managers and US West health professionals feel frustrated by this repetitive pattern observed in the same employees over many years. We realize that in our existing health plans, we have no appropriate place to refer these problem employees. We do not even have a very good system to communicate our professional concerns about an employee to the health plan administrators.

This pattern of frustration is seen within the medical system as well. Physicians like to succeed, and often these patients create interactions with little chance of success. Instead, physicians temporarily solve one problem only to have the patient reappear with a new and seemingly incapacitating complaint.

Finally, and most importantly, these employees are frustrated and unhappy. They feel dissatisfied with their doctor or their health plan because no one can find out what is "wrong" with them. They feel dissatisfied with their employer, who creates unrealistic job or performance expectations. And they feel dissatisfied with the health organization's medical case managers, who seem to constantly doubt their illness or second-guess their doctors. For this small but troublesome employee population, the situation could be described as "lose-lose-lose."

Solutions and Changes

Changes need to be made at several levels to adequately meet the problems posed by the high utilizer population. First, integrated primary care/behavioral health centers seem to be the ideal organizational model to manage these employees/patients. Essential elements of this model would include the evaluation and treatment of psychiatric disease and referral to the appropriate care system, if needed. Beyond this, a primary care/behavioral health model should focus on helping patients understand the underlying causes of perceived symptoms and recurring unsuccessful life behavior approaches, and to work on adopting new or more successful behavior skills. Recurring absence behavior would be identified and discussed, and new approaches to manage these behavior problems would be addressed.

Next, it seems imperative that employers and health plans communicate with each other and collaborate more effectively to manage these "difficult" employees. Communication channels between company health professionals and the primary care/behavioral health clinic are essential. Such communication must safeguard medical confidentiality. However, there must be active communication between the caregiver and the employer about observable behavior issues as manifested by documentable issues such as work attendance and performance. The employee involved should be fully aware of and involved in these communications. Obviously they are the focal point of these activities, and they should be considered a full partner in the process.

The challenge to business is to ensure that disability programs and attendance rules and regulations are designed to maximally reward appropriate behavior, while providing protection for true disability. In too many cases, existing disability and attendance policies reward inappropriate behavior and disability. Also, companies must administer their disability and attendance policies in a consistently fair way.

New Models

Our work with health plans to implement the two models briefly described below are only in the initial stages.

US West–HealthPartners Health Plan

Our trial plan is to identify US West employees with HealthPartners health plan who meet a defined threshold of high frequency for incidental, STD, and WC absence. HealthPartners determines high clinic utilizers among US West employees in their plans. A behavioral health intervention program such as Personal Health Improvement Program (PHIP; described fully in the second part of this chapter) would be offered on a voluntary basis within a clinic setting to employees who meet the high absence/high utilization criteria. Measurements of change such as increased/decreased absenteeism, clinic utilization, and changes in well being and physical and emotional distress will be used to assess the program's efficacy.

This program has not been implemented yet, primarily because both the company and the health plan wish to address some key issues within each group before entering into a collaborative project. Both parties espouse the concept, however, and a trial project should be underway soon.

US West–Group Health Cooperative of Puget Sound

As described above, the trial plan concept is to identify high risk employees/patients from certain employment and clinic indicators. These individuals would be enrolled in a disability registry. A new position would be created for a behavioral health clinician, who would serve as a liaison between the company and the primary care clinic. In a sense, this is another way of integrating behavioral health and primary care. Changes in behavioral approaches to life would again be emphasized with these high-risk individuals. Joint funding of this project is currently being explored.

Unanswered Issues

There is a new understanding of the problem presented by high utilizers to a large business. The search for solutions raises additional issues for consideration and extends initial concepts in new directions. Some of these issues include costs, exclusivity, and extension of models.

Costs

Who will pay for these new integrated models of care? Can companies expect health plans to routinely offer these options, or should they be included for an additional cost?

Exclusivity

Typically, employees of a business in a single geographic location may belong to one of several health plans offered by the company. If a single health plan offers an integrated primary care/behavioral health model, can it be accessed or utilized by high risk employees and family members not covered by that plan? From the purchaser or employer perspective, this issue could influence future plan selection if the integrated model proves successful and if costs are positively influenced.

Extension to General Population

If integrated models of primary care/behavioral health clinics prove successful in managing the high risk employee/patient, should the same integrative model be extended to the general "healthy" population?

Employer Perspective Revisited

By examining our own experiences with employees, we have identified a small percentage of the workforce who contribute disproportionately to absence and other related business and healthcare costs. Current methods of dealing with these employees, both from a business and a healthcare plan perspective, are not working. An integrated primary care/behavioral health model offers the best chance for success in managing these individuals, and will ultimately be supported by employer purchasers.

Part II: The Personal Health Improvement Program

One of the solutions to the high utilizer problem under consideration by US West is the Personal Health Improvement Program (PHIP), developed and owned by Harvard Pilgrim Health Care (HPHC) and marketed by Procter & Gamble (P&G). The PHIP is a clinically proven patient education program targeted to patients who overutilize the healthcare system. The remainder of this chapter is devoted to a description of this program and the preliminary results of its use.

The program's goal is to teach patients with unexplained general physical or psychological complaints—including those with chronic underlying medical disorders who are not coping well with their disease—how to manage their non-disease-related symptoms such as back pain, headache, and fatigue. The results have been shown to decrease healthcare utilization and increase patient and provider satisfaction.

Background

Ways to Wellness: A Precursor to the PHIP

HPHC found that the disease model for healthcare failed to address many health concerns of ambulatory patients with common complaints such as headache, fatigue, chronic pain, and insomnia. The diagnostic and therapeutic strategies of the disease model focused on organic causes, rather than psychosocial factors.

Building on current theories in neurobiology, linguistics, and philosophy, Matthew A. Budd, M.D., an internist at Harvard Community Health Plan (now Harvard Pilgrim Health Care), and his HPHC colleagues proposed a new model for working with patients experiencing physical and emotional distress in their day-to-day existence. The model, later named Ways to Wellness, incorporated an active, hands-on approach to help patients learn that how they go about their daily lives can affect their health. This approach stimulated new questions for the patients about the relationship between their orientation to life and their health.

Ways to Wellness was not based on psychology, nor was it simply about changing negative thinking to positive moods. It was based on studies in three areas: 1) the biology of human cognition (the act or process of knowing, including both awareness and judgment), 2) the history and philosophy of how humans understand their life and their bodies, and 3) speech-act theory from the field of linguistics.

These areas of research provided the basis for an interactive learning program that showed patients, through use of concrete examples from their own lives, that the ways in which we see ourselves affects our health and may generate physical symptoms and even illness. This is not to say that the patient causes his or her disease, or that "it is all in your head." The patient acts through habit, which may include behaviors and associated moods that produce suffering.

A fundamental premise of the program is that some patients experience a cognitive gap between what "is" and what patients would like reality to be. This experience is exacerbated when patients do not see that they can take steps to close the gap. Understanding how or why patients interpret life events the way they do does not magically stop the suffering. Helping these patients free themselves from their old behaviors involves teaching them to pay attention to their automatic reactions and increasing their awareness of the issues.

As patients learn to observe themselves, they can begin to change their automatic reactions and substitute new behaviors. This may involve asking for something they have had difficulty asking for in the past, or saying "no" in situations they previously accepted. A new intervention was needed to teach the skills for designing new behaviors that lead to the development of dignity, autonomy, trust, and self-efficacy. Patients must learn to be observers in the situation, assessing their life goals and making decisions about which actions to take, and completing them without alienating others. Building such a behavioral style enables trusting and mutually satisfying relationships with others in all areas of life. These "life skills" are an integral part of a strong and flexible foundation for health and well-being.

Procter & Gamble and the Harvard Pilgrim Health Care Collaboration

The Healthcare Division of Procter & Gamble Company (P&G) approached Harvard Pilgrim Health Care in 1991 regarding an interest in working together on projects of mutual benefit. Commercialization of the Ways to Wellness program was selected as the primary collaboration project. From both parties' perspectives, the project fit well with their interests and competencies. P&G's leveraged core expertise is in consumer understanding, marketing, and providing innovative strategies to lower total systems costs for its customers. HPHC continued its leadership role in developing, implementing, and integrating innovative behavioral medicine interventions into primary care settings. Following review and enhancement of program materials—incorporating adult learning principles and a revamping of the "train the trainer" methodology—a new, enhanced intervention was developed by HPHC: the Personal Health Improvement Program. The clinically proven core elements and underpinnings of Ways to Wellness were unchanged; essentially the information delivered was made more consumer-friendly, and the ability to deliver sufficient trainers for commercialization was made feasible. The collaboration continues today via innovative marketing and sales strategies to make PHIP more efficiently available to patients (P&G), on-going facilitator training and quality assurance programs (HPHC), and research and development projects investigating disease-specific applications (HPHC), and more efficient screening of target populations (P&G and HPHC).

Target Population

The Personal Health Improvement Program is targeted to patients who demonstrate chronic somatizing behavior. Barsky and Borus define *somatization* as "the propensity to experience and report somatic symptoms that have no pathophysiological explanation, to misattribute them to disease, and to seek medical attention for them."[1] Somatizing behavior may be chronic or acute, and it may or may not be associated with an underlying disease process.[2] Barsky and Borus further note that the current sociocultural environment reduces the individual's tolerance to mild medical and psychological infirmities and lowers the threshold for seeking medical care.

The magnitude of somatization in a managed care environment is shown by studies demonstrating that 38 percent to 60 percent of primary care patients present with symptoms that, following evaluation, have no serious medical or psychiatric basis.[3-9] The impact of this population on the healthcare system is extraordinary; patients who somatize chronically show elevated levels of hospitalization, emergency and ambulatory medical visits, and overall total health system costs, compared to nonsomatizing counterparts.[10-15]

The PHIP is not appropriate for individuals with unstable, acute medical illness requiring treatment, active alcohol or drug dependence, or those with psychological distress that would interfere with their participation in a learning, interactive environment. In addition, individuals exhibiting malingering behavior are not candidates for PHIP.

Elements of the PHIP

PHIP is a six-week intervention, with weekly two-hour sessions and home study exercises between sessions. It accommodates 15 to 25 participants at a time. The course is led by a trained facilitator, supplemented with a participant workbook and audiotape. The format is interactive and educational.

The course is designed to teach patients how to pay attention to their recurrent moods and behaviors. Through structured in-class exercises, dialogues with the facilitator, home study reading and writing exercises, and meditation, patients build awareness of thoughts, moods, and bodily reactivity, and their effects on health. Topics include:

- Coordinating life with others through requests and promises, fundamental human behaviors

- The role of history, culture, and traditions in shaping our beliefs, perceptions, and reactions in daily life
- The role of language—in particular, our interpretations and judgments on the moods we have, the possibilities we see, and the actions we take
- Self-monitoring and management of health-inhibiting moods

The program was designed as a group intervention to provide an environment for learning which emphasizes that people can learn new actions through active participation (experience) and practice. In the classroom, learners are asked to participate in small group exercises that are simple simulations of life situations. These might involve an action such as requesting a dollar from someone. The experiential model for learning is emphasized, because human bodies get "triggered" to the emotional/physical responses they have learned throughout their life, but the triggered responses are so automatic that we cannot see how we respond over and over. If the responses repeatedly involve anger, anxiety, helplessness, panic, depression, or despair, an individual's health can be affected.[8]

Following the small-group exercise, participants report what they observed about their automatic response (i.e., body sensations, thoughts, moods, emotions, judgments, etc.) during the exercise. The discussions are not intended to be for shared feelings, individual therapy work, correcting the patient's problem, or explaining what happened. Instead, the facilitator has the task of listening and carefully assisting the learners in recognizing their whole body response by using the distinctions of the course for observing. A learner who reports that the exercise created nervousness may need help recognizing his or her body response.

Once learners can see what they could not see before, due to the automatic response, the facilitator can ask further questions to build awareness. Questions such as "Can you now think of other times in your life when this is your response?" and "What effect could your response have on others?" are presented. The response is a body reaction triggered in the exercise, just as a knee jerk is a response to a hammer tap on the knee. The body does not distinguish that the event is simply an exercise.

Because of the group setting, the value of the exercise is intensified. Learners obtain evidence of their automatic patterns by seeing their own reactions. In addition, learners have the opportunity to see that all people do not respond in the same way. Classroom exercises provide grounding for the claim that our responses to everyday events are due in part to what we have learned in our individual life experiences.

Implementation

Table 1 outlines the major milestones involved in successfully implementing PHIP. The entire process could be accomplished in a minimum of four months, given that several tasks can be executed concurrently. Experience to date suggests that six to nine months is a more realistic timetable.

Marketing

Dr. Budd estimates that only a tiny fraction of the patients in a managed care population who could benefit from the course are actually referred. A state of "cognitive blindness" to mind-body issues, or the unwillingness of clinicians to discuss

TABLE 1. MILESTONES INVOLVED IN THE SUCCESSFUL IMPLEMENTATION OF PHIP

Major Milestone	What	Who	Comment	Timing
Obtain organizational buy-in	Conduct customer assessment	P&G/Customer		8–12 weeks
	Presentation to key decision makers	P&G/Customer		
	Management agrees to proceed	Customer		
	Contract	P&G/Customer		
Establish project implementation team	Identify: • Corporate champion • Medical champion • Project manager	Key customer decision makers/ P&G	Candidate profiles provided to guide selection process	6 weeks
Develop plan and allocate budget	Write project scope document including: • Problem definition • Target number of patients • Budget needs • Detailed task summary	Project Implementation Team	Determine involvement of mental health carve out	4 weeks
Identify, recruit and train facilitators/ coordinator	Six-day intensive course at Harvard Pilgrim Health Care	Identify and recruit: Medical and corporate champion Training: HPHC instructors	Candidate profiles provided to guide selection process	3 weeks
Set up foundation for referral process	Determine vehicle for generating referrals Set up toll-free number Conduct research	Project Implementation Team	See Marketing section for details	Ongoing
Teach the course	Six-week course Once a week for 2 hours 15-25 participants	PHIP facilitators		6 weeks
Evaluate results	Quality assurance module Patient surveys	Facilitators, champions, HPHC		4 weeks

"personal matters," are factors in the low utilization of such programs. Additionally, resistance of the patient to a nonmedical solution or fear of being labeled "crazy" are sometimes present. Clinician skill in addressing and allaying these fears, and in building trusting partnerships with patients, helps lessen these barriers (unpublished data).

Because of these factors, primary marketing strategies have been developed to identify appropriate patients with somatizing behavior, assure referral or interest in the course, and ensure completion of the course.

Direct to Physician

The primary care physician, as gatekeeper of medical care, is on the front line where this population is exhibiting care seeking behavior. The physician is in a perfect position to recognize high-utilizing, somatizing behavior. Generally, these patients frustrate the PCP, and are themselves frustrated with their physician and their health plan. For many patients, a recommendation from their physician adds substantial credibility to the program. However, the PCP must describe the relatively complex intervention in the context of a brief office visit. The following strategies increase awareness of the program among providers and drive the referral process:

- A speaker's program providing education about behavioral medicine, somatization, and PHIP
- A five-wave direct mail program with clinical reprints and a videotape instructing providers on referral protocols
- One-on-one direct selling of the program
- Dissemination of ongoing PHIP-specific and general behavioral medicine information at managed care conventions and professional meetings

Direct to Patient

This strategy recognizes that the patient is a full partner with his or her physician. It empowers the patient to actively take control of his or her health, without waiting for the provider to initiate the often awkward discussion of somatization. In addition, it follows the current healthcare trend of self-management of illness. However, a more rigorous screening process linked to their primary care provider may be necessary to screen out inappropriate referrals. The following strategies increase patient awareness:

- Direct-to-patient mail program, waiting-room patient brochures
- Newsletters from managed care organizations, capitated medical groups, behavioral care carve-outs, and patient advocacy groups
- Patient testimonials

P&G, HPHC, and other organizations are collaborating on identifying/developing psychographic-based screening tools to target potentially appropriate candidates.

Direct to Employer

This strategy focuses on self-insured employers interested in improving the quality of health and satisfaction of their employees regarding their medical benefits plan, while assuring continued fiscal stability. Self-insured employers retain the financial benefits that result from this program. This can provide for a data-driven approach to the identification of appropriate employees through measures such as high absenteeism, high medical claims, and/or performance and safety problems. Issues of confidentiality and privacy need to be managed in this approach. Marketing strategies include company communications, work-site bulletin boards, lectures, electronic media, and human resource workshops and videotapes.

Quality Assurance Program

Quality assessment developed by HPHC is a PHIP element that is undertaken to maintain and improve the quality of the PHIP course and to evaluate the impact of the course on patient well-being and system utilization. Data is evaluated by HPHC from the first 50 of every 1,000 patients who take the course at a particular organization. Patient well-being and satisfaction are assessed through questionnaires, which are administered three times: 1) before the course at the first session, 2) after the course at the last session, and 3) six months after the course by mail. Patient satisfaction is measured at times 2 and 3, asking patients to rate the helpfulness of the course as well as the importance of the course on a five-point Likert scale.

Basic information included in the first data packet includes questions on demographics, presenting complaint, and a checklist of chronic illnesses. The following three instruments are used to assess well-being.

Brief Symptom Inventory™ ® (BSI)

This psychiatric symptom checklist consists of 53 items, which are rated by the respondent for level of distress. It is derived from a longer instrument, the Symptom Checklist 90 Revised (SCL-90R).[9] Both the BSI and the SCL-90R are standard outcomes measures for psychological distress and have been used in multiple treatment evaluation studies. They yield nine scales, including somatization, anxiety, and depression; high scores on these three have been associated with high medical utilization. Extensive studies for validation of the establishment of norms have been conducted.[16,17]

Health Status Questionnaire 2.0

This is a health survey designed for use in clinical research and health policy evaluations. Its 36 items assess eight health concepts: 1) limitations of physical activity because of health problems, 2) limitations of social activity because of health problems, 3) limitations in usual role activities because of physical health problems, 4) bodily pain, 5) general mental health, 6) limitations of usual role activities because of emotional problems, 7) vitality, and 8) general health perceptions. A variety of forms and questions are used.[11] It has been extensively validated on patients in the Medical Outcomes Study.[18]

Medical Symptom Checklist

This is a checklist of common physical symptoms that are rated by the respondent on a four-point scale for degree of distress. It has been used in several studies evaluating the Ways to Wellness program.[19,20]

Summary of Results

Randomized, controlled studies and clinical trials in varied settings have repeatedly shown the efficacy of PHIP or Ways to Wellness.

Hellman, Budd, Borysenko, et al in 1990, investigated the effectiveness of two group behavioral medicine interventions for primary care patients experiencing physical symptoms with a psychosocial component. A total of 80 volunteers from a health maintenance organization in Greater Boston participated in a randomized, prospective study. Both interventions focused on the mind/body relationship and used didactic material, relaxation-response training, awareness training, and cognitive restructuring. The two behavioral medicine intervention groups were compared with a group that focused exclusively on information about stress management and its relation to illness. Visits to the HMO and distress from physical and psychological symptoms were measured before the intervention and again six months afterward. At the six-month follow-up, patients in the Ways to Wellness group showed significantly greater reductions in visits (5.7 compared to 1.8 visits for the six-month period) to the HMO and in discomfort from physical and psychological symptoms than the patients in the stress management information only group. The author suggested that when the relationship among thoughts and behaviors and symptoms of patients with psychosomatic dysfunction is actively addressed, the patients' discomfort level and cost of medical care can be reduced.[21]

McClelland, McLeod, and Budd conducted a randomized, controlled study of a six-week behavioral medicine intervention to examine the effectiveness of a behavioral medicine course designed to treat problems of somatization in primary care.[22] A total of 82 adult volunteers with stress and mood-related physical complaints were referred from PCPs (38 in the treatment group and 44 in the wait-list group). After data collection, patients in the Ways to Wellness group showed significantly greater improvement in physical symptoms, depression, and somatization than the wait-list group. Those in the treatment group also showed a marginally significant decrease in anxiety compared with the wait-list group. Within the treatment group, the decreases in physical complaints, somatization, anxiety, and depression were all statistically significant, and were maintained at six-month follow-up. The authors concluded that the Ways to Wellness course was effective in treating mood and stress-related illnesses.

In 1994 McLeod and Budd conducted a study to validate the effectiveness of the PHIP in the treatment of prevalent physical and psychological symptoms in primary care.[23] A total of 171 volunteer participants in 21 PHIP courses completed questionnaires at the beginning and end of the course, and three months later. Medical charts were reviewed to obtain clinical data. Participants reported statistically significant reductions in physical distress, psychological distress, and overall functional status. They also reported high levels of satisfaction, both immediately after the course and at three months' follow-up. Participants demonstrated significant reduction in mean number of healthcare visits (from 6.7 to 3.7 visits over the six-month period before and after PHIP, respectively). The authors concluded that PHIP effectively treated physical complaints resistant to traditional biomedical treatment alone, increasing quality of care and patient satisfaction and leading to better allocation of healthcare resources.

In 1996 McLeod conducted an observational study evaluating the effectiveness of the PHIP in treating emotional and stress-related physical complaints in primary care patients (unpublished data, September 1996). Again, participants demonstrated statistically significant improvements in overall physical distress, psychological distress, and overall functioning at six months' follow-up. Seventy-eight percent of patients reported the course to be moderately to extremely beneficial after six months. The author concluded that the important role of PHIP in the treatment of patients with stress-related complaints is reproducible outside of Harvard Pilgrim Health Care.

The outcome studies continue to demonstrate the effectiveness of PHIP in four statistically significant areas:

- Decreases in emotional and physical distress
- Increases in positive mood and functional status
- Patient satisfaction with the program
- Decreased use of medical resources after a pattern of high utilization

In addition, these improvements were maintained at follow-up.

PHIP: The Future

HPHC and other organizations are beginning to use PHIP for disease-specific applications such as panic disorders, irritable bowel syndrome, and asthma. Such approaches include offering courses for patients with the same underlying chronic medical conditions, with or without additional educational program information specific to diseases such as diabetes, asthma, irritable bowel syndrome, and others. Other organizations are interested in incorporating PHIP as the behavioral intervention component of a broader wellness program including modules on nutrition, exercise, and alternative/complementary medical therapies. There is ample opportunity for ongoing outcomes research comparing the different approaches.

Efforts are underway to develop ways of more efficiently and reliably identifying appropriate high-utilizing candidates for PHIP in the physician's office and in the workplace. A brief but predictive six- to ten-question screening tool identifying individuals with high-utilizing complaints and behaviors would be invaluable.

In conclusion, one of the most interesting potential uses of PHIP is as an organizational tool for primary care integration. Because PHIP is by its nature holistic and grounded in the mind-body connection, its implementation by an organization provides for paradigm shifts and testing infrastructure changes that integrate primary medical and mental health services. Change is costly; immense organizational inertia exists in the absence of concrete improvement in quality of care or cost savings. Tools like PHIP may produce the results in quality improvement, patient satisfaction, and medical cost offset that fuel support of integration.

References

1. Barsky A, Borus JF: Somatization and medicalization in the era of managed care. JAMA 274:24, 1995.
2. Lipowski ZJ: Somatization: The concept and its clinical application. Am J Psychiatry 145: 1358–1368, 1988.
3. Garfield SR, Collen MF, Feldman R, Soghikian K, Richart RH, Duncan JH: Evaluation of ambulatory medical care system. N Engl J Med 294:426–431, 1976.
4. Backett EM, Heady JA, Evans JCG: Studies of a general practice, II: The doctor's job in an urban area. BMI 1:109–115, 1954.

5. Van der Gagg J, van de Ven W: The demand for primary health care. Med Care 26:299-312, 1978.
6. Pilowsky I, Smith QP, Katsikitis M: Illness behavior and general practice utilization: A prospective study. J Psychosom Res 31:177-183, 1987.
7. Cummings NA, Vanden Bos GR: The twenty-year Kaiser-Permanente experience with psychotherapy and medical utilization: implications for national health policy and national health insurance. Health Policy Q 1:159-175, 1981.
8. Follette WT, Cummings WA: Psychiatric services and medical utilization in a prepaid health plan setting: part II. Med Care 6:31-41, 1968.
9. Hilkevitch A: Psychiatric disturbance in outpatients of a general medical outpatient clinic. Int J Neuropsychiatry 1:371-375, 1965.
10. Escobar JI, Golding JM, Hough RL, Karno M, Burnham MA, Wells KB: Somatization in the community: Relationship to disability and use of services. Am J Public Health 77:837-840, 1987.
11. Katon W, Von Korff M, Lin E, et al: Distressed high utilizers of medical care: DSM-III-R diagnoses and treatment needs. Gen Hosp Psychiatry 12:355-362, 1990.
12. Lipowski ZJ: Somatization: a borderland between medicine and psychiatry. Can Med Assoc J 135:609-613, 1986.
13. Bass C: Somatization: Physical Symptoms and Psychological Illness. Blackwell Scientific Publications Inc., Oxford, England, 1990.
14. Regier DA, Narrow WE, Rae DS, et al: The de facto US mental and addictive disorders service system. Arch Gen Psychiatry 50:85-94, 1993.
15. McFarland BH, Freeborn DK, Mullooly JP, et al: Utilization patterns among long-term enrollees in a prepaid group practice health maintenance organization. Med Care 23:1211-1233, 1985.
16. Derogatis L: SCL-90-R Administration, Scoring, and Procedures Manual. Clinical Psychometric Research, Towson, MD, 1977.
17. Derogatis L: The brief symptom inventory: an introductory report. Psychol Med 13:595-605, 1983.
18. McHorney CA, Ware JE, Raczek AE: The MOS 26-item short-form health survey (SF-36): II. Psychometric and clinical tests of validity in measuring physical and mental health constructs. Med Care 31:247-263, 1993.
19. McLeod C: Report: Findings from the Ways to Wellness research project. Harvard Community Health Plan Behavioral Medicine, Boston, MA, 1993.
20. McLeod C: Report: Ways to Wellness at the Chelmsford Center. Harvard Community Health Plan Behavioral Medicine, Boston, MA 1993.
21. Hellman CJC, Budd M, Borysenko J, et al: A study of the effectiveness of two group behavioral medicine interventions for patients with psychosomatic complaints. Behav Med December: 165-173, 1990.
22. McClelland DC, McLeod C, Budd MA: Psychological changes induced by a behavioral medicine intervention which predict better mental health six months later. MindBody Medicine (In press, 1997).
23. McLeod CC, Budd M: Treatment of somatization in primary care. J Gen Hosp Psychiatry (In press, 1997).

Chapter 11

The Group Practice Model: Allina Health System

Michael Trangle, M.D.

The Allina Health System is a not-for-profit regional, integrated health system serving people living in Minnesota, western Wisconsin, and eastern North Dakota and South Dakota. Health maintenance organizations (HMOs) and other managed care arrangements have long been part of the medical and mental health scene in this area. The state of Minnesota, which licenses and regulates HMOs, has some unusual and even unique requirements. As a condition of licensure, HMOs are required to be owned by a non-profit corporation and are required to have significantly greater financial reserves in Minnesota than in most states. According to Abrams, this prevents corporations from paying out "unreasonably" large payments to management companies, executives, providers, or others.[1] A Minnesota HMO is not allowed to maintain a net worth equal to more than two months of expenses. It must spend any monies over this figure on internal operations, contributions to charitable foundations, premium reduction, and so on.

In addition, a number of large and influential regional corporations have taken special interest in the medical care offered to their employees. A number of these corporations have banded into coalitions (such as the Buyers Health Care Action Group). These self-insured groups have taken a long-term view of promoting the quality and value of the mental health services offered to their employees. Recently they have designed and implemented new initiatives to promote direct contracting with organized care systems made up of primary care physicians (PCPs), specialists, hospitals, and other providers, and to minimize the role of intermediary insurance companies.

The Allina system came into being as a result of a series of mergers and acquisitions. Essentially, groups of physicians and clinics merged into a larger grouping, which in turn combined with a previously merged group of hospitals. This entity, in its turn, merged with a health insurance company (which also had several previously combined components). The resultant system went through a phase where it acquired a number of primary care practices and vigorously pursued strategic alliances with independent physicians and clinics in long-term arrangements, with varying levels of shared risks. Allina also agreed to management contracts with other hospitals and entities within the region. During this phase, nine mental health clinics that had been "carved out" and created to serve HMO patients on a capitated basis were also acquired.

Currently the system's group practice consists of about 550 providers, most of whom are PCPs, who work in 65 Allina-owned clinics in nearly 40 communities. Allina owns 12 hospitals, manages seven others, and either owns or manages seven nursing homes. The insurance arm of Allina Health System covers approximately one million subscribers—about one-third of the population of the state of Minnesota—and contracts with approximately 9,000 physicians and other providers.

Throughout Allina's various mergers and acquisitions, it has clung steadfastly to its vision: to create a continuous learning environment wherein providers relentlessly pursue the quality of the medical services provided, yet still value customer service, innovation, partnership, stewardship, and integrity.

The insurance arm of the system offers an array of health plans and options. These range from less expensive options where the mental health coverage is limited, to a network that consists of a group of clinics that exclusively work with capitated HMO patients. In this situation, all patients are expected to attend these clinics unless there is a need for specialty services or access is difficult, at which point they are referred out to a broader network. Other patients have chosen a health plan wherein it is less expensive for them to receive services in our restricted group of clinics, but they can opt to go outside for a greater out-of-pocket cost. There are a number of other plans with various gradations, where the customer can pay more to have greater freedom of choice.

Integration Model

So how does the system make sense of this complex series of relationships? How do we integrate our mental health services with the primary care component of our healthcare? Essentially we have divided ourselves into three regions and have analyzed the composition of the primary care groups in each region. We then designed our mental health services to complement the regional groups.

Site-based Integration

In one of our regions, the primary care group has carefully structured itself so that the care delivery system and its management is site-based. Hiring decisions, continuous quality improvement (CQI) initiatives, and many of the financial decisions are made by site-based personnel. Such clinics typically start with a core provider constituency of PCPs. At that stage, mental health referrals are usually made to private practice mental health clinicians in the community or, if the patients are in health plans with a more restricted network, to the nearest Allina clinic in that network. When the referral stream reaches a "critical mass," a mental health clinician is hired to work at the site. A critical mass is difficult to define; there is no quantitative formula to predictably determine this situation. For example, a four-member obstetrics/gynecology group where the physicians are sensitive to and sophisticated about mental health issues has generated more than enough referrals to keep a full-time practitioner busy. There have been other examples of larger groups, but if they do less case finding and referral for mental health treatment, a full-time practitioner is not needed.

Integration has been difficult to achieve when a mental health practitioner is primarily based in one clinic, but spends one to two days per week in a new clinic. The practitioner is not fully integrated into the interpersonal flow and patient flow in the new clinic. A better solution has been to hire a full-time Ph.D.-level psychologist to "anchor" the mental health services in the new clinic. The clinician is hired primarily by the PCPs in the clinic, although other mental health professionals catalyze and aid this process. The monies generated by this new clinician are merged in the revenue stream with the other physicians in the primary care clinic. The group must feel that the new psychologist shares the same risks and benefits as the other providers based in that clinic. The income stream for these clinics is varied (partly capitated, partly directly contracted, and partly from indemnity insurance companies).

Given the constraints of Medicare and medical assistance, it is simpler in this model to hire Ph.D.-level psychologists who are eligible to see patients from all insurance sources. As the referral stream grows, more psychologists are added. With appropriate supervision criteria, we have added graduate-level clinicians (psychologists, marriage and family therapists, or M.S.W.s). After two or three therapists are present, we consider adding a psychiatrist to the group. Again, the final decision is made by the physicians on the site.

Once the mental health contingent reaches this size, there is a natural tendency to achieve efficiencies of scale by having them share office space (near each other), receptionists, waiting areas, and other support services. The risk exists for this to become a "mini-department" and to be moved out of the mainstream of the clinic. The ideal balance seems to be to have several colleagues for stimulation and support, yet still be rubbing elbows with the PCPs, having curb-side consults, and attending all clinic-wide meetings.

This site-based system works quite well in terms of meeting patient needs and integrating the mental health services into primary care clinics in a seamless fashion. There is a need for some "extra clinic" involvement to either perform or consult with the lead physician at the clinic for quality improvement projects and for recruiting. A regional mental health director has taken an active role in performing these functions. When psychiatrists have split their time between these clinics and inpatient psychiatric units, the results were not always positive. In many ways, the increased intensity of work and collegiality of the hospital has made it difficult for them to consider the outpatient clinic their primary base.

Large Multispecialty Group Model

In another region, the primary care group is structured as a large, multispecialty medical clinic with a number of smaller satellites. In this system, the mental health group began as a department in the large group. The primary care administrators hired doctorate- and master's-level therapists to meet the needs of their patients. In addition, the group arranged for a limited amount of psychiatric time from clinicians who were not considered members of the group and who were not integrated with the other mental health providers in the department. When the group was acquired by Allina, the first goal was to hire full-time psychiatrists to join the group, thus providing the full range of mental health disciplines and services. An outpatient psychiatrist was initially added, followed by a psychiatrist who split his time between the clinic, inpatient chemical dependency work, and consultations at an Allina-based hospital. Our third psychiatrist spent half of her time performing outpatient work in the clinic and the other half performing inpatient psychiatric work at a different Allina hospital.

This plan successfully integrated the outpatient services with the acute care services (as represented by inpatient, partial, and residential psychiatric and chemical dependency services), and also integrated the psychiatrists and the various specialty physicians in the group. On the other hand, the transition created tension and mixed feelings within some of the original members of the mental health department. There was a sense that the case mix changed, focusing more on servicing patients who had more crises, were more severely disturbed, and were potentially more dangerous. Because a majority of these patients were shared between the psychiatrists and therapists, everyone was affected by the shift of focus.

More emphasis was placed on access, which affected the consistency and predictability of the therapists' schedules. In addition, there was a sense of "creeping medicalization" of the department. A retreat with an outside facilitator was held to process these feelings and direct them toward a constructive outcome. There was a small amount of personnel turnover, including both the psychiatric and therapist providers, but eventually an equilibrium was reached. The clinicians became more comfortable with the new group identity, and there was a sense of mutual respect.

Ongoing Integration Efforts

In another of our regions, there was *no* dominant medical group. Instead, there were disparate, not very well integrated medical groups, which were initially small. At the same time, Allina had some of its own carve-out mental health clinics in this region. These clinics thrived under the previous ownership of one of the hospitals.

One clinic consisted primarily of Ph.D.-level psychologists and neuropsychologists. Another was mainly a psychiatric group that performed substantial hospital work but also had three outpatient sites. Gradually, the psychology-only clinic has come to share more and more functions with the psychiatric group, to their mutual benefit. They are undergoing a planned, delicate merger of operations. In the first phase of this merger, the administrative, business, and support staff functions were integrated. Currently, the intake, supervision, and quality/utilization management functions are being merged.

Concurrently, the small primary care clinics in the region were merging into larger entities. We are establishing mental health clinicians at those sites, typically when the number of PCPs reaches at least 10. We have experimented with placing a psychiatrist, a master's-level therapist, and a doctoral-level psychologist there first. Ultimately, having a Ph.D. psychologist in the primary care group as the anchor person seems to best balance the need for clinical expertise with cost effectiveness in this system. The hiring process for the psychologists and psychiatrists placed in the primary care clinics is a joint process. Most recruitment efforts are performed by administrative psychiatrists. The PCPs then interview the final candidates.

Because the psychiatrists' and psychologists' salaries and revenues flow through the dominant psychiatric group in this region, they are not viewed as truly part of the primary care clinic. Rather, they are viewed as fellow corporate employees who do not share all the risks and benefits of the PCPs, depending on the finances of the clinic.

Former Carve-out Mental Health Clinics

Finally, we have a different class of clinics that were acquired within the last year. These clinics were created to serve the mental health needs of capitated HMO patients from a contract that had formerly been "carved out" from our own insurance company. These clinics are not set up to perform billing or documentation services that are needed for the entire array of insurance companies. Therefore clinicians in these clinics cannot see the entire spectrum of patients treated by our PCPs. Instead, they are only seeing patients on the health plan owned by our corporation.

Through CQI endeavors, these clinics have improved written communication with PCPs. We can document that written communication has occurred with the PCP 90 percent of the time, and the remaining 10 percent of patients have chosen not to have their PCP contacted. We are currently meeting and establishing better referral relationships with our primary care clinics in the regions, but until these clinics can see the entire array of patients, it will be difficult to cement strong and habitual referral patterns.

Summary

The Allina Health System is viewed as an integrated health system, which indeed it is. However, a more accurate description would be that it is an *integrating* health system, and a work in progress.

Reference

1. Abrams DR: A league of its own: HMO law according to the State of Minnesota. Minnesota Physician 10 (January 1997).

Chapter 12

The Quality Improvement Model of Behavioral Health Group Practices

Allen S. Daniels, Ed.D.

The integration of behavioral health and primary care is a process in rapid evolution. This is due, in part, to the redesign of reimbursement systems to increased risk-sharing agreements, and the development of delivery systems that span the spectrum of primary and specialty care providers. There has also been increased attention to quality improvement and the accountability of delivery systems.

In behavioral healthcare there has been a movement from solo practitioners to group practices. Behavioral groups may exist as freestanding practices, or as a part of integrated multispecialty medical systems. The Council of Behavioral Group Practices (a part of the Institute for Behavioral Healthcare) has defined a group practice as having the following 11 characteristics:

1. full economic and operational integration
2. business structure as a single-specialty behavioral group, or the mental health department within a multispecialty medical group
3. professional management and administration in place to facilitate claims processing, patient communication, contract management, risk management, and program development
4. computerized management and medical information system
5. a strong commitment to advanced training and leadership in managed behavioral healthcare
6. ten or more full-time equivalent behavioral health practitioners with psychiatrists fully integrated into the practice
7. active involvement in the provision of managed behavioral healthcare services
8. cost-effective and flexible treatment programs that use multidisciplinary treatment teams, which are linked to a continuum of care delivery system
9. 24-hour access and an emergency response system
10. an active quality assurance and/or quality management program
11. an active care management and continuity of care system

The spectrum of behavioral healthcare is provided only to a limited extent by specifically trained mental health and chemical dependency providers. However, many of these services are provided in primary care settings, in schools or other systems, or by clergy or other social service agencies. For this reason, it has become increasingly important for behavioral health providers to create a liaison among the broad spectrum of providers of behavioral healthcare services. One of the key areas in which this has been most evident is in the integration between behavioral healthcare providers and primary care systems.

For those providers interested in integration, accountability issues are critical. The National Committee for Quality Assurance (NCQA) has recently developed guidelines for the accreditation of managed behavioral health organizations to facilitate accountability. The following are the principal areas of organizations reviewed for accreditation:

- Quality assurance and quality plan
- Access, availability, referral, and triage
- Members' rights and responsibilities
- Utilization management
- Credentialing
- Prevention
- Clinical records

These standards are guidelines for the evaluation and review of a behavioral health system. In addition, they can be used to examine the evolving relationship between behavioral group practices and primary care delivery systems.

Each of the seven areas of NCQA standards for the accreditation for managed behavioral health organizations can serve as a tool for examining the principles and models for the integration of primary care and behavioral health. This system of accountability also provides a framework to chart the evolving course of behavioral health utilized in primary care. Because NCQA also accredits health plans, it will have a significant impact on the course of primary care and the overall healthcare delivery systems.

Quality Improvement

The NCQA guidelines stipulate the existence of a quality improvement plan with tracking of quality indicators and reporting of findings. Behavioral group practices are focusing on the development of quality improvement programs that meet the NCQA guidelines and also foster the integration of primary care resources. Historically, behavioral groups have had little formal programming in the area of quality improvement. Existing programming focuses on patient satisfaction rather than clinical outcome, and case supervision rather than a systematic review of clinical delivery processes.

The more sophisticated behavioral group practices have become directly involved in managed care contracting and have been required to develop quality improvement programs and plans. These groups have developed quality indicators to track and monitor the plan. Indicators that have been monitored often focus on tracking risk-based incidents like rehospitalization within a designated time frame, or the process of entry into care. In addition, these quality improvement indicators call for the existence of standard policies and procedures for the notification of primary care providers and their integration into the treatment process.

The value of a comprehensive quality improvement plan for a behavioral group practice is in its ability to create standard operational principles and track compliance with these guidelines. It also affords the group an opportunity to identify certain key aspects of their practice and to explore the relationship of these indicators to the effectiveness and efficiency of the care provided over time. As the integration of behavioral health and primary care becomes ever more prevalent, it provides an opportunity to coordinate quality indicators between behavioral health and primary care systems.

In some groups who share an ownership structure with a larger delivery system, the quality improvement program may already exist with the primary care practice. An example might be the treatment of major depression across the healthcare continuum. For an integrated delivery system, there is customarily a quality improvement program with representative membership from all participatory disciplines or clinical departments. This committee develops, monitors, and reviews the quality indicators and the findings of the ongoing work plan.

An important aspect of any quality improvement program is the cost associated with this process. A quality program requires clinicians to divert time from direct clinical service to practice operations. As the reimbursement for behavioral health is declining, there is a growing trend towards examining the costs associated with the quality improvement process to determine if they can be reduced. As quality improvement programs are linked to the overall healthcare delivery system, it will be necessary and important for behavioral health practices to foster the inclusion of these quality indicators to measure the cost offset indicators found in joint integration projects. The costs will more than pay off if outcomes and quality improvement are documented.

Access, Availability, Referral, and Triage

In the standards of access, availability, referral, and triage, NCQA stipulates that there must be a defined system of monitoring the resources for the initiation of behavioral healthcare. For the integration of behavioral health and primary care this is also a central issue. The design of the access system will likely be determined by the nature of the ownership of the delivery system. In a freestanding behavioral group practice, the access to care is less likely to be formally linked to primary care systems. However, in an integrated delivery system, there may be a common access path for all care, such as a physician referral service or a central access phone number.

Through the advent of managed care, some health plans require a primary care "gatekeeper," thus creating a more formal pathway for entry into care. In addition, it has long been the contention of many primary care physicians (PCPs) that they have not been aware of what course of treatment has been undertaken in the behavioral health system. This lack of communication is due to several factors. The main issue has been confidentiality. Historically, behavioral health providers have been reluctant to share much information with PCPs about the course of treatment, for fear that this information will be disclosed in inappropriate ways.

A number of approaches are currently in place among behavioral group practices to address the issue of a PCP's notification and inclusion in the course of care. These include standard protocols for the notification of a patient's PCP at the initiation of care and at designated points throughout the treatment process. An example might be a notification at the time of any medication initiation or change. (See Chapter 7 for further discussion of these issues.) In addition, some groups who are actively involved in outcomes evaluation are routinely providing PCPs with baseline and follow-up health status measures, with the patient's consent.

In an attempt to facilitate collaboration and integration of care, a number of large group practices and comprehensive systems are placing behavioral health providers in primary care offices. This facilitates a liaison among providers, and ready access to care for patients. Providers who work in integrated sites report a greater level of satisfaction in the management of all aspects of care. Principles that guide this practice include respect among practitioners, collaboration between behavioral health providers and all levels of the primary care staff including nurses and front office personnel, clear communication, and flexibility to facilitate practice patterns between professionals.

Members' Rights and Responsibilities

The NCQA standards stipulate that managed behavioral health organizations have established policies and procedures for the rights and responsibilities of their members. For behavioral group practices, there should also be a published set of rights and responsibilities. In some cases groups will have written standards for this, including the therapists' rights and responsibilities. Common features among the rights of patients include confidentiality, timeliness of service, and respect in the treatment process, as well as the responsibility to notify the therapist in the event of a canceled appointment and to pay for services in a timely manner.

The rights and responsibilities of patients are somewhat more complicated within integrated delivery systems that include both primary care and behavioral health. Issues of confidentiality are less secure in an environment that shares scheduling functions, control of viewing patients' appointments and medical records, and billing accounts.

Utilization Management

In managed behavioral healthcare, the role of utilization management is central to the quality of care delivered. For NCQA, behavioral health organizations are required to have established standards for the utilization management process. These guidelines indicate a process by which all care is to be reviewed through established criteria by appropriately trained professionals. Most managed care systems will have a utilization management division, with a designated medical director. However, behavioral health is not consistently a part of this process. In some organizations the benefits for behavioral health may be carved out to another company or organization. Therefore, the integration between behavioral health and primary care is limited.

There are a number of approaches to facilitate the integration of behavioral health and primary care in utilization management. This can be accomplished through established standards for integration in the utilization management program plan, with regular review by the quality improvement committee. Many managed behavioral health groups and organizations with delegated utilization management responsibilities will have a joint liaison committee that monitors and provides oversight for this integration. A key component is the regular communication between medical directors and program directors, leading to a common understanding of the issues of medical necessity review and adherence to covered benefit services.

Credentialing

Credentialing services apply primarily to managed care companies. However, the activities involved require a considerable amount of time from clinicians and group practices to meet the credentialing standards of the managed care organizations. In addition, physicians are required to meet the privileging requirements of hospitals. Recently, integrated delivery systems have attempted to consolidate the credentialing functions required of them by managed care companies and hospitals.

In an attempt to contain costs, managed care companies have begun to delegate credentialing functions to practice entities that meet the established NCQA standards. Through this process the managed care company establishes a formal relationship with the delivery system to provide these services. This may be to a designated group practice or to an entire network management system. It is less common for a single behavioral group, unless they have other delegated functions for utilization management, quality, or risk.

A common approach for delivery systems with delegated credentialing functions is to consolidate the data collection functions. These can be provided through an internal credentialing unit or purchased from a service bureau. In organizations with a spectrum of responsibilities including hospital and physician organizations, it is common to share the data collection functions. These entities serve as central verification offices, and they coordinate the assembly of primary source data and other documentation. Provider data files are then made available to the requisite quality and credentialing committees for review. In any instance in which functions are delegated, an audit process is necessary to review the consistency of the units functions.

Although it is not always a part of a behavioral health or primary care clinical practice, credentialing can be a useful tool for a provider. The consolidation of these functions as an internal process can facilitate the membership in managed care programs. Standards for the development of a credentialing system are an important part of the behavioral health and primary care quality plan.

Prevention

Behavioral health group practices and primary care systems are collaborating in many ways to develop prevention activities. These prevention services can be at the primary, secondary, or tertiary level. Although these services have traditionally had a low reimbursement by health plans, data clearly show that prevention can have a profound effect on health outcomes. Also, attention has recently focused on medical cost offset from behavioral health intervention. These are the savings in general health costs, when the necessary behavioral health treatment requirements are met (see Chapter 5).

Several examples of prevention exist in delivery systems with various levels of integration between behavioral health and primary care. These are often focused on the high utilization diagnostic categories such as major depression, anxiety, substance abuse, or somatization. The development of treatment algorithms, pathways, and/or clinical protocols are an attempt to facilitate the coordination of care in cases where there is likely to be some overlap in treatment between primary care and behavioral health. These protocols serve as a model for the routine care and referral of these clinical conditions.

Another form of prevention occurring in large multispecialty systems is the redesign of the treatment process. In these centers, providers from a spectrum of disciplines are coming together to examine the components of treatment and implement new frameworks and models of intervention. Such treatment models often go beyond the customary level of care and may bring together new clinical resources to address the treatment of designated disorders.

In behavioral group practices, a spectrum of prevention activities can be seen. Examples may include time-focused groups for stress management, parenting, or adjustment to a certain clinical diagnosis. These may be provided as part of the initial evaluation process, as an adjunct to treatment, or as aftercare following an intervention process.

Clinical Records

The NCQA standards for clinical records address the content and review of a patient's record. Many small behavioral group practices do not have a well-documented set of policies and procedures for their medical records. They may lack consistency and are rarely peer reviewed. For practices that are not medically based, they may also fail to meet minimum practice standards. Clinical records are considered legal documents, however, and require established standards for their maintenance and review. The relevant issues of confidentiality have already been reviewed.

For large behavioral health practices that are a part of integrated delivery systems, clinical records are maintained both jointly and separately, depending on the system. There are inherent problems with either method. If the records are separate, the integration of care is compromised by the lack of direct communication in keeping two records. For systems with a common patient record, the anonymity of patients receiving care services may be compromised.

In any clinical delivery system, the form and content of a clinical record must be established. This format should require that all care which could affect another level of care (for example primary care) must be documented and communicated. It is imperative that collaboration and communication be part of the treatment and documented in the clinical record.

Conclusion

For the behavioral healthcare industry, this is a time of rapid evolution and change. General health systems are facing similar issues. One of the keys for adaptation to these changes must be the integration of behavioral healthcare and primary care. This can be achieved through a common ownership structure or by collaboration between the disciplines. However, at the core of this process must be a commitment on all sides to an integrated quality improvement system.

The standards for the accreditation of managed behavioral health organizations have been used as a framework to examine some significant aspects of the integration of primary care and behavioral health. The map or standard model for how this must occur is in a state of evolution. However, the standards for quality and accountability can serve as a guide for primary care/behavioral health integration.

Part IV.
WORKING IN PRIMARY CARE SETTINGS: WHAT YOU NEED TO KNOW

Chapter 13

The Primary Care Perspective: Culture and Reality

Michael D. Cirigliano, M.D. and Mary F. Morrison, M.D.

Primary care providers are constantly challenged by time limitations, managed care related issues, mountains of paperwork, and in many instances, difficult patients. Patients with psychosocial problems requiring inordinate amounts of time and energy can exhaust a busy clinician who, at the start of the day, may have a waiting room full of patients with a variety of medical ailments ranging from renal insufficiency to chest pain, and in between, a patient with depression or panic disorder. Such is the culture of the primary care physician (PCP) in the late twentieth century.

In most instances, patients are expected to be seen every 15 minutes, but some require much more time than has been allotted. Many patients do not fit into the biomedical model of illness and healthcare that dominates the training of PCPs.[1] Studies have shown that many PCPs are not skilled at recognizing psychiatric disorders meeting diagnostic criteria, and many go undiagnosed.[2] In addition, some mental health practitioners are unavailable or poorly responsive to the needs of the PCP, which makes the care of the psychiatric patient in the primary care setting a formidable task.

Differentiating Medical from Psychiatric Illness

Historically, psychiatric care and general medicine have not been integrated. Factors such as insufficient psychiatric training of PCPs and the stigma associated with mental illness have kept psychiatry out of the general medical setting.[3] Primary care providers have been known to be concerned about patient response to psychiatric questioning. This is unfortunate, given the prevalence of psychiatric illness in general medical practice. Many common medical complaints may, in fact, be rooted in psychiatric illness. Fatigue, for instance, is one of the most common presenting complaints in primary care. Some studies indicate that up to 40 percent of patients with this complaint actually suffer from depression.[4] Insomnia has also been shown to be related to psychiatric disorders in up to two-thirds of patients.[5]

By developing long-term relationships with patients, differentiating medical from psychiatric illness can become easier. General medicine practitioners should realize that patients with chronic medical conditions such as arthritis, diabetes, hypertension, and emphysema have a significantly increased prevalence of psychiatric disorders.

Although improved and increased training is required to aid PCPs in recognizing and treating mental illness, keeping these issues on the differential diagnostic list may assist in formulating an accurate diagnosis. To help PCPs ask the right questions efficiently, the American Psychiatric Association published the *Diagnostic and Statistical Manual of Mental Disorders*, Fourth edition, for primary care *(DSM-IV-PC)*, which groups psychiatric disorders by their presenting symptoms. Although helpful, this resource requires significant time for PCPs to use in practice. Other screening tools for use in primary care include the PRIME-MD (Primary Care Evaluation of Mental Disorders) and the Psychosocial Review of Systems (PROS).[6,7] PROS was designed to include selected psychosocial variables essential in evaluating every new patient in the primary care setting. Because of time constraints, physicians cannot adequately administer all the key questions. They must therefore develop skills of active listening and recognize manifestations of disorders such as anxiety, depression, and other psychiatric conditions.

Time Limitations

With changes in healthcare management and delivery occurring almost on a daily basis, the primary care provider's daily schedule has become ever more hectic and stressful. The time spent with a patient in the past was certainly less harried and might last up to an hour for a new patient. The advent of managed care, however, has decreased this time to a usual 15 minutes per patient for follow-up visits, or roughly four encounters per hour.[8]

The challenge is managing both the medical problems and the mental health issues presented by the patient. However, questioning of patients about psychosocial issues is time consuming and therefore uncomfortable. All too often the result is that patients have underdiagnosed and misdiagnosed psychiatric disorders. These misdiagnosed patients are sometimes told that their symptoms are "all in your head" and hurriedly prescribed an antidepressant or anxiolytic agent.[9] This can have long-term and significant consequences for the patient and emphasizes the importance of properly diagnosing and treating these patients in the primary care setting.

Billing for Time Spent Counseling

As managed healthcare continues to pervade medical practice, reimbursement for time spent on psychological counseling has changed. Most plans, including Medicare and traditional indemnity coverage, do partially reimburse the PCP for counseling patients individually, as long as it is well documented and includes the patient's history, diagnosis, and disposition. Some managed care plans will not reimburse for treating chronic mental illnesses that require long-term treatment. Few managed care or indemnity plans pay for marriage or family counseling, even if prescribed by the PCP. Additionally, managed care and indemnity plans limit the number of covered days per year, based on medical necessity. Many studies have shown that proper psychiatric care can actually reduce overall long-term healthcare costs and improve the effectiveness of medical treatment.[10] For the most part, third-party payers consider addressing psychosocial issues to be a standard part of medical care. Generally, managed care organizations expect the primary care practitioner to initially provide this form of care. This may be accomplished in the typical 15-minute time slot by using the techniques described below.

Improving Recognition of Psychiatric Disorders in Primary Care

It is often difficult to ascertain whether a patient presenting with physical symptoms has a true medical problem or a psychiatric disorder. If testing and clinical evaluation do not reveal an organic cause, psychiatric illness should then be entertained. Psychological causes of illness are suggested by a patient with a family member who has similar physical complaints or who may exhibit learned illness behavior. In addition, if there appears to be secondary gain for the patient by being ill, the likelihood of psychogenic illness is increased. Sometimes the patient may need to return for subsequent visits to help elucidate a psychological illness.

Screening Instruments

Despite the fact that most people with mental disorders seek care in the general medical setting, studies have shown that primary care practitioners have a low detection rate for many mental disorders. Several tools have been developed to aid PCPs in diagnosing mental illness in the primary care setting. However, these new tools have not yet become a routine part of most office practices. The *DSM-IV-PC* is a manual developed by both PCPs and psychiatrists to diagnose mental disorders in the general medical setting.[11] This manual was designed to facilitate diagnosis by focusing on mental conditions important to the primary care setting. The two screening instruments developed for primary care use are the PRIME-MD and the Symptom Driven Diagnostic System for Primary Care (SDDS-PC).[6,12,13]

The PRIME-MD evaluates five groups of mental disorders (mood, anxiety, somatoform, alcohol, and eating disorders). It has a 26-item questionnaire that is completed by the patient before seeing the physician. The physician uses a structured interview form to obtain more clinical information related to the positive responses only. The average time to administer the PRIME-MD in the initial utilization studies was 8.4 minutes.[6] A new, briefer version of the PRIME-MD (the Patient Problem Questionnaire) is also under development (see Appendix 4).

The SDDS-PC has a 16-item questionnaire that can be used to evaluate six mental disorders: depression, generalized anxiety disorder, panic disorder, obsessive compulsive disorder, suicidal ideation, and alcohol abuse and dependence (see Appendix 3).[13] The paper version of the SDDS-PC utilizes a physician-administered diagnostic interview to further assess positive results. The physician module for each of the six disorders is designed to be administered in less than five minutes. However, in the initial pilot study 26 percent of the physicians found the procedure to be too time consuming. In response to this, a new computer-assisted telephone interview was developed.

Stuart and Lieberman have developed a protocol to aid the PCP in eliciting information about the patient's emotional health using the acronym BATHE.[8] This entails asking several simple questions during the office visit as follows:

Background: "What's been happening in your life?"
Affect: "How do you feel about that?"
Trouble: "What is it about this situation that troubles you most?"
Handling: "How are you handling that?"
Empathy: "That must be very difficult for you."

In summary, structured screening for mental disorders is not common in primary care practices, despite the fact that the majority of mental disorders are seen in this setting. Other possible uses of these screening instruments include the initial diagnostic work-up, screening high-risk populations (people with family history of mental disorder, certain medical disorders with high psychiatric comorbidity, frequent physician visits for the patient's burden of medical illness), or as an educational tool for medical students, residents, and practicing physicians.

Establishing a Therapeutic Relationship

The Primary Care Culture

The primary care setting enables a long-term relationship between patient and physician to develop. Over time, the physician is able to become intimately knowledgeable about a particular patient's medical and psychosocial background. Those physicians who understand the psychosocial milieu of their patients can develop a more comprehensive picture of the patients' health and well-being. If the physician approaches patients in a trusting, caring, and compassionate way, there is a greater likelihood that patients will be amenable to discussing underlying psychosocial issues.

Cultural Diversity

Primary care providers have to be comfortable treating culturally diverse populations. The doctor-patient relationship differs, depending on the cultural backgrounds of both doctor and patient. Some educational programs are encouraging medical residents to become familiar with an array of cultural variations. In providing care for a diverse patient population, the physician must always be cognizant of possible stereotypes and biases based on race, gender, and/or age.[14] In addition, communication can be a major problem and may require the presence of an interpreter. Finally, different cultures may view medicine and mental illness in different ways with varying belief models.[14] The PCP should always attempt to understand and appreciate a patient's particular cultural needs and mores.

Personal Discussions after Intimate Exams

In the general medical office, it is often common to greet the patient while he or she is dressed in a gown. After a brief interview, the patient is examined, sometimes involving intimate pelvic and genital evaluations. This is followed again by a brief discussion with recommendations. Many patients complain that there is not enough time to have questions answered. Also, the environment is not conducive to discussing intimate psychological and psychosocial issues.

An improvement on this process is having the patient dress after the physical examination and return to the physician's office. This may foster an improved environment of trust and comfort when discussing sensitive issues. Trust is also promoted when the physician accepts sensitive information without being judgmental, controls inappropriate reactions to difficult patients, and takes patient concerns seriously. Clear communication of treatment options and prognosis further complement the doctor-patient relationship. Patient accessibility to the physician is a necessity.

Discussing Bad News

One of the most difficult situations PCPs encounter is discussing negative news. This situation is often fraught with emotion and tension, which can result in anger and hostility focused on the physician simply because he or she has delivered the information. Many physicians may appear cold and indifferent, further contributing to this hostility. Robert Buckman, M.D., in his book *How to Break Bad News* recommends a six-step approach to discussing bad news.[15]

The physician should start by shaking hands and making sure all participants are present for the discussion. Buckman then recommends finding out how much the patient knows about the condition and ascertaining how much the patient wants to know. Once this is accomplished, he recommends sharing the information by educating the patient at his or her level without using medical jargon. Additionally, the physician should respond to the patient's feelings by identifying and acknowledging the patient's reaction to the bad news. Finally, he identifies the importance of planning and organizing follow-through and arranges a contact for the future, making sure that the patient has been listening and picked up the main concerns and issues of the discussion.

Physician Stress

Physician stress and burnout is high. Threat of lawsuits, managed care, mountains of paperwork, and difficult patients all take a toll on the physician. Many studies have cited a perceived lack of value of their work as a major cause of both stress and burnout among physicians.[16] Research also shows that stress and burnout may occur in those physicians with personal characteristics that leave them vulnerable to burnout. To help prevent this, healthcare professionals must take time to exercise regularly, pursue hobbies, and utilize supports such as family and friends. Counseling is also a viable option if stress appears to be escalating without relief. These are only a few measures that may help prevent burnout.

Common Mental Disorders in the Primary Care Setting

Psychiatric disorders are present in high rates in primary care and other medical settings. Mood disorders, anxiety disorder, somatization disorders, and substance abuse problems are the most common mental health disorders seen in primary care. Each of these disorders will be discussed in detail in the next four chapters. In addition to these common disorders, there are other illness types and mental health problems that require discussion.

Suicide

Suicide is seen infrequently in the general medical practice, but does represent a significant problem. Some researchers have found an incidence of 0.3 deaths per general practitioner per year and found that only 3 percent of deaths were preceded by parasuicidal behavior in the previous 12 months.[17] Many of these patients have presented with somatic complaints that the primary care provider failed to recognize. As the sole provider of care for many, the general practitioner has to be able to detect changes in behavior or family concerns that may prompt further questioning and evaluation. (For a detailed discussion of suicide, see Chapter 14.)

Violence Victims

Some studies have shown that up to 37 percent of general medicine patients were victims of violence as children or victims of domestic violence as adults.[18] Often it is the PCP who first detects signs of abuse and/or violence, such as unexplained bruises, fractures, or lacerations. In a study of battered women, results indicated that victims of spousal abuse had not only suffered physical harm but had subsequently more somatic complaints, a higher level of anxiety, and more depression.[19] It is imperative that the primary care provider actively ask pertinent questions and do a complete physical exam if violence is suspected. If confirmed, appropriate social and legal services can be contacted to assist the patient.

The Disability Patient

Some patients present with chronic complaints related to a work injury. Often these patients have been evaluated by multiple subspecialists and have sought the advice of an attorney. Back-related injuries are quite common. Patients often present with forms and documents related to workers' compensation and may request medical documentation of disability.

Some studies regarding low back pain have shown that a patient's cognitive coping strategies are the most powerful predictive variable in prognosis and resolution of chronic pain.[20] In some patients, persisting symptoms are due more to psychosocial influences than to medical factors. For some patients, the goal of disability plays a large role in prognosis. Some believe that labeling a person as disabled and giving income awards on the basis of disability provides disincentive to rehabilitation and encourages people to see injuries as opportunities for financial gain.[21]

In most systems, the inability to work must be based on a physiological, biochemical, or psychological aberration verified by clinical and/or laboratory diagnostic techniques. Unfortunately, the physician is often faced with a complaint such as chronic pain that may be harder to diagnose quantitatively. With these patients, the PCP must use his or her clinical judgment in determining disability. This can be difficult if pressure is put on the physician by not only the patient but by the patient's attorney as well. In many cases, patients who are malingering or are clearly interested in secondary gain from their illness can be ferreted out with the help of subspecialists. The final decision to deny disability or continue treatment may ultimately lead to the dissolution of the doctor-patient relationship, but must be carried out if honest medical judgment warrants such a decision.

The Litigious Patient

In the primary care setting, the risk of a lawsuit is certainly less than in the invasive subspecialties. While most patient encounters are positive experiences, occasionally one encounters a difficult patient. The one common denominator of patients who sue is anger.[22] Most experts agree that the risk of a lawsuit increases when physicians do not communicate with their patients. Because patients have high expectations and "expect" to be cured, bad outcomes can lead to angry patients. It behooves the physician to communicate and educate the patient as to all possible outcomes from a particular treatment or procedure. This helps prevent the patient from feeling surprised by a certain outcome.

In dealing with the hostile patient, many recommend using open-ended questions such as "What can I do to remedy the situation?" or "How can I be of assistance in this situation?" This encourages the patient to communicate and may diffuse a difficult situation. Office staff should be educated in detecting unhappy and/or angry patients.[22]

This might simply involve noticing an angry verbal comment or late bill payment. By calling a patient who has missed an appointment, arrangements can be made for follow-up care, and patient complaints can be dealt with quickly. In some cases, referral to a subspecialist or even another physician in the same field may be needed to avoid confrontation. If the physician is made aware of the details of the situation, he or she may be able to focus on the patient's concerns quickly, thereby reducing tension and anger. A final key point is the importance of documentation. The phrase "if it is not documented, it didn't happen" holds true. Every phone call and patient interaction should be carefully and legibly documented. Each patient chart should be regarded as a legal document and must stand up in court if reviewed by a jury. Also, no changes or alterations should ever be made in a medical record after the event.

The Nonadherent Patient

Physicians formerly used the term *compliance* to indicate the degree to which patients submit, yield, or acquiesce to the suggestions, recommendations, and pharmaceutical orders given by a physician. In the past, the doctor-patient relationship was more like a parent-child paternalistic role than an equal partnership. Today, this has been largely supplanted by the notion that the relationship between patient and physician is an equal partnership, which fosters patient adherence.[9] There are several techniques available to increase adherence among patients. A supportive and interested physician capable of providing encouragement promotes adherence. This can be fostered by improving listening skills and allowing the patient to do most of the talking.

A three-step problem-solving approach by Lieberman includes determining what the patient is feeling, noting what the patient wants, and educating the patient on what he or she can do to remedy the situation. By demonstrating an interest in patients' problems, regardless of the cause, and engaging them in the resolution of their problems, one can improve patient adherence.[9] By enabling patients to be responsible for their own health, adherence can be increased. If patients believe that you have their best interests at heart, adherence to medical recommendations is sure to increase.

Bereavement

Bereavement has been defined as a healing process to deal with loss and attempt to come to terms with it. Loss can take the form of a loved one, strength, a limb, or even health. Feelings of loss can have real consequences for health. In one study, 30 percent of close relatives had been admitted to the hospital and 12 percent had experienced major depression after the loss of a loved one.[23] Other studies have shown a seven-fold increase in mortality of the significant other.[24]

To help bereaved patients, one must first help patients admit their loss and then identify and verbalize their feelings.[25] The patient should be reassured that these feelings are normal and that, with time, healing will occur. The PCP may suggest frequent follow-up visits after the loss, with visits becoming less frequent as the patient adjusts to the loss. Office staff should be notified of a patient's death and correspondence to the deceased should be avoided. With the advent of computerized databases, this is becoming less of a problem. If the patient is religious, the family priest or rabbi can provide powerful sources of support and comfort, especially if there is a long relationship involved.

Interface Between Mental Health Professionals and Primary Care Providers

Currently the structure and reimbursement of care discourages linkages between primary care providers, and psychiatrists and other mental health professionals. In addition, there is some discomfort with the style of practice between these physician groups. Psychiatrists, concerned about confidentiality, have not communicated routinely with PCPs. Because of the stigma attached to the field and the changes in the health system, psychiatrists feel undervalued as colleagues and worry that PCPs will take over the treatment of their patients. However, the changes in healthcare structure offer an opportunity for both physician groups—as well as non-physician providers—to develop new models of collaborative practice that provide high-quality, coordinated, and efficient mental healthcare to patients. Primary care practitioners will improve their competency in detecting mental disorders in the general medical setting, resulting in an increase in patients with diagnosed psychiatric disorders. While many of these patients can be treated by PCPs, many others will require the assistance of mental health professionals. The following are some guidelines for referral to mental health professionals with an explanation of the training and strengths of each profession.

Psychiatrists

Patients with major mental illness or serious symptoms such as suicidality and unclear behavioral symptoms should be referred to a psychiatrist. Psychiatrists are qualified to evaluate patients with comorbid medical conditions and consider a full differential diagnosis. Primary care practitioners may want to occasionally refer to psychiatrists with subspecialty training such as child psychiatrists, geriatric psychiatrists, medical and consultation psychiatrists (comorbid medical conditions), neuropsychiatrists, and specialists in substance abuse.

Psychologists

Psychologists may have training at the doctoral or master's level. The level of training should be ascertained before referral. Clinical doctoral training will include expertise in psychotherapy and possibly psychological testing. The PCP should understand the model of therapy that the psychologist provides before referral. Most primary care patients require only short-term treatment, and an effective referral will be to a practitioner who provides therapy compatible with that goal. Cognitive therapy, behavioral therapy, and supportive therapy are examples of models of effective short-term treatment. Psychological testing that may be useful to the PCP can include neuropsychological assessment for specific neurological complaints such as memory difficulty. Psychologists' fees tend to be somewhat lower than those of psychiatrists. However, if patients are likely to need psychiatric medication, they will also need to be referred to a psychiatrist.

Social Workers

Most social workers in mental health practice are educated at a master's level. As such, their fees tend to be lower than those of a psychiatrist or psychologist. Some social workers may have special expertise in family or group therapy.

Nurses

In some medical communities, doctoral and master's level nurses may also provide psychotherapeutic treatment. Many nurse practitioners provide counseling services in medical and nonmedical settings. Expertise varies with clinical experience and training.

In summary, the system of mental health professionals is complex, with overlapping areas of expertise between mental health professions. Primary care physicians need to obtain information on the training and models of practice of the mental health professionals to whom they refer, because there can be substantial variation. Primary care physicians may want to consider collaborative practice models with psychiatrists and other mental health practitioners to better serve their patients.

Conclusion

The main problems facing the primary care provider when treating patients with psychosocial issues involve time restraints, inadequate training, poor coordination of cases with mental health practitioners, and the overall environment and "culture" of the primary care physician. It is easy to understand why many patients with psychiatric illness go undiagnosed. Additionally, the traditional training of physicians has involved a hospital-based biomedical model that does not foster the kinds of doctor-patient interactions required to make diagnoses in this area.

To rectify the situation, changes in education, improved integration, and better responsiveness of the behavioral healthcare team must occur. It is to be hoped that managed care organizations will see the benefits of compensating PCPs to recognize, diagnose, and treat psychiatric illness.

References

1. Novack DH, Goldberg RJ: Psychiatric problems in primary care patients. J Gen Intern Med 11:56–57, 1996.
2. Schulberg HC, Burns BJ: Mental disorders in primary care: epidemiologic, diagnostic, and treatment research directions. Gen Hosp Psychiatry 10:79–87, 1988.
3. Goldberg, MD: Psychiatry and the practice of medicine: the need to integrate psychiatry into comprehensive medical care. Southern Med Journal 88:260–267, 1995.
4. Kroenke K, Wood DR, Mangelsdorff D, et al: Chronic fatigue in primary care. Prevalence, patient characteristics, and outcome. JAMA 260:929–934, 1988.
5. Gillin JC, Byerley WF: The diagnosis and management of insomnia. N Engl J Med 322:239–248, 1990.
6. Spitzer RL, Williams JB, Kroenke K, et al: Utility of a new procedure for diagnosing mental disorders in primary care. The PRIME-MD 1000 study. JAMA 272:1749–1756, 1994.
7. Goldberg RJ, Novack DH: The psychosocial review of systems. Soc Sci Med 35:261–269, 1992.
8. Stuart MR, Lieberman JA III: The Fifteen Minute Hour: Applied Psychotherapy for the Primary Care Physician, Second edition. Praeger, Westport CT, 1993.
9. Lieberman JA III: Compliance issues in primary care. J Clin Psychiatry 57(suppl 7):76–82, 1996.
10. Strain JJ, Lyons JS, Hammer JS, et al: Cost offset from a psychiatric consultation-liaison intervention with elderly hip fracture patients. Am J Psychiatry 148:1044–1049, 1991.
11. Pincus HA, Vettorello NE, McQueen LE, et al: Bridging the gap between psychiatry and primary care. Psychosomatics 36:328–335, 1995.
12. Weissman MM, Olfson M, Leon AC, et al: Brief diagnostic interviews (SDDS-PC) for multiple mental disorders in primary care. Arch Family Med 4:220–227, 1995.

13. Broadhead WE, Leon AC, Weissman MM, et al: Development and validation of the SDDS-PC screen for multiple mental disorders in primary care. Arch Family Med 4:211–219, 1995.
14. Shapiro J, Lenahan P: Family medicine in a culturally diverse world: a solution-oriented approach to common cross-cultural problems in medical encounters. Family Med 28:249–255, 1996.
15. Buckman R: How to Break Bad News. A Guide for Health Care Professionals. The Johns Hopkins University Press, Baltimore MD, 1992.
16. Fields AI, Cuerdon TT, Brasseux CO, et al: Physician burnout in pediatric critical care medicine. Crit Care Med 23:1425–1429, 1995.
17. Diekstra RFW, van Egmond M: Suicide and attempted suicide in general practice 1979–1986. Acta Psychiatr Scand 79:268–275, 1989.
18. Wyshak G, Modest GA: Violence, mental health, and substance abuse in patients who are seen in primary care settings. Arch Family Med 5:441–447, 1996.
19. Jaffe P, Wolfe DA, Wilson S, Zak L: Emotional and physical health problems of battered women. Am J Psychiatry 31:625–629, 1986.
20. Kim Burton A, Malcom Tillotson K, Main CJ, Hollis S: Psychosocial predictors of outcome in acute and subchronic low back trouble. Spine 20:722–728, 1995.
21. Osterweis M, Kleinman A, Mechanic D (eds): Institute of Medicine. Committee on Pain, Disability, and Chronic Illness Behavior. Pain and Disability: Clinical, Behavioral, and Public Policy Perspectives. National Academy Press, Washington DC, 1987.
22. Kraushar MF: Recognizing and managing the litigious patient. Survey Ophthalmol 37:54–56, 1992.
23. Wilkes E: The Dying Patient: The Medical Management of Incurable and Terminal Illness. MTP Press, Lancaster, 1982.
24. Rees WD, Lutkins SG: Mortality of bereavement. BMJ 4:13–16, 1967.
25. Jones A: Bereavement counseling: applying ten principles. Geriatr Med 9:55, 1989.

Chapter 14

Depression in Primary Care: Assessment and Management

Steven Cole, M.D., Mary Raju, RN, M.S.N., and James Barrett, M.D.

The recognition and management of depressive disorders in primary care settings has received increasing attention as the true prevalence, and the related morbidity, of these disorders has become better understood and documented. Recognizing the importance of this issue, the MacArthur Foundation launched the Initiative on Depression in Primary Care. One focus of that Initiative was to develop tools and methods to change provider behavior concerning recognition and to improve the actual care that patients received. The material which follows in this chapter was developed as the resource manual for an eight-hour training program to improve the assessment and management of depressive disorders by primary care providers.

Major depression is a chronic, recurrent illness with a lifetime prevalence approximating 10 percent in men and 20 percent in women.[1] Dysthymic disorder (chronic depression) and other subthreshold depressive disorders (minor depressions) further increase this prevalence. Depressive disorders are associated with excessive utilization of medical services, marked morbidity, staggering economic costs, and significant mortality from suicide, as well as from associated comorbid general medical illnesses.[2-5] Despite a tendency to rationalize depressive symptoms as an expected consequence of life stresses or physical illnesses, the syndrome of major depression should be viewed as a serious complication warranting deliberate assessment and aggressive intervention.

Depression Is Common in Primary Care

Most individuals with mental disorders receive their mental healthcare from primary care physicians (PCPs), rather than from psychiatrists or other mental health professionals.[6] Depression is probably the most common mental disorder in primary care practice, as its prevalence increases from the community setting (2 percent to 4 percent), to outpatient care (5 percent to 10 percent), to inpatient medical units (6 percent to 14 percent).[7] Because depressed patients in primary care settings often present with somatic symptoms rather than complaints of depressed mood, clinicians must be proficient in assessing and managing depression. Skillful differential diagnosis of depressive symptoms is essential, because major depression commonly presents as an associated problem in patients with other physical illnesses.[8] In addition, 10 percent to 15 percent of all depressions may actually be caused by a physical illness or medication.[1]

Depression is Underdiagnosed and Undertreated

Despite the high prevalence of depressive symptoms and major depressive episodes in patients of all ages, numerous studies indicate that approximately half of all cases of major depression often go undiagnosed or are undertreated in primary care settings.[1] A careful review of the literature concerning under-recognition reported that depressive diagnosis may be missed in primary care in 10 percent to 50 percent of cases, depending on the setting studied and the severity of the symptoms reported.[9]

Several theories have been offered to explain these findings, such as health services issues (e.g., limited time), sociocultural barriers (stigma), and physician and patient knowledge level or skills.[10,11] Patient denial, cognitive impairment, lack of awareness of depressive symptoms, or inability to articulate symptoms compound the difficulty of detecting depression in primary care.

Even when diagnosed, depression may go untreated or partially treated. Katon and colleagues report that 55 percent of diagnosed patients in primary care receive no treatment, and 34 percent receive inadequate treatment.[7] Both physician and patient variables probably account for this finding. Patient nonadherence, resistance to diagnosis, and subtherapeutic dosages of antidepressants all contribute to insufficient management. Social forces, cultural factors, and low reimbursement rates also lead to inadequate treatment of depression. Because many employment, health, disability, and life insurance practices discriminate against individuals with mental illness, physicians and patients alike may avoid the diagnosis of depression.

Depression Causes Significant Morbidity and Mortality

Suicide is a very real and common consequence of unrecognized or inadequately treated depression. Regier reports that depressive disorders account for 16,000 deaths annually.[12] Approximately 15 percent of patients with severe depression lasting at least one month succeed in killing themselves. Half of those who eventually commit suicide see their physicians within the month preceding their death, underscoring the importance of prompt identification and treatment of depression.[13] Increased age is also a risk factor; it has been reported that 75 percent of elderly patients committing suicide had seen a PCP shortly before their death.[14]

Major depression is a risk factor for death in patients with general medical illnesses. Patients with major depression after myocardial infarction are three times more likely to die within the subsequent year than nondepressed patients; and depressed patients admitted to nursing homes are 56 percent more likely to die in the subsequent year than nondepressed nursing home patients, controlling for severity of other physical illnesses.[15,16]

Perhaps less obvious are the consequences of depression on personal lives and interpersonal relationships. Patients with depression may experience significant physical, social, and occupational difficulties. The Rand Medical Outcomes Study demonstrated that patients with depressive symptoms, with or without a major depressive disorder, had worse physical functioning, less social interaction, and spent more days in bed than patients with seven other general medical conditions such as arthritis, hypertension, and diabetes.[17]

The Economics of Depression

Depressive disorders represent a major national public health problem, costing approximately $43.1 billion annually. With only $7.7 billion attributed to direct treatment costs, the remaining expenses reflect reduced productivity, absenteeism, and mortality.[5] Depressed patients also contribute to escalating medical costs through extensive utilization of services, including outpatient visits, laboratory procedures, and hospitalizations.[2] In examining records of the top 10 percent of utilizers of primary care, Katon found evidence of recurrent depression in approximately one-third of the patients, and noted that over two-thirds of depressed patients made more than six visits per year to PCPs for somatic complaints.[18] Affective disorders, associated with increased rates of accidents and substance abuse, lead to even greater utilization of medical services.[1]

Signs and Symptoms of Depression

Patients and physicians often think of depression as a symptom of social maladjustment, personal weakness, or even divine retribution. This accounts for the stigma still attached to this disorder. Depression actually represents a clinical syndrome with associated biologic changes, characterized by a specific cluster of signs and symptoms that form the basis for diagnosis. Depression presents in three distinct forms: 1) major depression; 2) chronic depression, or "dysthymia" in the *Diagnostic and Statistical Manual of Mental Disorders*, Fourth edition *(DSM-IV)*; and 3) minor depression, called "adjustment disorder with depressed mood" or "depressive disorder not otherwise specified (NOS) in *DSM-IV*.[19]

Major Depression

There are nine signs and symptoms of major depression identified in *DSM-IV*, which can be categorized into four groups:

1. *Depressed mood most of the day, nearly every day.* Subjective feelings of sadness or emptiness, or observed tearfulness
2. *Anhedonia.* Markedly diminished interest or pleasure in all or almost all activities
3. *Physical symptoms.* Fatigue or loss of energy, significant appetite or weight change, sleep disturbances (either insomnia or hypersomnia), and psychomotor retardation or agitation
4. *Psychologic symptoms.* Feelings of worthlessness or inappropriate guilt, diminished ability to concentrate or indecisiveness, and recurrent thoughts of death or suicidal ideation

For a diagnosis of major depression, the patient must have exhibited either a depressed mood or a markedly diminished interest in pleasure or activities, and four other symptoms; three, if *both* depressed mood and diminished pleasure are present. These symptoms must be present for at least two weeks, occurring most of the day, nearly every day.

Chronic Depression (Dysthymia)

Chronic depression, or dysthymia, is characterized by persistent depressed mood present for more days than not, for at least two years. Depressed mood must be accompanied by two of the other depressive symptoms listed above. These symptoms must be present for at least two years, with no major depressive episode. Thus, dysthymic disorder does not represent a major depressive episode in partial remission. Many patients have experienced dysthymia for their entire adult lives, and may have come to accept depressed mood as a part of life.[20]

Minor Depression

Sadness is an appropriate response to stressful life events, such as job loss, death of a family member, loss of a close friend, health impairment, marital difficulties, or financial hardship. When the reaction appears excessive or continues for an inordinate amount of time, these patients are considered to have an adjustment reaction with depressed mood. Other patients may have mixed depressed mood and anxiety symptoms, some of which recur on an intermittent basis. Patients with one of these depressive disorders that do not fit well into any other category can be diagnosed with the syndrome of minor depression. These minor forms of depression are distinguished from major depression by absence of the full complement of five depressive symptoms, and from chronic depression by their shorter duration. If at any time, however, the symptomology changes, the diagnosis and management strategy should be adjusted accordingly.

Management Strategies

Once identified, depression can almost always be treated successfully, either with medication, psychotherapy, or a combination of both. Not all patients respond to the same therapy, but a patient who fails to respond to the first treatment plan is likely to respond to a change in strategy. Management depends largely on the severity of functional impairment, as judged by both the clinician and patient. Establishing a partnership with the patient promotes adherence to the treatment plan. Realistic goals can be set when patient preferences are respected. Enlisting the support of significant others also enhances the efficacy of mutually agreed-upon management strategies.

Major Depression

Mild forms of major depression, found in patients who meet criteria for major depression but who lack significant functional impairment, may respond equally well to psychotherapy or pharmacotherapy. Moderate to severe depression, however, should be treated with pharmacotherapy. A combination of pharmacotherapy and psychotherapy may be superior to either approach alone and proves particularly useful in patients with significant psychosocial problems.

Chronic Depression

Supportive, regularly scheduled visits with the PCP may be helpful for the management of chronic depression. A cautious trial of pharmacotherapy may be undertaken; however, data supporting the efficacy of drug therapy in chronic depression is still limited. The syndrome of dysthymia can be very frustrating to manage because of its chronicity and the tenacity of symptoms. Referral to a mental health specialist should be considered for patients who do not improve after initial management efforts.

Minor Depression

Because most cases of minor depression are self-limiting, a period of one to two months of watchful waiting may be sufficient for patients with mild impairment. If symptoms do not improve or impairment continues, regular supportive visits with the physician may be beneficial. Patients with moderate or severe impairment may be referred for mental health consultation. Despite the fact that no adequate scientific studies have been completed to support the efficacy of pharmacotherapy in patients with adjustment disorder or depressed mood NOS, anecdotal clinical experience suggests that a cautious trial of antidepressant medication may be beneficial.

Pharmacotherapy

In most cases, major depression is treated in primary care with a combination of patient education and antidepressant medication, or in combination with supportive office counseling. Efficacious antidepressants have been available for over 40 years, but newer agents offer the advantage of fewer side effects, resulting in greater patient acceptance. Older heterocyclic antidepressants (tricyclics, maprotiline, and amoxapine) are often associated with troubling side effects, including anticholinergic (dry mouth, constipation, urinary retention, etc.), antihistaminic (sedation), antiadrenergic (postural hypotension), and cardiac (quinidine-like delayed conduction). Because of a low therapeutic index, they are often lethal in overdose. In addition, older antidepressants often need to be titrated, rendering them more problematic for a PCP to use due to time limitations.

Consequently, the new agents have become increasingly popular for the first-line pharmacotherapy of depression, despite their generally higher cost. If cost factors become paramount, or there is no response to new agents, heterocyclic agents retain importance in the treatment arsenal. The two most useful older agents are nortriptylene (Pamelor or Aventyl), which has an established therapeutic window (blood level) with relatively less postural hypotension than other tricyclics, and desipramine (Norpramin), which has the lowest level of anticholinergic side effects of the tricyclic drugs.[1]

The introduction of the selective serotonin reuptake inhibitor (SSRI), fluoxetine (Prozac), in the late 1980s heralded a new era in the pharmacotherapy of depression. For the first time, a medication with fewer side effects became available for treatment of depression in medical practice. More than 19 million individuals throughout the world have now been treated with fluoxetine. Five other similarly effective new agents have now been introduced in the United States. Two of these five are SSRIs: paroxetine (Paxil), and sertraline (Zoloft). The other new agents, buproprion (Wellbutrin), venlafaxine (Effexor), and nefazodone (Serzone) have different chemical structures and mechanisms of action (Table 1).

In comparison to the heterocyclic agents, the new antidepressants are relatively free of dangerous side effects, are not lethal in overdose (when not combined with other medications), and are, for the most part, better tolerated. Despite their higher

TABLE 1. ANTIDEPRESSANTS: DOSAGES AND SIDE EFFECTS

Antidepressants	Sedating Effect	Anticholinergic Effect	Orthostatic Effect	Effective Dosage Range
Heterocyclic Antidepressants				
Tricyclics				
Amitriptyline (Elavil)	+++	+++	+++	75–300 mg
Desipramine (Norpramin)	+	+	+	75–250 mg
Doxepine (Sinequan)	+++	+++	+++	75–300 mg
Imipramine (Tofranil)	++	+++	+++	75–300 mg
Nortriptyline (Pamelor)	++	++	+	50–150 mg
Protriptyline (Vivactyl)	+	++	+	10–40 mg
Trimipramine (Surmontil)	+++	++	++	75–300 mg
Other Heterocyclics				
Amoxapine (Asendin)	++	++	++	150–600 mg
Maprotiline (Ludiomil)	++	+	++	150–225 mg
Trazodone (Desryl)	+++	0	++	200–600 mg
New Agents				
SSRIs				
Fluoxetine (Prozac)	0	0	0	20–80 mg
Paroxetine (Paxil)	0	+	0	20–50 mg
Sertraline (Zoloft)	0	0	0	50–200 mg
Other New Agents				
Buprorion (Wellbutrin)	0	0	0	150–450 mg
Venlafaxine (Effexor)	+	0	0	75–375 mg
Nefazodone (Serzone)	+	0	0	300–600 mg

0 = None, + = Slight, ++ = Moderate, +++ = Marked

per unit cost, they may be cost-effective compared to heterocyclic drugs due to fewer side effects, better patient adherence, and fewer follow-up visits to titrate dose and monitor side effects. The most common side effects of SSRIs are agitation, gastrointestinal distress, insomnia, and sexual dysfunction (decreased libido or difficulty reaching orgasm). These generally occur in less than 20 percent of patients and require discontinuation of medication in less than 5 percent. Despite the small incidence of agitation or insomnia, these agents can be used in depressed patients with anxiety or insomnia, since SSRIs usually lead to improved sleep and decreased anxiety within two to three weeks. Adjuvant agents, such as hydroxyzine, diphenhydramine, or lorazepam, can be used in the short term to manage underlying or treatment-emergent anxiety or insomnia.

The side effects of venlafaxine and buprorion are similar to the effects of SSRIs. In high doses, venlafaxine can cause persistent blood pressure elevation, and buproprion (in high doses) is associated with an increased risk of seizures. Buprorion is generally safe, but should not be used in patients at risk for seizures, and no single dose should exceed 150 mg. This drug, however, can be a good choice for patients with sexual side effects secondary to SSRIs. The newest agent, nefazodone, is a proserotonergic agent (not an SSRI) that may cause fewer sexual side effects but may be slightly sedating, although clinical experience is still limited.

Patient Follow-up

While all depressed patients need regularly scheduled appointments, it is especially important for those who have initially been prescribed an antidepressant. The physician should see the patient within two weeks to monitor effects of the medication, to check for adherence, and to offer support. Patient response can best be evaluated approximately six weeks after reaching a therapeutic dose of the antidepressant agent (which may take several weeks, depending both on the drug and the patient's response). The use of a physician and/or patient outcome assessment instrument is suggested to help physicians evaluate the magnitude of response (Figure 1). An increase in dose or the introduction of a new medication may be indicated if response to the original agent is insufficient. After attaining an adequate antidepressant response, the patient should be re-evaluated in another six weeks to ensure that remission has been sustained. Psychiatric evaluation may be appropriate at this time, if the response to treatment is inadequate.

Physician encouragement is particularly important in the interval between beginning treatment and evaluating outcome. The hopelessness that accompanies depression can interfere with the patient's ability to note improvement, although progress may be apparent to others. In the absence of support by the physician and significant others, depressed patients may see a perceived lack of progress as further evidence of their inadequacy, thereby exacerbating their hopelessness and perhaps triggering nonadherence.

Psychologic Approaches

Patients with minor depression, chronic depression, and mild to moderate major depression may benefit from a short course—approximately 8 to 12 weeks—of counseling or psychotherapy. Two forms of psychotherapy have proven effective in the treatment of depression: cognitive behavioral therapy and interpersonal therapy. These therapies are time-limited, focused on current problems, and aimed at symptom resolution rather than personality change. While supportive office counseling by the PCP has never been empirically tested, many physicians treating depression combine this intervention with pharmacotherapy and achieve seemingly beneficial results.

Cognitive Behavioral Therapy

Many depressed patients view themselves, the world, and the future with recurrent negativism. Cognitive behavioral therapy focuses on revising maladaptive processes of thinking, perceptions, attitudes, and beliefs. Emphasis is placed on identifying positive experiences, experimenting with new behaviors, and gradually progressing to more difficult situations. By challenging negative interpretations and reinforcing positive experiences, the therapist facilitates internalization of a more positive outlook on life.

Patient Name: _____

DSM-IV Checklist
Flowsheet

Symptom Ratings: 0 Absent   1 Mild   2 Moderate   3 Severe

	Date	Date	Date	Date	Date
Medication(s)/Dose(s): _____ _____ _____	___ ___ ___	___ ___ ___	___ ___ ___	___ ___ ___	___ ___ ___
I. Depressed mood					
II. Anhedonia					
III. Physical Symptoms					
A. Sleep disorder					
B. Appetite or weight change					
C. Low energy					
D. Psychomotor change					
IV. Psychological Symptoms					
A. Poor concentration					
B. Low self-esteem or guilt					
C. Suicidal ideation					
DSM-IV Score Sum of the nine symptoms above					
Comments:					

Figure 1

Interpersonal Therapy

Interpersonal conflict and social isolation can be associated with depression. Interpersonal therapy is a time-limited approach to the clarification of interpersonal difficulties such as role disputes, prolonged grief reactions, or role transitions. The therapist and patient define the nature of the problem, identify solutions, and utilize skills to reach a resolution.

Supportive Office Counseling

Supportive office counseling is based on empathic listening to patients' perceptions of life stresses. It focuses on managing current difficulties by emphasizing the patient's strengths and available resources. Discussing practical approaches to daily living can simply be a matter of making commonsense suggestions, such as discouraging patients from assuming new stresses, and encouraging them to engage in pleasurable activities. Physicians can remind patients that negative thinking passes as the depression improves. In order to reap the benefit of increased social support, patients should generally be encouraged to increase their contacts with family, friends, and community groups.

Specialist Referral

At the time of diagnosis, patients should be prepared for the possibility of referral to a mental health specialist, with reassurance that consultation is not evidence of personal failure or rejection by the PCP. Conditions warranting psychiatric evaluation include the presence of suicidal ideation, psychosis, severe functional impairment, and treatment failure. Referral is also indicated when the physician is unsure of the diagnosis or feels unable to provide recommended treatment.

Mastering Communication Skills

Open-ended Questions

Physicians should allow patients to describe their chief complaints without interruption. This can be facilitated by using open-ended questions that cannot be answered with a simple "yes" or "no." Introductory open-ended questions (e.g., "How can I help you today?") should be followed by other open-ended questions or facilitation techniques, as described below. This allows patients to present their problems in their own words. Unfortunately, studies show that physicians tend to interrupt their patients, on average, within the first 18 seconds of the interview.[21] These interruptions lead to premature closure, diagnostic errors, and inefficiency.

Facilitation Techniques

Patients describing their concerns may need prompting to speak freely. The physician can facilitate additional commentary by using nonverbal cues, such as head nodding and silence, or verbal phrases such as "Tell me more about it," or "Go on, please." Sometimes it is helpful to repeat the last phrase of the patient's sentence or simply nod, while saying "uh-huh." The silence that follows may facilitate further discussion. A truly loquacious patient may need help staying focused. A gentle interruption, such as "I'm glad your Aunt Thelma is doing so much better, but right now I'm concerned about your headaches, and I'd like to hear a little more about them," can be used.

Surveying

Sometimes initial complaints divert attention from more significant underlying concerns. Divulging issues loaded with personal embarrassment, shame, or fear requires a level of comfort with the physician. Thus, after the patient's presenting complaint has been addressed, the physician should encourage patients to discuss any other concerns. For example, "Before we go into further discussion about your headaches, I'd like to hear about anything else that may be bothering you." This open-ended statement is more productive than the closed version, "Are there any other problems?," which may lead to patient denial. Many patients view physicians as providers of traditional medical services, and may need some prompting to discuss depressed mood or related concerns.

Physicians may be apprehensive that a surveying question might lead to a plethora of complaints. Opening a Pandora's box of emotional issues can occupy time that the physician simply does not have. To the contrary, however, surveying can avoid the troublesome "door knob" or "Oh, by the way, doctor..." question that is time-consuming and distressing. These interactions may occur in 20 percent of all physician-patient encounters.[22] Surveying and clarifying issues in early stages of the interview actually saves time and decreases frustration. Furthermore, such techniques may be instrumental in drawing attention to the patient's most distressing problems.

Assessing Mood, Anhedonia, and Other Depressive Symptoms

Physicians should inquire directly about mood, using open-ended questions and facilitation techniques. "How's your mood been lately?" may be more productive than the closed question, "Have you been depressed?" The latter requires patients to understand depression and to make their own diagnosis. Furthermore, fear of social stigma may invite denial, defensiveness, or irritation in response to direct questions about depression. Patients often prefer terminology such as feeling "down," "irritable," or "not myself lately," because depression is so commonly viewed as a sign of personal weakness.

Patients who deny a depressed mood should be screened for anhedonia. This is particularly important in anxious patients not cognizant of an underlying depressed mood, in patients with chronic general medical illness, and in those recently subjected to acute stresses. Examples of screening questions for anhedonia include, "What are you doing for fun?" "Does your pain/anxiety/grief keep you from golfing/bowling/gardening/seeing the grandchildren?"

An indication of either depressed mood or anhedonia signals the need to screen for other symptoms of major depression. The physician might ask, "How's your energy level been lately?" "How have you been sleeping?" and "How's your appetite been?" Direct questions can be used to assess loss of self-esteem ("Have you been down on yourself or feeling guilty?"), lack of concentration ("How's your concentration been lately?"), and suicidal thoughts.[23]

Assessing Functioning

Patients should be asked in what ways their symptoms have caused physical, social, and role impairment; for example, "How has your pain affected your ability to work?" or "Has the pain affected your sexual life?" Querying patients about function in this way encourages discussion of underlying emotional distress and facilitates the efficient diagnosis of mental disorders. Once depressive symptoms have been revealed, questions about function also help the physician evaluate the severity of a depressive syndrome.

Assessing Patient Expectations

Asking patients about their expectations of care can reveal underlying reasons for visits, helps detect emotional causes for complaints, and promotes partnership between physician and patient. Understanding patient expectations enables physicians to better satisfy patients, facilitates patient acceptance of diagnoses, and promotes mutual agreement on treatment plans.

Responding to Patients' Emotions

By accepting intense feelings of sadness, anger, and anxiety in a nonthreatening manner, physicians build rapport and establish a trusting relationship with depressed patients. Failure to address emotions reflects lack of physician concern, leading patients to feel distant and defensive. Two techniques that are useful in responding to patients' emotions are reflection and legitimation.[24]

Reflection

Reflection acknowledges the patient's emotion by naming it in a nonaccusatory, nonjudgmental way. For example, "It seems that talking about this pain you've been having upsets you," or "Sounds like a pretty frustrating situation for you." These statements convey physician empathy, build rapport, and elicit further information about crucial issues that may be causing emotional distress.

Reflecting comments used during the course of an interview can change in character and intensity. Choose familiar phrases, use nonthreatening words, and avoid overstating the emotion. Patients more easily hear that they seem to be frustrated or are feeling down than that they are angry or in despair. If the emotions are understated, the patient can amplify: "I'm not just frustrated, I'm angry." Inappropriate labeling of an emotion can create barriers to effective communication by evoking feelings of shame, guilt, or defensiveness. A patient's unwillingness to pursue a subject should be acknowledged and respected.

Legitimation

Legitimation refers to statements that signal physician acceptance of the patient's feelings. "I can understand that your pain is tiring and upsetting to you." Or, "It makes sense that after losing a good job you'd be anxious and worried." Another form of legitimation puts the patient's experience within the context of a universal response. "Many people would feel that way." "I've had lots of patients go through what you've described."

Assessing Suicidal Ideation

Studies indicate that approximately 80 percent of seriously depressed patients think about suicide. Patients suspected of suicidal ideation should be directly but sensitively questioned about thoughts of hurting themselves, with a gradual progression toward more focused questioning. Begin by asking several questions to ascertain the presence of hopelessness. "How does the future look to you?" "Do you think things will get better for you?" Although seriously depressed patients often express a deep sense of hopelessness, not everyone with a feeling of despair contemplates suicide. Differentiating the suicidal patient requires focused questioning: "Living with pain/anxiety/illness can be very difficult. Do you sometimes wish your life was over?" "Do you ever have thoughts of hurting yourself?" "Do you sometimes wish you were dead?"

There is no evidence to suggest that raising the issue of suicide will suggest the idea or provoke the patient to action. Discussing the subject may actually relieve some of the anxiety patients have about suicidal thoughts, and may reduce their risk of suicide.[25]

Assessing Suicide Risk

Patients with an equivocal response to questions about suicidal ideation should be probed for evidence of specific plans. "Tell me if you've thought about how you might hurt yourself." "What methods have you considered?" Patients with specific plans are at greater risk than those who only think about suicide or express reservations because of the impact their death will have on family or significant others. In addition, other risk factors for suicide include social isolation, history of a previous suicide attempt, alcoholism, chronic physical illness, and age.

Patients judged to be at risk should be referred immediately to a mental health professional. When this is impossible, the physician may ask patients to enter into a "no suicide contract," whereby they agree to contact the physician if they feel unable to control suicidal impulses. Patients who refuse to enter into the agreement or who are unconvincing are candidates for immediate hospitalization or involuntary commitment.

Presenting the Diagnosis and Treatment Plan

Before presenting the diagnosis, the physician should determine the patient's understanding of depression in order to allay fears and educate the patient relative to his or her perceptions. Patients may need encouragement to reveal their fears, but addressing those views can increase the efficiency of the interview and acceptance of the diagnosis.

Providing the Diagnosis

Statements used in presenting the diagnosis should be simple and succinct. Patients are anxious at the time of diagnosis and should only be given small, discrete blocks of information. Once they have accepted the diagnosis, it is appropriate to explain the diagnosis in greater detail.

Responding to Patient Emotions

After communicating the diagnosis, pause and allow the patient to react and to ask questions. The stigma associated with mental disorders may cause patients to become angry, frustrated, or teary, and may sometimes cause them to reject the diagnosis of depression. Those who do not verbalize their emotions may exhibit facial expressions, hand gestures, body movements, and other nonverbal cues indicating their distress. Verbal and nonverbal expressions of emotion should be directly acknowledged (reflection) and validated (legitimation).

Communicating the Treatment Plan

The physician should stress that depression is a medical illness involving a chemical imbalance, and that it is highly treatable. It is not a sign of personal weakness. Recommendations for treatment should be offered, with the caveat that pharmacotherapy may take several weeks to take effect, and patients will need to follow the regimen for several months to ensure a full, sustained recovery.

Up to 50 percent of depressed patients in primary care will stop treatment within three months of starting.[26] Seven specific physician interventions have been identified with improved patient adherence to antidepressant treatment plans. They include 1) asking about prior use of antidepressants; 2) instructing patients to take medication daily; 3) explaining that it may take two to four weeks to notice an effect of treatment; 4) advising patients to engage in pleasant activities; 5) reminding them to continue taking medication even if they are getting better; 6) asking patients to call if they are about to stop taking the medication; and 7) informing patients what to do if they have questions.[26]

After providing the patient with an opportunity to respond and ask questions, review agreed-upon treatment plans to assess patient understanding and to increase the likelihood of adherence.

Referral Skills for Specialty Consultation

Patients who are severely disabled, psychotic, suicidal, or refractory to treatment will generally require a psychiatric referral. Patients with psychosocial issues too complex to manage in a primary care setting may also benefit from mental health evaluation. Patient acceptance of the referral is greater if this possibility has been broached at the time of initial diagnosis. Patients should be informed that a physician's request for psychiatric assessment is for consultation and improved care, just as similar referrals are made to other specialists, such as cardiologists or gastroenterologists.

Summary

Depression is a medical disorder commonly seen in primary care. Despite its significance as a major public health problem, it is often underdiagnosed and undertreated. Effective treatment of depression requires a compassionate approach, skillful care, long-term follow-up, and very often, active pharmacotherapy. Bolstered by a positive attitude toward its diagnosis and management, effective communication skills, and appropriate psychiatric back-up, the primary care practitioner can confidently assess and manage this highly treatable disorder.

References

1. Rush AJ, Golden WE, Hall GW, et al: Depression in Primary Care: Clinical Practice Guidelines. Agency for Healthcare Policy and Research. AHCPR Publication no. 93-0550. U.S. Department of Health and Human Services, Rockville MD, 1993.
2. Simon GE, Von Korff M, Barlou W, et al: Healthcare costs of primary care patients with recognized depression. Arch Gen Psychiatry 52:850–856, 1995.
3. Broadhead WE, Blazer DG, George LK, et al: Depression, disability days, and days lost from work in a prospective epidemiologic survey. JAMA 264:2524–2550, 1990.
4. Conti DJ, Burton WN: The economic impact of depression in a workplace. J Occup Med 36:983–988, 1994.
5. Greenburg PE, Stiglin LR, Finklestein SN, et al: Depression: a neglected major illness. J Clin Psychiatry 54:419–424, 1993.
6. Regier D, Narrow W, Rae R, et al: The de facto US mental and addictive disorders service system. Arch Gen Psychiatry 50:85–94, 1993.
7. Katon W, Schulberg H: Epidemiology of depression in primary care. Gen Hosp Psychiatry 14:237–247, 1992.
8. Cohen-Cole SA, Kaufman K: Major depression in physical illness: diagnosis, prevalence, and antidepressant treatment (a ten year review: 1982-1992). Depression 1:181–204, 1993.
9. Barrett JE: The role of psychiatry in the management of depressive disorders in primary care. In: Michels R, et al (eds) Psychiatry. JB Lippincott, Philadelphia PA (in press).
10. Shulberg HC, McClelland M: A conceptual model for educating primary care providers in the diagnosis and treatment of depression. Gen Hosp Psychiatry 9:1–10, 1987.
11. Cohen SA, Raju M: Overcoming barriers to integration of primary care and behavioral healthcare: focus on knowledge and skills. Behavioral Healthcare Tomorrow 5:30–35, 1996.
12. Regier D, Hirschfield R, Goodwin F, et al: The NIMH depression awareness, recognition, and treatment program: structure, aims, and scientific basis. Am J Psychiatry 145:1351–1357, 1988.
13. Barraclough B, Bunch J, Nelson B, et al: A hundred cases of suicide: clinical aspects. Br J Psychiatry 125:355–373, 1974.
14. NIH Consensus Development Panel on Depression in Late Life: Diagnosis and treatment of depression in late life. JAMA 268:1018–1024, 1992.
15. Frasure-Smith N, Lesperance F, Talajic M: Depression following myocardial infarction: impact on 6-months survival. JAMA 270:1819–1825, 1993.
16. Rovner BW, German PS, Brant LJ, et al: Depression and mortality in nursing homes. JAMA 265:993–996, 1991.
17. Wells KB, Stewart A, Hayes RD, et al: The functioning and well-being of depressed patients: results of the medical outcomes study. JAMA 262:914–919, 1989.
18. Katon W: The epidemiology of depression in medical care. Int J Psychiatry Med 17:93–112, 1987.
19. American Psychiatric Association: Diagnostic and Statistical Manual of Mental Disorders, Fourth edition. American Psychiatric Association Press, Washington DC, 1994.
20. Kocsis JH, Klein DN, (eds): Diagnosis and Treatment of Chronic Depression. The Guilford Press, New York NY, 1995.
21. Beckman HB, Frankel RM: The effect of physician behavior on the collection of data. Ann Intern Med 101:692–696, 1984.
22. White J, Levinson W, Roter D: "Oh by the way...": the closing moments of the medical visit. J Gen Intern Med 9:24–28, 1994.
23. Cohen-Cole SA, Brown F, McDaniel JS: Assessment of grief and depression in the medically ill. In: Psychiatric Care of the Medical Patient. Edited by A Stoudemire and B Fogel. Lippincott, New York NY, 1993.

24. Cohen-Cole SA: The Medical Interview: The Three-Function Approach. Mosby, St. Louis MO, 1991.
25. Cohen-Cole SA, Mance R: Evaluating the suicidal patient. In: The Medical Interview: Clinical Care, Education, and Research. Edited by M Lipkin, S Putnam, and A Lazare. Springer-Verlag, New York NY, 1995.
26. Lin E, Von Korff M, Katon W: The role of the primary care physician in patient's adherence to antidepressant therapy. Med Care 33:67-74, 1995.

Chapter 15

Anxiety Disorders in Primary Care

Mack Lipkin, Jr., M.D.

Anxiety disorders vex primary care clinicians more than most mental disorders because they most often present in primary care as physical symptoms. In addition, they often require prescription medications that make generalists uneasy, such as benzodiazepines. Since anxiety often presents with physical manifestations, the patients believe their problem is a physical disease. Attempts to make referrals to mental health professionals often anger patients and cause at least some to leave the practice or the health plan.[1]

Like most major categories of mental disorder, the anxiety disorders are truly biopsychosocial. They are complex diseases with biological, psychological, and social components and complications. The seven anxiety disorders are panic disorder, generalized anxiety disorder, adjustment disorder with anxious mood, post-traumatic stress disorder, obsessive-compulsive disorder, simple phobia, and social phobia. The first five of these commonly present in primary care. Simple and social phobias are often first detected by the primary care practitioner (PCP) but are seldom brought up spontaneously, so that awareness of them and their crippling manifestations can empower the primary care clinician to prevent future problems.

Modern primary care approaches to the seven anxiety disorders have three treatment components: 1) recognizing and diagnosing the disorder early and accurately; 2) tailoring specific treatment to the diagnosis; and 3) preventing long-term complications such as agoraphobia, work disruption, and suicide.

Diagnosis and Description

The anxiety disorders are seven groups of conditions that share common symptoms and physical complaints (Table 1). They also include feelings of agitation, derealization ("Am I real?" "Is this real?") and depersonalization ("Am I really here?"); panic or fear; and tension or arousal.[2]

Panic Disorder

This disorder is characterized by spontaneous and often terrifying "attacks," lasting from 10 to 60 minutes and including four or more of the symptoms in Table 2. The person must either have four attacks or one attack followed by the persistent fear of future attacks. Without treatment, persons with panic disorder may develop *agoraphobia*, a fear of leaving one's home that can be totally disabling. Some literature suggests that persons with panic disorder are at heightened risk of suicide.

TABLE 1. ANXIETY SYMPTOMS, DIFFERENTIAL DIAGNOSES, AND TESTS

Symptom	Differentials	Tests
Lump in throat	Dysphagia	Manometry
	Cancer of the esophagus	Barium swallow
	Esophageal obstructions	Multiple tests
Tachycardia	Arrhythmias	Holter monitor
	Thyroid disease	Thyroid function tests
	Medications	
Diarrhea	Bacterial infection	Stool smear, culture
	Viral infection	Stool smear, culture
	Parasitic infection	Stool for ova/parasites
	Inflammatory bowel disease	Sigmoidoscopy
		Bowel biopsy
		Barium enema
Muscle aches	Myositis	CPK enzymes
	Musculoskeletal pain	Orthopedic/sports consult
Dry mouth	Dehydration	Specific gravity
	Medication	
Frequent urination	Bacterial infection	Culture and sensitivity
	Chemical cystitis	Urology consult
		Cystoscopy
Shortness of breath	Cardiac disease	Cardiac work-up
	Pulmonary disease	Pulmonary work-up
Dizziness	Pre-syncope	Holter monitor
		Tilt table
		EEG

Generalized Anxiety Disorder (GAD)

This disorder involves the presence of almost constant anxiety symptoms. It can vary in intensity and is associated with major psychological and social disruption. If the disorder goes undetected, patients may exhibit a downward spiral of desperate behavior intended to correct the problem. Such patients often respond quickly and completely to adequate doses of anxiolytics; thus, they may appear to suspicious PCPs to be seeking sedatives.

Adjustment Disorder with Anxious Mood

This disorder is one of the most common psychiatric diagnoses among patients with serious physical illness. In contrast to panic disorder and GAD, adjustment disorder with anxious mood has a specific precipitant, occurs shortly after the incident, and is of brief duration. It differs from normal grief or adjustments in being more specifically anxious in nature and pathological in extent.

Post-Traumatic Stress Disorder (PTSD)

This disorder is always precipitated by an event or series of events that constitute the "trauma." While the Vietnam veteran has become stereotypical of the condition in recent years, the trauma is more commonly caused by surgery, a major illness, rape, or abuse.

Obsessive-Compulsive Disorder

Persons with this disorder have frequent episodes of socially and/or psychologically disruptive thoughts (obsessions) or behaviors (compulsions). There is partial evidence of an organic cause in these patients; most have some response to pharmacologic intervention.

Simple Phobia

Simple phobia is excessive fear and anxiety of some specific normal object or situation, such as the elevator, airplane, snakes, or small places. These patients also show heightened anxiety when approaching their feared object.

Social Phobia

This phobia is an abnormally intense fear of speaking or performing in groups or social situations. Persons with this condition may not perform up to their mental capacity in school (when grading depends on class participation) or at work. They may select isolating interests and careers. The specific fear often involves being shamed or humiliated in front of others.

Cost Considerations

Anxiety disorders contribute substantially to overall medical costs because they are often approached as diagnoses of exclusion, resulting in unnecessary medical testing. Without proper diagnosis, there is also an increase in morbidity and mortality due to the anxiety disorder or other medical conditions. Consider the following case: A 45-year-old Caucasian man with a history of stable, chronic active hepatitis C and cardiac ventricular arrhythmia presented to the emergency room with chest pain, dizziness, sweating, and fear of death. In the emergency room he received an electrocardiogram, cardiac enzymes, liver enzymes, intravenous electrolytes, narcotic analgesics, chest x-ray, and cardiology consult. The cardiologist recommended admission to intensive care, thallium stress testing, and cardiac catheterization. Additionally, he recommended a gastrointestinal consult, due to the patient's history of chronic active hepatitic C; in turn, this consultant recommended liver biopsy and viral titers. The liver biopsy was complicated by bleeding, which required an additional two-day stay in the hospital. The total cost of his treatment was $13,000. Four days after discharge, the patient had another episode of chest pain and was referred to a different PCP who diagnosed panic disorder and prescribed an appropriate medication (costing only $1 per day). The symptoms resolved. This example is typical of the average patient with

TABLE 2. SYMPTOMS AND SIGNS ASSOCIATED WITH PANIC ATTACKS

Chest pain or discomfort
Shortness of breath or smothering
Palpitations, pounding heart, tachycardia
Sweating
Chills or hot flashes
Choking sensation
Nausea or abdominal distress
Trembling or shaking
Numbness or tingling (paresthesias)
Feeling dizzy, unsteady, faint, light-headed
Derealization or depersonalization
Fear of losing control and/or going crazy
Fear of dying

panic disorder, who sees approximately 10 physicians before diagnosis, each of whom performs testing and procedures.

Anxiety Disorders in the Primary Care Setting

The patient with an anxiety disorder usually presents to the PCP with a physical complaint. These complaints (Table 1) may include a lump in the throat, a speeding heart, sweaty palms or feet, weakness in the knees, diarrhea, nausea and vomiting, abdominal pain, shaking or trembling, twitching, fainting, feeling "uptight," inability to relax, muscle tension or pain, dryness of the mouth, frequent urination, inability to focus or concentrate, insomnia, and irritability. In Table 1, sample differential diagnoses of some of these symptoms and their work-ups are illustrated.

Anxiety disorders must be detected early if cost-effective treatment is to be provided. However, detection will remain difficult until PCPs learn more about these disorders, develop a high index of suspicion, and know how to make the diagnosis. There are several screening instruments that can detect common anxiety disorders with adequate sensitivity and specificity. However, they may be too cumbersome to administer in a busy primary care practice. Two instruments, the SDDS-PC and PRIME-MD, were developed for use in primary care (see Appendix 3 and Appendix 4).[4] They include screening questions for anxiety disorders. However, some studies suggest that even when practitioners are given screening test results, they do not change their treatment plan unless they receive specific education on these disorders and their management (see Chapter 13).

Assessment and Treatment of Specific Disorders

The assessment of the patient with possible anxiety disorder begins with clinical observation. Does he or she demonstrate signs of anxiety—nervousness, agitation, hand wringing, obsessive behaviors, or fearfulness? Does the patient complain of strange feelings or of not being himself or herself? Are there symptoms in multiple organ systems? When present, these constellations may suggest the patterns of panic disorder, GAD, adjustment disorder, post-traumatic stress disorder, or obsessive-compulsive disorder. These are described below. Often, screening questions are problematic in the patient with anxiety disorder, because these patients may already have been told that their symptoms are "all in their heads," and they will be sensitive to rejection or to having their symptoms dismissed again.[5,6]

Panic Disorder

Panic disorder has a lifetime prevalence of 1.5 percent, although many believe that a more realistic prevalence is closer to 3 to 4 percent.[7] Two-thirds of those with panic disorder are women. Of all the anxiety disorders, panic disorder is most likely to produce extensive and unnecessary work-up, misdiagnosis, and increased costs.

The diagnosis of panic disorder, or even a single panic attack, depends on the multiplicity of symptoms from different organ systems, usually a lack of precipitants (such as fear or stress), and the prominence of fear of another attack. Convincing a patient that the problem is panic disorder may be difficult. It is important to explain that the problem is a common biological problem with psychological manifestations, and that it responds well to treatment.

Effective treatment of panic disorder is critical, because patients have elevated levels of secondary depression and suicide attempts and completions. Clinicians can consider selective serotonin reuptake inhibitors (SSRIs), benzodiazepines, monamine oxidase inhibitors, and tricyclic antidepressants. Although paroxetine is currently the only SSRI approved by the Food and Drug Administration (FDA) for use in panic disorder, the others (sertraline and fluoxetine) are also effective. The starting dose of paroxetine for an adult should be 5-10 mg to avoid precipitating a panic attack. Dose should be increased slowly, if necessary, to control symptoms.

Benzodiazepines, such as lorazepam, clonazepam, and alprazolem are also effective. Many prefer to use the longer-acting lorazepam or clonazepam, because of the more gradual onset of action and the lower potential for abuse. The likelihood of benzodiazepine abuse is minimal if prescribed for patients with no prior history of substance abuse, and use is monitored. Monamine oxidase inhibitors, newer antidepressants, and tricyclic antidepressants (such as imipramine) are also effective in controlling symptoms. Most physicians start with benzodiazepines or SSRIs.

It is imperative to treat patients with adequate doses of medication for an appropriate period of time. Pharmacologic therapy should be continued for a minimum of three to six months. Those who stop taking medication within three months experience a 70 percent relapse rate. Most patients require two years or more of therapy before medication can be successfully discontinued.

Patients with phobic elements to their illness often require behavioral therapy to decrease disabling anxiety. These treatments, which utilize relaxation techniques and cognitive-behavioral therapy, help provide the patient with tools to manage their anxiety. If symptoms are untreated, they may progress to agoraphobia, for which desensitization may be needed. Some patients experience a chronic relapsing course with persistence of intermittent symptoms for years. Self-help groups can be helpful and rehabilitative in this population.[8]

Generalized Anxiety Disorder

The lifetime prevalence of GAD is less than 0.3 percent.[9] The cause and precipitants of this disorder are relatively unknown, but many patients have a specific life stress precipitant. The following case illustrates a typical presentation. A 25-year-old white female executive secretary presented at a free clinic in a disheveled and frightened state, demanding Valium. She stated that, while in college, she had experienced a gradual onset of intense anxiety with excessive worries about school and her future, accompanied by chest and abdominal pain and palpitations. She sought medical care, had numerous evaluations, and was hospitalized for chest pains. In the hospital she was prescribed a benzodiazepine for sleep, which caused her symptoms to almost disappear for a few hours, only to gradually return. The physician refused to prescribe Valium for her, resulting in her discharge against medical advice and her purchasing of Valium on the street. On a self-administered dose of 10 mg. every six hours, she was able to graduate college with honors. However, she later lost her source for Valium and began to experience the same symptoms. She later found a physician who was willing prescribe this dosage, and she improved once more.

The hallmark of GAD is continuous cognitive anxiety, accompanied by varied physical symptoms. Patients have excessive worry about two or more life problems and six symptoms from the groups of motor tension (trembling, tensions and aches, fatigue, etc.), autonomic hyperactivity (palpitations, sweating, frequent urination, etc.), vigilance or scanning (on edge, startles easily, irritable and impatient, etc.). There is no pharmacologic or disease precipitant (see Table 3). The usual patient has a worried presentation, but more severe cases may be anxious about the return of physical and emotional symptoms.[10]

These patients often need long-term anxiolytic therapy with either benzodiazepines or other anxiolytic drugs such as buspirone.[11] While the onset of action of buspirone is generally two to four weeks, it does not impair memory or coordination and is not associated with abuse. Antidepressants such as trazodone and imipramine have also been shown to be effective. Patients may also need supportive therapy and cognitive-behavioral techniques while transitioning back to higher functioning. Other therapies may include relaxation and other "self-regulatory" training.[12] The prognosis for patients with GAD is unclear, but the disorder is often chronic and may fluctuate in intensity and severity. Educating patients about this disorder, including the variations in their illness, may alleviate reactive anxiety resulting from having a chronic disease.

Adjustment Disorder with Anxious Mood

Adjustment disorder with anxious mood is an anxious response that is beyond normal in the extent, variety, or disruptiveness of symptomology to a life event. It occurs within three months of the event and lasts less than six months (although one can speak of a chronic adjustment disorder if the response lasts longer than six months). It does not meet criteria for another anxiety disorder, and no confounding medical condition is present.[13] Estimates of the frequency of this disorder are inconsistent, but it is believed to be common. Prognosis of adjustment disorder is extremely good.

TABLE 3. COMMON MEDICAL CONDITIONS THAT MIMIC ANXIETY

Cardiac diseases
    Acute myocardial infarction
    Angina pectoris
    Congestive heart failure

Thyroid disease
    Graves disease
    Hashimoto's thyroiditis

Endocrine conditions
    Pheochromocytoma
    Hypoglycemia (insulin reactions)
    Hypoglycemia (insulin-secreting tumors)

Substance abuse
    Cocaine use
    Amphetamine excess
    Marijuana intoxication
    Halucinogen abuse

Caffeine excess

Medication side effects or overdose

Partial complex seizures

The disorder is illustrated in the case of a 41-year-old Hispanic woman who presented feeling faint, dizzy, and having abdominal pain of two weeks' duration. She was restless, jittery, and startled when her name was called in the waiting room. She had been in good health and was using no medications. Four weeks previously she had a spontaneous miscarriage, after seven years of attempting to become pregnant. She stated that she had experienced similar feelings when her younger brother died 35 years ago.

The key factor in making the diagnosis is eliciting the history of the stressor. Stressors most often involved are those most valent in a given population or subgroup. When available, these are reflected in the Holmes and Rahe scale for the specific community.[14] Death of a spouse, divorce, moving, death of other family members, illness, injury, violence, marriage, pregnancy, job change, and many others are among the stressful life events to be considered. Risk factors for an adjustment disorder include a history of prior adjustment disorder, divorced or separated marital status, past mental illness, and low socio-economic status.

Treatment should involve supportive counseling. It is essential to reassure the patient about the time-limited nature of the disorder and to encourage the verbalization of feelings about the precipitant event. Adjunctive treatments include relaxation methods, support groups, and continued supportive counseling. Medication is only needed when symptoms are disabling or disruptive. In these cases, the short-term use of benzodiazepines may be indicated.

Post-Traumatic Stress Disorder

The frequency of post-traumatic stress disorder, using stringent criteria, is estimated to be approximately 1 percent. However, 10 to 15 percent of the population experience some symptoms of this disorder. For example, an entrepreneur who was married with two teen-aged children developed chest pain, diaphoresis, pallor, anxious restlessness, and feelings of dread one day while playing tennis. He was rushed by ambulance to the hospital, where it was determined that he was having a significant myocardial infarction. As thrombolytic therapy was administered he lost consciousness while thinking that he was dying. He later awoke to find himself in intensive care, connected to myriad tubes and wires, with lights flashing and monitors beeping. After his emergency cardiac catheterization and bypass surgery, he recovered uneventfully and left the hospital after seven days. Three weeks later, he awoke imagining himself still in the recovery room, still in pain and dying. He had frequent and disruptive flashbacks to scenes from the hospital. Thoughts of the heart attack and surgery intruded often, and he began to withdraw from his family, from work, and from his former recreational pursuits. He became irritable, vigilant, and easily startled. These events continued for months. Eventually he lost his job and his marriage ended.

This case illustrates post-traumatic stress disorder in a medical setting.[15,16] The precipitants are often serious disruptions in life events, including severe illness, surgery, rape, physical violence, bodily integrity, natural disasters, and mass disasters (earthquakes, floods, plane crashes, war, etc.).[17] The patient described above illustrates the classic description of post-traumatic stress disorder. He experienced flashbacks, nightmares, intrusive thoughts, fear and avoidance of similar situations or settings, and overall feelings of numbness. This led to estrangement from others and from his work.

Mild cases often spontaneously resolve with time and supportive therapy, including discussion of the patient's feelings of loss of control, responsibility, or regret for actions not taken. More severe patients often require case management, psychiatric consultation, group therapy, vocational rehabilitation, and other team approaches to treatment. Relaxation training and education of family members may be of benefit.

Pharmacologic treatment may help with sleep and controlling obsessive thoughts. The most useful medications include tricyclic antidepressants (i.e., imipramine), SSRIs (i.e., fluoxetine), and monoamine oxidase inhibitors (i.e., phenelzine).[18] Support groups aimed at preventing or intervening in drug abuse or other maladaptive behaviors can also be effective. The majority of patients respond well to these interventions and recover substantially in six to twelve months. Others may progress to substance abuse, depression, and self-destructive outbursts that can be fatal.

Obsessive-Compulsive Disorder

This disorder has a 2.5 percent lifetime prevalence, with women affected 1.5 times more frequently than men. An illustrative case history is provided by a 22-year-old medical student who became upset during a lecture in which numerous infectious diseases were discussed. She found herself imagining situations in which she might contract one of these diseases. She began to wash her hands often, avoid classmates, and soon stopped going to lectures and places where she would have to mingle with large crowds. It became difficult for her to finish examinations because of her need to wash her hands. While she recognized that these concerns were irrational, she was unable to stop the behavior. Fearing that she would fail her classes, she went to her advisor who referred her to professional help.

These patients often present with complaints about their compulsive behavior only after it has become significantly disruptive. Ninety percent of patients have both obsessions and compulsions. The problem behavior (whether thought or action) must consume significant time (an hour or more each day), cause disruptive social or psychological functioning, and be upsetting.[19] The most common obsessions include fear of making mistakes, being humiliated or shamed, hurting other people, or being unclean. Common compulsions include cleaning, washing, counting and repeating, checking, arranging, making lists, organizing, and hoarding.

In recent years, pharmacologic treatment with clomipramine and SSRIs have become the mainstays of pharmacologic care. Studies suggest that while the SSRIs have better side effect profiles, they are not more effective than clomipramine.[20] Behavior therapies such as aversive conditioning, flooding, desensitization, response prevention, or implosion therapy may be used in primary care by adequately trained professionals. The essential techniques are to teach patients to expose themselves to the things they fear, to extinguish their disruptive thoughts, and to reduce or prevent the compulsive actions.

Up to 40 percent of patients do not respond to the initial treatment.[21] Few recover completely, but most benefit from medication combined with behavior therapy and support groups. Failing this, combination therapy with the addition of buspirone or fenfluramine may result in improvement, as can the combination of clomipramine and fluoxetine.

Simple Phobias

The lifetime prevalence of both simple and social phobias is approximately 12.5 percent, with women experiencing phobias twice as often as men. Presentation of a simple phobia is illustrated by the following case. Following the death of her pet dog, a 34-year-old woman journalist began to notice that her lifelong aversion to snakes had become an intense fear. For example, when she heard that someone on the bus had seen a person with a boa constrictor, she stopped taking public transportation. When she thought about snakes, she became diaphoretic, short of breath, and had palpitations. When she actually saw snakes in the window of a pet store, she hyperventilated and became so anxious that she was unable to go to work that day.

Phobias may be well circumscribed and handled by simple avoidance until the fear becomes severe enough to be dysfunctional and maladaptive. In the case described above, a psychologist trained in desensitization (teaching self-calming techniques and then introducing gradual exposure to the feared object) helped her reduce her anxiety toward snakes in ten weeks. Although she has relapses, she uses relaxation methods to induce remission of symptoms. When necessary, pharmacologic treatment can include a brief course of low doses of beta blockers (propanolol) and benzodiazepines for symptomatic anxiety reduction.

Social Phobias

A 28-year-old medical resident, who was regarded as a fine doctor, was required to make a series of conference presentations. He began missing some conferences, did not speak when he did attend, and seemed anxious. In contrast, he was vivacious and very effective when engaged in a one-on-one interaction. He had avoided group speaking and group activities since adolescence. He recognized that this was an incapacitating disability but felt humiliated discussing the problem.

Social phobias are more complex to treat; they usually require approaches that include cognitive and other behavior therapies. These involve teaching of social skills, flooding and desensitization, and relaxation techniques.[22] Anxiolytics, including benzodiazepines, beta blockers, monoamine oxidase inhibitors, and buspirone (in higher doses) may be useful adjuncts in social situations that induce fear.[23]

Additional Considerations

Differential Diagnoses

One of the principle reasons that physicians must be involved in the initial assessment and care of patients with anxiety disorders is that there are a substantial number of serious conditions that present with anxiety symptoms. Some of these are listed in Table 3.

Providing Treatment

The question of who should treat patients with anxiety disorders often depends on the training of the practitioner, the financing of healthcare systems, and the time available to the provider for ongoing care. Primary care practitioners are uniquely positioned to evaluate patients, as patients present to them first. Most primary care clinicians have an established rapport with their patients, many of whom will not accept a mental health referral. For these reasons, PCPs must begin to identify, diagnose, and provide appropriate treatment and referral for these complex disorders.

References

1. Lipkin M, Levinson W: The medical interview. In: Primary Care and General Medicine, Nobel J (ed). Primary Care Medicine. Mosby, St. Louis, MO, 1996, pp. 2–8.
2. DSM-IV-PC. American Psychiatric Association, Washington, D.C., 1995.
3. Friedman S, Jones JC, Chernen L, Barlow DH: Suicidal ideation and suicide attempts among patients with panic disorder: a survey of two outpatient clinics, Am J Psychiatry 5:680–685, 1992.
4. Spitzer et al: Utility of a new procedure for diagnosing mental disorders in primary care. The Prime-MD 1000 study. JAMA 242:1749–1756, 1994.
5. Lipkin M Jr., Kaplan C, Clark W, Novack DH: Teaching medical interviewing: the Lipkin model. In: The Medical Interview: Clinical Care, Education, and Research. Springer-Verlag, New York, NY, 1995.
6. Putnam SM, Lipkin M Jr., Lazare A, Kaplan C, Drossman D: Personality styles. In: The Medical Interview: Clinical Care, Education, and Research. Springer-Verlag, New York, NY, 1995.
7. Katon WJ, Von Korff M, Lin E: Panic disorder: relationship to high medical utilization. Am J Med 92:75–115, 1992.

8. Katon WJ: Panic disorder in the medical setting. American Psychiatric Press, Washington, D.C., 1991.
9. Robins LN, Regier DA (eds): Psychiatric disorders in America. Macmillan, New York, NY, 1991.
10. Goldberg D: Detection and assessment of emotional disorders in a primary care setting. Int J Ment Health 8:30-48, 1979.
11. Shader RI, Greenblatt DJ: Use of benzodiazepines in anxiety disorders. N Engl J Med 329:1398, 1993.
12. Benson H: The Relaxation Response. Morrow, New York NY, 1975.
13. Andreasen NC, Wasek P: Adjustment disorder in adolescents and adults. Arch Gen Psychiatry 37:1166-1170, 1980.
14. Holmes TH, Rahe RH: The social readjustment rating scale. J Psychosom Res 31:389-392, 1987.
15. Pilowski I: Cryptotrauma and "accident neurosis." Br J Psychiatry 147:310-311, 1985.
16. Kestrel RC, Sonnega A, Bromet EA, et al: Post-traumatic stress disorder in the National Comorbidity Study. Arch Gen Psychiatry 52:1048-1060, 1995.
17. Davidson JRT, Book SW, Colker JT, et al: Assessment of a new self-rating scale for post-traumatic stress disorder. Psychol Med 1997 (in press).
18. Davidson JRT: Post-traumatic stress disorder in primary care: diagnosis and pharmacologic treatment. Primary Psychiatry 4:23-29, 1997.
19. Karno M, Golding J, Sorenson S, Burnham MA: The epidemiology of obsessive-compulsive disorder in five U.S. communities. Arch Gen Psychiatry 45:1094-1099, 1988.
20. Kelly A: Selecting a serotonin reuptake inhibitor for obsessive-compulsive disorder. Primary Psychiatry 4:61-70, 1997.
21. Fein S: Combined treatment strategies in resistant anxiety disorders. Primary Psychiatry 3:52-60, 1996.
22. Heimberg RH, Dodge CS, Becker RE: Social phobias. In: Michelson L, Ascher LM (eds). Anxiety and Stress Disorders: Cognitive-behavioral Assessment and Treatment. Guilford, New York NY, 1987.
23. McGlynn TJ, Metcalf HL (eds): Diagnosis and Treatment of Anxiety Disorders: Physician's Handbook. American Psychiatric Press, Washington, D.C., 1989.

Chapter 16

Clinical Presentation, Screening, and Treatment of Substance Abuse in the Primary Care Setting

Thomas Horst, M.D., M.P.H.

Alcohol and drug problems are relatively common in the U.S. population, and even more common in most primary care settings. The primary care physician (PCP) sees many patients with substance abuse problems, but identifies only some of these and treats or refers even fewer.[1] The reasons for this low identification and treatment rate are the result of provider attitudes about patients with substance abuse, knowledge of the conditions and how best to handle them, lack of financial incentives, and best use of provider time.[2]

Attitudes of physicians about substance abuse are strongly shaped by their exposure to patients with the conditions that the average medical school program provides—generally involving late stage alcoholics and intravenous drug abusers with infections. Exposure to middle class and professional people with alcohol or drug dependence may occur for some physicians, especially for more recent graduates, but it has not been the mainstream approach to education about these conditions. Knowledge about the medical management of patients with these conditions has been limited to a few hours in most training programs, and management of the patient beyond the period of detoxification and into recovery is seldom emphasized. Due to this lack of exposure and experience with successfully recovering patients, the average PCP may have a sense of futility when confronted with a substance abuse patient. The physician may feel that inadequate supports exist to help manage such a patient, therefore screening for these conditions is not justified.

Finally, patients with substance abuse may have exhausted some or all of their insurance coverage for treatment, so arrangements for definitive treatment are often less than ideal. However, the patient with these conditions is often at high risk for exposure to human immunodeficiency virus (HIV) and thus to acquired immunodeficiency syndrome (AIDS), and the potential spread of these conditions along with the direct and indirect burden of human suffering are compelling reasons to screen for substance abuse, and to give patients appropriate counseling about abstinence and safety issues regarding drug use.

One additional factor that has probably contributed to provider confusion about appropriate management in this area is the growing awareness that the majority of people experiencing problems with alcohol and drug use are not alcohol or drug dependent, but rather at-risk users who drink too much and/or use too many drugs.[3] The relationship between health and alcohol or other drug use is complex, and not subject to easy division into diseased and nondiseased states.[4] Studies of clinical prevalence, which allow clinicians to compare treatment practices, are more easily comparable if standard definitions are used for clinical terms. The following definitions have been suggested by the National Institute on Alcohol Abuse and Alcoholism to provide such comparability.[5]

At-risk Drinkers

These are defined as men who drink 15 or more drinks a week, women who have 12 or more drinks a week, and men or women who drink 5 or more drinks per occasion one or more times a week. Groups who may be at risk at lower levels of use include operators of hazardous machinery, women who are pregnant or trying to conceive, children and adolescents, patients using some types of medications, and older adults.

Problem Drinkers

These are persons who drink three or more drinks per day, or who have one or more problems related to their alcohol use. At-risk or problem drinking is reported by 10 percent of adult men and 2 percent of adult women in community studies.[6]

The diagnosis of alcohol dependence is based not on quantity and frequency of use, but rather on the consequences of use. *The Diagnostic and Statistical Manual,* Fourth edition, *(DSM-IV)* outlines clinical criteria for individual diagnoses.[7] These include loss of control, compulsion to use, physical withdrawal, and repeated consequences of use in social, employment, legal, financial, or medical areas. Community prevalence rates are around 5 percent for men and 1 percent for women, using these criteria.[1] Prevalence in primary care settings of all alcohol-related conditions is even higher.[8]

The definitions of *drug abuse and dependence* outlined in *DSM-IV* use similar concepts of repetitive consequences and compulsion to use, but not all drugs of abuse have a clear-cut abstinence syndrome. Community prevalence of illicit drug use is age-dependent, with the highest use in persons 18 to 21 years old (18 percent), declining to 1 percent in those 50 or older. No studies have been performed in primary care settings on the prevalence of illicit drug use.

To Screen or Not to Screen

Clinical presentation should be the first guide in screening for substance abuse problems. The patient who presents with a complaint of an alcohol or drug problem deserves careful evaluation and planning for follow-up, as the long-term management of these disorders involves the care and coordination skills of the PCP. The patient with symptoms in other areas, however, deserves a conservative clinical approach: first, do no harm. Most PCPs would agree that to justify the effort, screening and therapy must be shown to cause greater reduction in morbidity and mortality at an early point in the disease than therapy applied after symptoms appear. Because this criterion has been partially established, it is suggested that the PCP screen as many patients as possible.[9] Patients seen for preventive care exams, pregnancy, problems with anxiety or depression, hypertension, dyspepsia or peptic ulcer conditions, and trauma are a reasonable first level of screening, since the screen fits logically into the clinical interchange, and substance abuse issues are clearly relevant to these diagnostic areas (Table 1).

Patients who use tobacco are also a high-risk group and deserve screening; according to the 1995 National Household Survey on Drug Abuse, 13 percent of smokers are heavy drinkers, and 14 percent are illicit drug users. Patients presenting with other

TABLE 1. PRESENTING CONDITIONS THAT SHOULD PROMPT SCREENING FOR SUBSTANCE ABUSE

Preventive care exams
Pregnancy
Anxiety or depression
Hypertension
Dyspepsia or peptic ulcer disease
Trauma (acute or follow-up visit)
Tobacco use

complaints should be screened if the provider has time to act, at the time of screening or at follow-up, on the clinical information obtained. Because early symptoms of substance abuse are in social areas, the provider should be alert for problems in the patient's life aside from standard medical symptoms, and apply screening tools when such problems are brought to light by the patient or, occasionally, by a family member. Screening should not occur when the provider has no working relationship with the patient and no intention of using the data obtained (i.e., urine toxicologic drug screens to check for drug use, in the absence of time for a detailed clinical interview with the patient and a family member).

Screening Instruments: How Useful Are They?

The first criterion of effectiveness of a primary care screening approach is the accuracy of screening tools used for identification. The gold standard for diagnosis in substance abuse areas is the long clinical interview, which is impractical for use in primary care situations. Brief screening instruments that show good sensitivity and specificity for alcohol use problems have been designed and tested in primary care settings. *Sensitivity* is the proportion of persons with a condition who correctly test "positive" when screened, and high sensitivity minimizes the problem of missing individuals with the disorder of interest: false negatives. *Specificity* is the proportion of persons without the condition who correctly test negative when screened, and high specificity minimizes the problem of healthy people being incorrectly identified as having the disorder: false positives.[10]

The original Michigan Alcoholism Screening Test has 25 items, and several variations have been studied in primary care settings.[11] Despite its sensitivity, even the brief versions seem to be too long for routine use in primary care screening.

The CAGE instrument has been well studied in primary care settings, contains only four questions, and has good sensitivity and specificity for alcohol dependence

> C: "Have you ever felt you ought to **Cut** down on your drinking?'
> A: "Have people **Annoyed** you by criticizing your drinking?"
> G: "Have you ever felt bad or **Guilty** about your drinking?"
> E: "Have you ever had a drink first thing in the morning to steady your nerves or get rid of a hangover (**Eye-opener**)?"
>
> Figure 1. The CAGE questionnaire.[12] A score of two or more positive responses is suggestive of alcohol dependence or abuse.

(Figure 1).[12] It is probably too insensitive to screen for nondependent problem drinkers, however. To address these concerns, the ten-item Alcohol Use Disorders Inventory Test (AUDIT) was developed.[13] It has been shown to perform with good sensitivity and specificity in primary care settings (Table 2). However, this screening instrument may be too long for daily clinical use for the provider who has no special interest in this area. Shorter instruments using as few as two questions have recently been described, and if shown reliable in further studies may offer a more practical alternative with similar effectiveness.[14] For now, the combination of questions used at Group Health Cooperative of Puget Sound is recommended, and are listed in Table 2.

Pregnant women and adolescents are special populations that require modified screening instruments for detecting at-risk drinking and other alcohol and drug problems.

TABLE 2. THE ALCOHOL USE DISORDERS INVENTORY TEST (AUDIT). A SCORE OF GREATER THAN 8 (OUT OF 41) IS SUGGESTIVE OF PROBLEM DRINKING AND INDICATES NEED FOR MORE IN-DEPTH ASSESSMENT.[13]

Question	Score				
	0	1	2	3	4
How often do you have a drink containing alcohol?	Never	Monthly or less	2-4 times a month	2-3 times a week	4 or more times a week
How many drinks do you have on a typical day when you are drinking?	None	1 or 2	3 or 4	5 or 6	7 to 9
How often do you have six or more drinks on one occasion?	Never	Less than monthly	Monthly	Weekly	Daily or almost daily
How often during the last year have you found that you were unable to stop drinking once you had started?	Never	Less than daily	Monthly	Weekly	Daily or almost daily
How often during the last year have you failed to do what was normally expected from you because of drinking?	Never	Less than monthly	Monthly	Weekly	Daily or almost daily
How often during the last year have you needed a first drink in the morning to get yourself going after a heavy drinking session?	Never	Less than monthly	Monthly	Weekly	Daily or almost daily
How often during the last year have you had a feeling of guilt or remorse after drinking?	Never	Less than monthly	Monthly	Weekly	Daily or almost daily
How often during the last year have you found that you were unable to remember what happened the night before because you had been drinking?	Never	Less than monthly	Monthly	Weekly	Daily or almost daily
Have you or someone else been injured as a result of your drinking?	Never	Yes, but not during the last year (2 points)		Yes, during the last year (4 points)	
Has a relative, doctor, or other health worker been concerned about your drinking or suggested you cut down?	Never	Yes, but not during the last year (2 points)		Yes, during the last year (4 points)	

System Supports for Provider Screening

Brief screening instruments are more likely to be incorporated into clinical practice compared to longer instruments, and alcohol and drug problems are only one of many conditions that PCPs are expected to address in nearly every adult patient. Provider behavior seems to most closely approach the ideal when the format of the provider visit suggests the use of screening (more screening is done at preventive care visits), and especially when the clinical forms that providers use have screening material built in. At the Group Health Cooperative of Puget Sound (GHC), the adult physical exam form has contained the CAGE questionnaire since 1984. In addition, the revised Adult Health Questionnaire has two quantity/frequency questions about alcohol that are included immediately after the CAGE (see Table 3). There is also a screening question regarding illicit drug use in the same section. Primary care physician training is currently focused on maximizing use of clinical data gathered from the form and from the subsequent clinical interview with the patient. The intent of such screening is to provide brief interventions in the primary care setting for at-risk and problem drinkers or drug users, with consultation and referral when needed for the dependent drinker or drug user.

Other clinical documents designed for use in primary care, such as the Group Health Cooperative depression guideline (to be implemented in primary care in 1997), and the long interview form designed for adolescent preventive exams, have screening questions regarding alcohol and drug use built into the format of the questionnaire to use with patients.

The second component of system support is counselors trained in the area of chemical dependency who work closely with the PCP office to allow direct clinical interface between providers. At Group Health Cooperative we have a spectrum of co-location arrangements, from part-time liaison counselors at PCP offices to full-time chemical dependency counselors who share space with PCPs. We are increasing such mutual location wherever possible, because our internal referral data show the highest

TABLE 3. THE ADULT HEALTH QUESTIONNAIRE SECTION, WHICH INCLUDES ALCOHOL AND DRUG QUESTIONS, IS EMBEDDED IN THE MIDDLE OF THE QUESTIONNAIRE, AFTER QUESTIONS ABOUT NUTRITION AND SMOKING*

17. Have you ever felt you ought to cut down on your use of drugs? yes or no
18. Have you ever felt you ought to cut down on your drinking? yes or no
19. Have you ever felt annoyed by criticism of your drinking? yes or no
20. Have you ever felt bad or guilty about your drinking? yes or no
21. Have you ever had a drink first thing in the morning to steady your nerves or get rid of a hangover? yes or no
22. Do you often have more than 2 alcoholic drinks a day? yes or no
23. How often do you have six or more drinks on one occasion? never, less than monthly, monthly, weekly, daily or almost daily.
24. Do you ever drive or ride when the driver may have had too much alcohol or drugs? yes or no

*Any yes answer, or monthly or more for the six drink question, is an indication for further screening for at risk drinking or substance abuse. The tools to perform such further screening are available to providers on the Group Health Cooperative webspace at http://www.ghc.org. Enter the clinical home page, and then follow the path via the Adult Health Questionnaire to the drug and alcohol questions.

levels of interaction between PCPs and chemical dependency providers when they share physical space.

The third component of system support is smooth access of patients and providers to chemical dependency services. Primary care practitioner access to specialists in addiction medicine has been an important focus of our chemical dependency program, to promote the use of outpatient detoxification when appropriate, and the use of inpatient observation and detoxification services when needed.

The final component of system support is clinical feedback regarding chemical dependency treatment issues to the PCP, tailored to the interests of the provider. Our chemical dependency program is currently using several different formats of provider feedback, including periodic written clinical summaries and voicemail between chemical dependency counselors and physicians, to improve mutual clinical work.

Screening for Drug Abuse

The routine use of screening instruments or laboratory tests has not yet been proven effective in reducing harmful drug use.[15] In particular, toxicologic tests do not distinguish between occasional users and persons who are impaired by their drug use. However, questions about drug use and potential adverse consequences in interviews with adolescents and adults may be justified on other grounds, such as high prevalence and serious consequences of use and the spread of HIV (not just from intravenous drug users sharing needles, but from any patient who is high and makes bad decisions about risky behaviors). The clinician should look for signs of trouble in patients who use drugs, and explore substance use in a confidential manner with patients who report drug use. Concerns about adverse consequences such as problems at school or work should prompt detailed evaluation for drug dependence: exploring frequency/quantity patterns of drug use, arguments with family members about use, neglect of expected obligations related to use, use while operating an automobile or machine, any change in tolerance in the past year, efforts to cut down or control use, and compulsion to use. The "three Cs" of dependence include loss of control, compulsion to use, and continued use despite adverse consequences.

Effectiveness of Early Detection: Interventions in Primary Care

A second screening criterion is the effectiveness of the clinical intervention aimed at the designated conditions identified as a result of screening.

Nondependent Drinkers

Brief interventions have shown effectiveness in reducing levels of at-risk drinking by 32 percent over nine months in men compared to 10 percent in controls, and 30 percent for women in both intervention and control groups.[16] Effectiveness seems to hold true for interventions as brief as a single five-minute interview with a concerned provider. The essential components of brief interventions can be summarized by the acronym FRAMES: Feedback to the patient about the need for change, Responsibility of the patient for the change, Advice about what changes should be considered, a Menu of choices for the patient to take action, Empathy from the provider, and a Self-efficacy message that the patient has the ability to make the required change.[17]

Pregnancy and Alcohol

There is uncertainty about the effects of interventions during pregnancy. Uncontrolled trials have shown significant reductions in drinking, but trials with control groups showed similar reductions in intervention groups and controls. The U.S. Preventive Services Task Force summarized the data by stating "it is difficult to determine precisely the benefit of screening and counseling during pregnancy."[9] However, screening seems justified by the potential of adverse effects of alcohol on the fetus. Optimal screening methods are still being explored, but a brief questionnaire called the TWEAK (Tolerance, Worry, Eye-opener, Amnesia, and Kut [sic] down) was recently shown to be sensitive to the risk of drinking in at least some obstetric patient populations.[18]

Adolescents

Despite a wide variety of approaches to adolescents with substance abuse problems, there have been no controlled studies of treatment outcomes for this population.[19] Until more information is available from future studies, the clinician must make decisions about treatment based on advice from their appropriate local chemical dependency consultant.

Alcohol-dependent Patients

A 1990 comprehensive review of treatment for alcohol dependence concluded that a variety of treatments were effective, no single superior treatment modality exists, and few treatments were effective for the majority of patients.[3] A recent employee referral study showed better outcomes at two years after an inpatient treatment with mandatory Alcoholics Anonymous (AA) follow-up than after mandatory AA only.[20] Alcoholics Anonymous may have some independent treatment effect, however, and no control arm (i.e., a group receiving no treatment) was included in this study. Studies on the treatment of alcohol dependence continue, but specialized treatment does seem to work much better than no treatment.

Drug Abuse

Brief intervention principles have not yet been studied in primary care regarding drug abuse, but the brevity of the approach warrants use until better information on treatment becomes available. A recent employee assistance program study on alcohol and cocaine dependence suggests that matching of services to specific multidimensional problems improves outcomes.[21] Another recent evaluation showed the number of sessions in treatment (treatment length and intensity) is more important than the type of addiction treatment for crack cocaine users.[21]

Integrated Care

The interventions or specialized treatment of the patient with substance abuse problems should be seen by both the provider and the patient as a logical extension of the usual work done in primary care. When providers do an intervention for problem or at-risk drinking, they should also take responsibility for follow-up of the effects of the intervention. When the patient is referred for more specialized treatment, the PCP plays an important role in the recovery phase of the patient's illness.[23]

Referral for Specialized Treatment

Although the current emphasis in chemical dependency clinical management is on intensive outpatient treatment for alcohol and drug use disorders, some patients need comprehensive evaluation and treatment in more specialized settings that have access to inpatient medical monitoring. Patients with physical withdrawal that cannot be managed in the outpatient setting, patients with serious alcohol or drug-related health problems such as alcoholic hepatitis and gastritis with gastrointestinal bleeding, and patients with psychiatric disorders such as active bipolar disorder or severe depression with suicidal ideation should all be referred for specialized evaluation and treatment. Patients who fail to change their at-risk use of alcohol or other drugs with the brief intervention approach (advice of a physician) also need evaluation for treatment in a more intensive environment than the primary care setting.

The Role of Pharmacotherapy

It is not usually recommended that the PCP treat patients with alcohol and drug dependence outside the context of a comprehensive treatment program. However, certain medications have proven effectiveness as adjuncts to primary therapy. Disulfiram (Antabuse) has been the traditional adjunctive treatment by the PCP for the patient with alcohol dependence, especially when binge drinking behavior is present. However, many patients refuse to consider it as part of their treatment plan, and recent review has raised doubts about its effectiveness in actual clinical use.[1]

Naltrexone (Revia) has been found to be effective in the short-term treatment of alcohol dependence, in which it reduces not only total days of drinking but reported craving and the intensity of drinking in patients who relapse to alcohol use.[24] Some evidence suggests that its effectiveness may persist for some patients beyond three months, and investigation into the role of this medication continues in several centers. In our experience at GHC, naltrexone can be helpful in selected cases of alcohol dependence, where the patient expresses problems with craving and is willing to use medication to improve his or her chances of continued sobriety. Naltrexone has also been shown to be an effective treatment in patients with opiate dependence who need an abstinence-based treatment program.[25]

Methadone and buprenorphine have been established as effective and safe maintenance agents for opioid dependence. Their use is currently restricted to federally approved clinics, however, and they are not directly available for use by PCPs. The comparison of maintenance agents with abstinence-based treatment for opioid dependence is complex. Physicians are urged to discuss such treatment options with their local chemical dependency expert, and use patient history and preference as a guide to such treatment decisions.

The Importance of Follow-up

Alcohol and drug disorders frequently become more severe over time, and the physician working with the patient in primary care can use this progression to aid in diagnostic screening and referral. Patients who attain significant recovery often view the PCP as their ally in maintaining improved health and are, in turn, usually much easier to work with in future clinical events.

Integration of Substance Abuse Services in Primary Care

There are four key components to the successful integration of substance abuse services in the primary care setting. These include mutual location, collaborative treatment plans, consultant/liaison function, and system support tools.

Mutual Location

This is defined as shared or integrated treatment space with the presence of behavioral health professionals alongside PCPS. As noted above, referral rates by physicians are much higher for evaluation and treatment when architectural barriers are removed, and the other components of integrated care are facilitated.

Collaborative Treatment Plans

Although there may be convincing reasons, such as legal or confidentiality issues, for the behavioral health and primary care providers to have separate charting, the treatment plans implemented by each provider need to be developed with the knowledge and input from the other disciplines.

Consultant/Liaison Function

The function of the behavioral health counselor changes character in the primary care setting. Although a full evaluation for chemical dependency can be performed in the primary care office, there are often regulatory requirements or statutory limitations restricting aspects of the treatment of chemical dependency to certain specialized settings. When the patient does not have obvious disease in the area of substance abuse, the provider may obtain consultation with a chemical dependency counselor regarding the optimal approach for management.

System Support Tools

System support tools that can be built into the primary care work flow include the use of screening tools in everyday clinical forms; computer support for the PCP that clarifies management of clinical data when the provider needs a reminder; mutual discussion of patients by behavioral health and primary care providers, with treatment plans that reflect multidisciplinary planning; and easy access to consultation with a physician specialist in addiction medicine when needed.

Summary

The PCP has important roles to play in the management of patients with substance use disorders: identification of patients with alcohol and drug dependence, screening for patients in high-risk diagnostic categories for dependence and abuse, and screening for at-risk and problem drinkers. Fortunately, the screening tools and brief interventions that target these patients are simple, short, and shown to be surprisingly robust and effective in primary care settings. The value and power of longitudinal follow-up in primary care practice are important secrets of integrated care. Continued care for patients in recovery and patients who have not yet entered definitive treatment is also an important link to improved health for patients and their families. Appropriate system support and clinical information exchange can reduce frustration for providers and increase their effectiveness in management of patients with substance abuse problems.

References

1. National Institute on Alcohol Abuse and Alcoholism: Alcohol and health: eighth special report to the US Congress from the Secretary of Health and Human Services. NIH Publication no. 94-3699. US Department of Health and Human Services, National Institutes of Health, Rockville MD, 1993.
2. Group Health Cooperative of Puget Sound: Internal Group Health Cooperative ADAPT survey of primary care providers, 1996.
3. Institute of Medicine: Broadening the basis of treatment for alcohol problems. National Academy Press, Washington DC, 1990.
4. Vinson DC: Alcohol is not a dichotomous variable. J Fam Practice 44:147-149, 1997.
5. National Institute on Alcohol Abuse and Alcoholism: The physician's guide to helping patients with alcohol problems. NIH Publication no. 95-3769. National Institute on Alcohol Abuse and Alcoholism, Bethesda MD, 1995.
6. Substance Abuse and Mental Health Administration: National Household Survey on Drug Abuse: Population Estimates 1993. Publication no. SMA-94-3017. US Department of Health and Human Services, Substance Abuse and Mental Health Administration, Rockville MD, 1994.
7. American Psychiatric Association: Diagnostic and Statistical Manual of Mental Disorders, Fourth edition. American Psychiatric Association, Washington DC, 1994.
8. Bradley KA: The primary care provider's role in the prevention and management of alcohol problems. Alcohol Health Res World 18:97-104, 1994.
9. Chapter 52, Problem Drinking. In: U.S. Preventive Services Task Force. Guide to Clinical Preventive Services: Report of the U.S. Preventive Services Task Force, Second edition. Williams & Wilkens, Baltimore MD, 1996.
10. Riegelman RK, Hirsch RP: Studying a Study and Testing a Test: How to Read the Medical Literature, Second edition. Little, Brown & Co, Boston MA, 1989.
11. Selzer ML: The Michigan Alcoholism Screening Test: the quest for a new diagnostic instrument. Am J Psychiatry 127:1653-1658, 1971.
12. Ewing JA: Detecting alcoholism: the CAGE questionnaire. JAMA 252:1905-1907, 1984.
13. Saunders JB, Aasland OG, Babor TF, et al: Development of the Alcohol Use Disorders Identification Test (AUDIT): WHO collaborative project on early detection of persons with harmful alcohol consumption - II. Addiction 88:791-804, 1993.
14. Brown RL, Leonard T, Saunders LA, Papasouliotis O: A two-item screening test for alcohol and other drug problems. J Fam Practice 44:151-160, 1997.
15. Chapter 53, Drug Abuse. In: U.S. Preventive Services Task Force. Guide to Clinical Preventive Services: Report of the U.S. Preventive Services Task Force, Second edition. Williams & Wilkens, Baltimore MD, 1996.
16. WHO Brief Intervention Study Group: A cross-national trial of brief interventions with heavy drinkers. Am J Public Health 86:948-955, 1996.
17. Miller WR, Rollnick S: Motivational Interviewing. Guilford Press, New York, 1991, pp 30-35.
18. Russell M, Martier SS, Sokol RJ, et al: Detecting risk drinking during pregnancy: a comparison of four screening questionnaires. Am J Public Health 86:1435-1439, 1996.
19. Kaminer Y: Adolescent substance abuse. In: American Psychiatric Press Textbook of Substance Abuse Treatment. American Psychiatric Press Inc, Washington DC, 1994; pp 415-435.
20. Walsh DC, Hingson RW, Merrigan DM, et al: A randomized trial of treatment options for alcohol-abusing workers. N Engl J Med 325:775-782, 1991.

21. McClellan AT: Dose-response studies of psychosocial services during substance abuse treatment. In: Problems of Drug Dependence 1994: Proceedings of the 56th Annual Scientific Meetings. Edited by LS Harris. National Institute on Drug Abuse, Rockvflle MD, 1995, 152:73.
22. Hoffman JA, Caudill BD, Koman JJ, et al: Psychosocial treatments for cocaine abuse: treatment intensity as a predictor of long-term clinical outcomes. In: Problems of Drug Dependence 1994: Proceedings of the 56th Annual Scientific Meetings. Edited by LS Harris. National Institute on Drug Abuse, Rockville MD 1995, 152:72-73.
23. Del Toro IM, Thom DJ, Beam HP, Horst T: Chemically dependent patients in recovery: roles for the family physician. Am Fam Physician 53:1667-1673, 1996.
24. Volpicelli JR, Watson NT, King AC, et al: Effect of naltrexone on alcohol "high" in alcoholics. Am J Psychiatry 152:613-615, 1995.
25. O'Connor PG, Waugh ME, Carroll KM, et al: Primary care-based ambulatory opioid detoxification: the results of a clinical trial. J Gen Intern Med 10:255-260, 1995.

Chapter 17

Clinical Presentation, Screening, and Treatment of Somatization Abuse in Primary Care

Steven E. Locke, M.D. and Katharine M. Larsson, RN, M.S., CS

In the changing healthcare environment, primary care clinicians (PCCs) face increasing practice demands. (We prefer the inclusive term *clinicians* because it subsumes physicians as well as mid-level clinicians such as nurse practitioners and physicians assistants.) PCCs need to provide more and higher quality care to a wider variety of patients and to achieve greater patient satisfaction within a context of increasing time pressures.

Maintaining patient satisfaction in this time-conscious milieu is challenging. Frequently, PCCs rely on diagnostic procedures for decision support, despite personal doubts that they will uncover an organic problem. These procedures are costly and rarely address the real causes of the elusive, recurrent, or chronic symptoms with which the majority of patients present.[1] Furthermore, patients themselves have become more interested in and accepting of mind-body approaches. Patients are also increasingly dissatisfied with costly and technical approaches to diagnosis and treatment. These changes have created a new opportunity to educate patients about somatization.

What Is Somatization?

Somatization is a mind-body process in which emotions or moods manifest as physical sensations in the body.[2] This universal phenomenon only achieves pathological significance under certain conditions.[3] The continuum ranges from normal somatization, such as blushing when embarrassed or sweating when anxious, to *somatization disorder,* a severe form of somatization representing 0.3 percent of the general population and 1 to 4 percent of all patients.[4,5] Somatization disorder is a chronic, relapsing condition that usually begins during adolescence or early adulthood. It is characterized by multiple unexplained somatic complaints of several years' duration, for which medical attention was sought, a resultant change in lifestyle occurred, or medication was required. Most somatizing patients who seek medical attention fall into the middle of this spectrum, a condition known as *subsyndromal somatization,* i.e., not meeting Diagnostic and Statistical Manual of Mental Disorders, Fourth edition, *(DSM-IV)* criteria for a somatoform disorder (Table 1).[6]

One of the challenges of primary care is to help these patients learn to determine when it is appropriate to see their physician. Many patients worry that their symptoms signal an underlying disease. Even when a careful history and physical examination reveal no demonstrable pathology, some patients are difficult to reassure. They may spend more time undergoing laboratory evaluations than discussing their concerns with their PCC. As a result, somatizing patients often report having too little

TABLE 1. SOMATOFORM DISORDERS IN THE *DIAGNOSTIC AND STATISTICAL MANUAL FOR MENTAL DISORDERS*, FOURTH EDITION

Somatization Disorder: (historically referred to as hysteria or Briquet's syndrome) is a polysymptomatic disorder that begins before age 30 years, extends over a period of years, and is characterized by a combination of pain, gastrointestinal, sexual, and pseudoneurological symptoms.

Undifferentiated Somatoform Disorder: is characterized by unexplained physical complaints, lasting at least 6 months, that are below the threshold for a diagnosis of somatization disorder.

Conversion Disorder: involves unexplained symptoms or deficits affecting voluntary motor or sensory function that suggest a neurological or other general medical condition. Psychological factors are judged to be associated with the symptoms or deficits.

Pain Disorder: is characterized by pain as the predominant focus of clinical attention. In addition, psychological factors are judged to have an important role in its onset, severity, exacerbation, or maintenance. Hypochondriasis is the preoccupation with the fear of having, or the idea that one has, a serious disease based on the person's misinterpretation of bodily symptoms or bodily functions.

Body Dysmorphic Disorder: is the preoccupation with an imagined or exaggerated defect in physical appearance.

Somatoform Disorder Not Otherwise Specified: is included for coding disorders with somatoform symptoms that do not meet the criteria for any of the specific somatoform disorders.

time with their clinicians, and they may feel that their symptoms are not taken seriously. At the same time, PCCs may feel discouraged because they cannot make a diagnosis, or they suspect that the symptoms represent somatization or a mental disorder but are too pressed for time to explore the issue. These patients, the so-called "worried well," easily become the object of blame. Treatment may become adversarial, to the patient's detriment. A thorough understanding of somatization and its treatment is important to provide optimal care in this population.

All definitions of somatization acknowledge the role of mind-body continuity.[3,7,8] Barsky and Klerman defined somatization as the expression of emotional and psychosocial distress in the language of physical or bodily symptoms.[7] McCleod and Budd believe that somatization consists of prevalent and ill-defined symptoms that have no organic or psychiatric cause, respond poorly to biomedical interventions, and are frequently associated with psychological distress.[8] The psychosomatic perspective, embodied in the biopsychosocial model proposed by Engel, accepts that the patient's symptoms are real, even when no organ pathology or abnormal physiology can be demonstrated.[9] However, the biomedical model still dominates Western medicine, and only gradually is the biopsychosocial model being incorporated.

It is important to distinguish between somatization as a psychological defense mechanism or process, and somatization *disorder* as a psychiatric condition. Somatic symptoms such as tachycardia, sweating, increased gastrointestinal motility, and even pain, often accompany psychiatric disorders such as anxiety without necessarily meeting the diagnostic criteria for somatization disorder. As described in the *DSM-IV*, somatization disorder refers to a specific condition in which symptoms include four distinct somatic areas (pain, gastrointestinal, sexual, and pseudoneurological). In addition, symptoms must meet temporal requirements (i.e., occur over a period of several years) and cause significant functional impairment (Table 2).

Other somatoform disorders can involve the mechanism of somatization, but additional specific diagnostic requirements must be met (see Table 1). Predisposing factors that contribute to somatization include *alexithymia* (a pattern of communication in which there is both impoverishment of fantasy and difficulty expressing feelings or describing inner states in emotional terms), psychic trauma, and poor social support. Therefore, all of these factors must be considered when trying to identify, understand, and treat somatization. Furthermore, there is considerable comorbidity among mental disorders that frequently present with somatic symptoms such as mood, anxiety, and somatoform disorders (Figure 1).

TABLE 2. DIAGNOSTIC CRITERIA FOR 300.81 SOMATIZATION DISORDER (FROM THE *DIAGNOSTIC AND STATISTICAL MANUAL FOR MENTAL DISORDERS*, FOURTH EDITION)

A. A history of many physical complaints beginning before age 30 years that occur over a period of several years and result in treatment being sought or significant impairment in social, occupational, or other important areas of functioning.

B. Each of the following criteria must have been met, with individual symptoms occurring at any time during the course of the disturbance:

   1. Four pain symptoms: a history of pain related to at least four different sites or functions (e.g., head, abdomen, back, joints, extremities, chest, rectum, during menstruation, during sexual intercourse, or during urination).

   2. Two gastrointestinal symptoms: a history of at least two gastrointestinal symptoms other than pain (e.g., nausea, bloating, vomiting other than during pregnancy, diarrhea, or intolerance of several different foods).

   3. One sexual symptom: a history of at least one sexual or reproductive symptom other than pain (e.g., sexual indifference, erectile or ejaculatory dysfunction, irregular menses, excessive menstrual bleeding, vomiting throughout pregnancy).

   4. One pseudoneurological symptom: a history of at least one symptom or deficit suggesting a neurological condition not limited to pain (conversion symptoms such as impaired coordination or balance, paralysis or localized weakness, difficulty swallowing or lump in throat, aphonia, urinary retention, hallucinations, loss of touch or pain sensation, double vision, blindness, deafness, seizures, dissociative symptoms such as amnesia or loss of consciousness other than fainting).

C. Either 1 or 2 below:

   1. After appropriate investigation, each of the symptoms in Criterion B cannot be fully explained by a known general medical condition or the direct effects of a substance (e.g., drug abuse, or a medication).

   2. When there is a related general medical condition, the physical complaints or resulting social or occupational impairment are in excess of what would be expected from the history, physical examination, or laboratory findings.

D. The symptoms are not intentionally feigned or produced (as in Factitious Disorder or Malingering).

Prevalence and Impact

Somatization accounts for at least 50 percent of the patients seen in primary care settings, with prevalence rates ranging widely from 20 percent to 92 percent of the primary care population.[10-12] Most experts concur that roughly one-half to two-thirds of all office visits involve patients with no demonstrable organic pathology.

The economic impact of somatization is difficult to calculate. In the workplace, somatization leads to reduced productivity and increased absenteeism. Patients who somatize are disproportionately high users of medical services, laboratory tests, and surgical procedures.[12] They have higher rates of ambulatory medical visits, hospitalization, and total health costs. They also are more likely to seek care simultaneously from multiple providers, fail to keep scheduled appointments, and frequently switch physicians. Furthermore, somatizing patients are often difficult to treat because they resent and reject any suggestion that psychosocial factors might play a role in the onset or course of their symptoms. These patients frequently resist referral to mental health clinicians; thus, they can be frustrating for the PCC.

Common Somatic Complaints

Eight common complaints—fatigue, back pain, headaches, dizziness, chest pain, dyspnea, abdominal pain, and anxiety—account for more than 80 million physician visits annually in the United States.[13] The most common somatic complaints brought to physicians can be grouped into five symptom categories: 1) gastrointestinal, 2) neurological, 3) autonomic, 4) cardiovascular, and 5) musculoskeletal (Table 3).[1,8,14] Many of these symptoms, however, are common to both anxiety and depression.

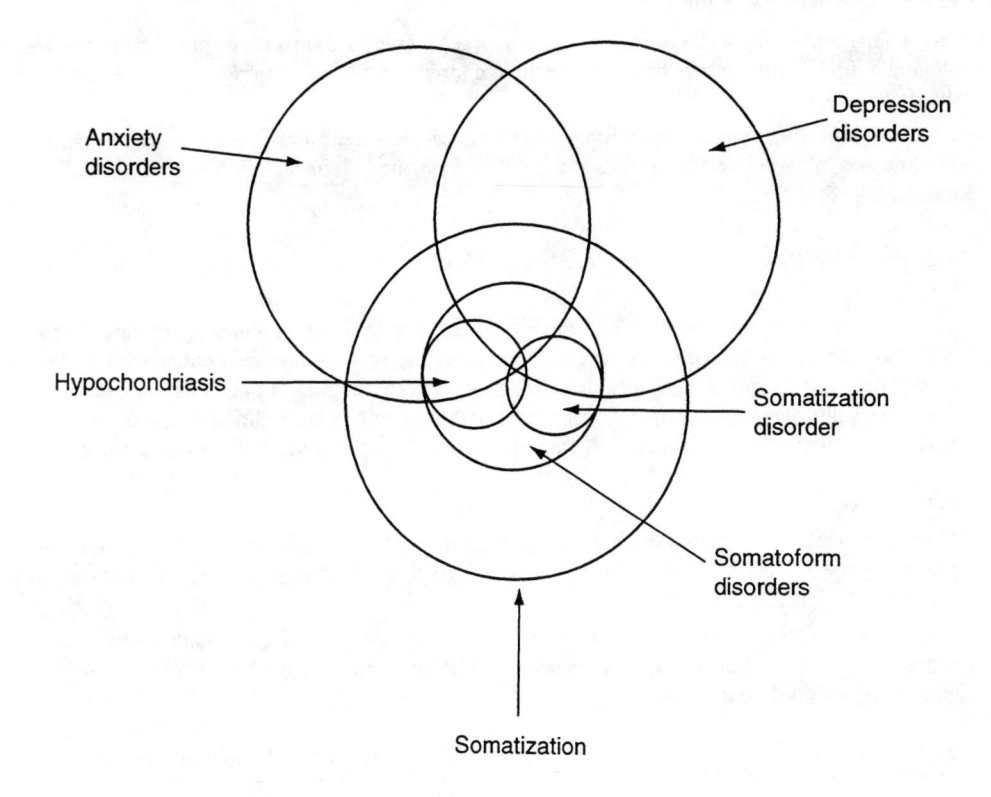

Figure 1

TABLE 3. THE MOST COMMON COMPLAINTS IN PRIMARY CARE PRACTICE

Gastrointestinal	Neurological	Autonomic	Cardiovascular	Musculoskeletal
Constipation	Dizziness	Impotence	Chest pain*	Back pain
Abdominal pain	Headache*		Edema	
Weight loss	Disturbed sleep*		Cough	
Nausea	Fatigue*		Dyspnea	
Diarrhea	Numbness			

*These symptoms tend to be least responsive to current biomedical treatments.[8]

Cultural Factors

As Western societies become more culturally diverse, healthcare providers must acquire a better understanding of the cultural significance of symptoms, especially for patients who somatize. Social scientists who study somatization find that expressing emotional distress somatically appears to be universal.[15] Patterns of expression, as well as the meaning attached to symptoms, may vary greatly with the culture. Recognizing this universality can lead to greater sensitivity on the part of clinicians.

Detecting Somatization

The intertwining of physiological and psychological features of somatization makes it difficult to detect and treat. Diagnosis and treatment are further complicated by the nature of the continuum, from normal somatization to pathological somatization disorder. For example, patients with chronic medical illnesses often seek care for concerns such as sleep or appetite disturbance, fatigue, pain, nausea, or other gastrointestinal complaints. Conversely, patients with psychiatric illnesses such as panic disorder may complain of shortness of breath, palpitations, sweating, and even chest pain.

Although understanding its role in both medical and psychiatric conditions is essential, somatization is not a diagnosis. Nevertheless, some clinicians make a "diagnosis" of somatization that can be misleading. If a patient does not meet *DSM-IV* criteria for somatization disorder, a different somatoform disorder diagnosis should be used. Another *DSM-IV* diagnosis that overlaps the phenomenology of somatization is Psychological Factors Affecting a Medical Condition. Unfortunately, lack of diagnostic precision can lead to the "diagnosis" of somatization based solely on the absence of identifiable pathophysiology. When patients are labeled as somatizers based on a diagnosis by exclusion, they often feel blamed for not producing verifiable pathology.[16]

Somatic symptoms of fluctuating or chronic medical illnesses, especially if they are susceptible to exacerbation by psychosocial stressors, may be indistinguishable from somatization in an otherwise healthy person. For example, an insulin-dependent diabetic might present with parasthesias and dizziness. These symptoms may represent either a stress-induced exacerbation of the disease, or a psychophysiological response to the stressor, reflecting increasing psychological distress.

Patient Self-Assessment

Patients with generalized anxiety disorder, panic disorder, and major depression frequently present with somatic complaints in primary care. This occurs in up to 80 percent of patients. Subsyndromal symptoms of anxiety and depression, along with somatization, are even more common.[17,18] One strategy to address this problem involves active case-finding approaches to identify such patients and triage them into appropriate behavioral, interpersonal, or pharmacologic treatments. It is not yet clear that this strategy is cost effective.

Using psychiatric screening tools in primary care is problematic. Physicians have been reluctant to use these measures, fearing discovery of new cases. Screening instruments that are too sensitive will generate extra work to evaluate newly detected "cases," impeding work flow and raising costs. Also, screening tools have been criticized for being too expensive, too time-consuming, and too general (i.e., screening for too many different diagnoses).

Despite these problems, screening can be a valuable tool in primary care, where there is a high prevalence of psychiatric disorders. If undetected, these disorders cause emotional distress and impaired functioning. Undiagnosed mental disorders and somatization have an adverse impact on health costs, as affected patients are often high utilizers of nonpsychiatric services.[19]

The first questionnaire used for screening in primary care populations was the Cornell Medical Index, introduced in 1956. Other one-stage screening instruments borrowed from the mental health setting followed, including the General Health Questionnaire, the Beck Depression Inventory, the Zung Self-rating Depression Scale, and the Hamilton Anxiety Scale.

Newer screening tools for case finding in primary care use a two-stage screening approach. They require the administration of a short questionnaire or computer administered interview. If results are positive, more specific follow-up questions are used to query the patient. Examples of these new two-stage measures are the PRIME-MD and the Symptom-Driven Diagnostic Symptom-Primary Care (SDDS-PC). (See Chapter 13 and Appendices for more information on these screening tools.)

In recent years, older measures such as the Beck Depression Inventory have been re-examined for use in primary care screening. Another useful one-stage screening tool is the Brief Symptom Index (BSI), a revised version of the Symptom Checklist (SCL-90R). Although expensive, the 53-item BSI is multidimensional, with nine symptom subscales that include somatization, depression, anxiety, phobic anxiety, obsessive-compulsive, hostility, interpersonal sensitivity, psychosis, and paranoia. There are also three summary scales measuring overall distress. These can help the clinician assess whether somatic symptoms represent an underlying psychiatric or medical disorder.

Building Collaborative Multidisciplinary Teams

Successful management of somatization requires the development of an integrated, multidisciplinary approach. This idea was pioneered by Lipsitt, who developed the Integration Clinic at Boston's Beth Israel Hospital in the 1960s (see Chapter 1).[20] Recently there has been a resurgence of interest in integrated care, with the ac-

TABLE 3. THE MOST COMMON COMPLAINTS IN PRIMARY CARE PRACTICE

Gastrointestinal	Neurological	Autonomic	Cardiovascular	Musculoskeletal
Constipation	Dizziness	Impotence	Chest pain*	Back pain
Abdominal pain	Headache*		Edema	
Weight loss	Disturbed sleep*		Cough	
Nausea	Fatigue*		Dyspnea	
Diarrhea	Numbness			

*These symptoms tend to be least responsive to current biomedical treatments.[8]

Cultural Factors

As Western societies become more culturally diverse, healthcare providers must acquire a better understanding of the cultural significance of symptoms, especially for patients who somatize. Social scientists who study somatization find that expressing emotional distress somatically appears to be universal.[15] Patterns of expression, as well as the meaning attached to symptoms, may vary greatly with the culture. Recognizing this universality can lead to greater sensitivity on the part of clinicians.

Detecting Somatization

The intertwining of physiological and psychological features of somatization makes it difficult to detect and treat. Diagnosis and treatment are further complicated by the nature of the continuum, from normal somatization to pathological somatization disorder. For example, patients with chronic medical illnesses often seek care for concerns such as sleep or appetite disturbance, fatigue, pain, nausea, or other gastrointestinal complaints. Conversely, patients with psychiatric illnesses such as panic disorder may complain of shortness of breath, palpitations, sweating, and even chest pain.

Although understanding its role in both medical and psychiatric conditions is essential, somatization is not a diagnosis. Nevertheless, some clinicians make a "diagnosis" of somatization that can be misleading. If a patient does not meet *DSM-IV* criteria for somatization disorder, a different somatoform disorder diagnosis should be used. Another *DSM-IV* diagnosis that overlaps the phenomenology of somatization is Psychological Factors Affecting a Medical Condition. Unfortunately, lack of diagnostic precision can lead to the "diagnosis" of somatization based solely on the absence of identifiable pathophysiology. When patients are labeled as somatizers based on a diagnosis by exclusion, they often feel blamed for not producing verifiable pathology.[16]

Somatic symptoms of fluctuating or chronic medical illnesses, especially if they are susceptible to exacerbation by psychosocial stressors, may be indistinguishable from somatization in an otherwise healthy person. For example, an insulin-dependent diabetic might present with parasthesias and dizziness. These symptoms may represent either a stress-induced exacerbation of the disease, or a psychophysiological response to the stressor, reflecting increasing psychological distress.

Patient Self-Assessment

Patients with generalized anxiety disorder, panic disorder, and major depression frequently present with somatic complaints in primary care. This occurs in up to 80 percent of patients. Subsyndromal symptoms of anxiety and depression, along with somatization, are even more common.[17,18] One strategy to address this problem involves active case-finding approaches to identify such patients and triage them into appropriate behavioral, interpersonal, or pharmacologic treatments. It is not yet clear that this strategy is cost effective.

Using psychiatric screening tools in primary care is problematic. Physicians have been reluctant to use these measures, fearing discovery of new cases. Screening instruments that are too sensitive will generate extra work to evaluate newly detected "cases," impeding work flow and raising costs. Also, screening tools have been criticized for being too expensive, too time-consuming, and too general (i.e., screening for too many different diagnoses).

Despite these problems, screening can be a valuable tool in primary care, where there is a high prevalence of psychiatric disorders. If undetected, these disorders cause emotional distress and impaired functioning. Undiagnosed mental disorders and somatization have an adverse impact on health costs, as affected patients are often high utilizers of nonpsychiatric services.[19]

The first questionnaire used for screening in primary care populations was the Cornell Medical Index, introduced in 1956. Other one-stage screening instruments borrowed from the mental health setting followed, including the General Health Questionnaire, the Beck Depression Inventory, the Zung Self-rating Depression Scale, and the Hamilton Anxiety Scale.

Newer screening tools for case finding in primary care use a two-stage screening approach. They require the administration of a short questionnaire or computer administered interview. If results are positive, more specific follow-up questions are used to query the patient. Examples of these new two-stage measures are the PRIME-MD and the Symptom-Driven Diagnostic Symptom-Primary Care (SDDS-PC). (See Chapter 13 and Appendices for more information on these screening tools.)

In recent years, older measures such as the Beck Depression Inventory have been re-examined for use in primary care screening. Another useful one-stage screening tool is the Brief Symptom Index (BSI), a revised version of the Symptom Checklist (SCL-90R). Although expensive, the 53-item BSI is multidimensional, with nine symptom subscales that include somatization, depression, anxiety, phobic anxiety, obsessive-compulsive, hostility, interpersonal sensitivity, psychosis, and paranoia. There are also three summary scales measuring overall distress. These can help the clinician assess whether somatic symptoms represent an underlying psychiatric or medical disorder.

Building Collaborative Multidisciplinary Teams

Successful management of somatization requires the development of an integrated, multidisciplinary approach. This idea was pioneered by Lipsitt, who developed the Integration Clinic at Boston's Beth Israel Hospital in the 1960s (see Chapter 1).[20] Recently there has been a resurgence of interest in integrated care, with the ac-

TABLE 3. THE MOST COMMON COMPLAINTS IN PRIMARY CARE PRACTICE

Gastrointestinal	Neurological	Autonomic	Cardiovascular	Musculoskeletal
Constipation	Dizziness	Impotence	Chest pain*	Back pain
Abdominal pain	Headache*		Edema	
Weight loss	Disturbed sleep*		Cough	
Nausea	Fatigue*		Dyspnea	
Diarrhea	Numbness			

*These symptoms tend to be least responsive to current biomedical treatments.[8]

Cultural Factors

As Western societies become more culturally diverse, healthcare providers must acquire a better understanding of the cultural significance of symptoms, especially for patients who somatize. Social scientists who study somatization find that expressing emotional distress somatically appears to be universal.[15] Patterns of expression, as well as the meaning attached to symptoms, may vary greatly with the culture. Recognizing this universality can lead to greater sensitivity on the part of clinicians.

Detecting Somatization

The intertwining of physiological and psychological features of somatization makes it difficult to detect and treat. Diagnosis and treatment are further complicated by the nature of the continuum, from normal somatization to pathological somatization disorder. For example, patients with chronic medical illnesses often seek care for concerns such as sleep or appetite disturbance, fatigue, pain, nausea, or other gastrointestinal complaints. Conversely, patients with psychiatric illnesses such as panic disorder may complain of shortness of breath, palpitations, sweating, and even chest pain.

Although understanding its role in both medical and psychiatric conditions is essential, somatization is not a diagnosis. Nevertheless, some clinicians make a "diagnosis" of somatization that can be misleading. If a patient does not meet *DSM-IV* criteria for somatization disorder, a different somatoform disorder diagnosis should be used. Another *DSM-IV* diagnosis that overlaps the phenomenology of somatization is Psychological Factors Affecting a Medical Condition. Unfortunately, lack of diagnostic precision can lead to the "diagnosis" of somatization based solely on the absence of identifiable pathophysiology. When patients are labeled as somatizers based on a diagnosis by exclusion, they often feel blamed for not producing verifiable pathology.[16]

Somatic symptoms of fluctuating or chronic medical illnesses, especially if they are susceptible to exacerbation by psychosocial stressors, may be indistinguishable from somatization in an otherwise healthy person. For example, an insulin-dependent diabetic might present with parasthesias and dizziness. These symptoms may represent either a stress-induced exacerbation of the disease, or a psychophysiological response to the stressor, reflecting increasing psychological distress.

Patient Self-Assessment

Patients with generalized anxiety disorder, panic disorder, and major depression frequently present with somatic complaints in primary care. This occurs in up to 80 percent of patients. Subsyndromal symptoms of anxiety and depression, along with somatization, are even more common.[17,18] One strategy to address this problem involves active case-finding approaches to identify such patients and triage them into appropriate behavioral, interpersonal, or pharmacologic treatments. It is not yet clear that this strategy is cost effective.

Using psychiatric screening tools in primary care is problematic. Physicians have been reluctant to use these measures, fearing discovery of new cases. Screening instruments that are too sensitive will generate extra work to evaluate newly detected "cases," impeding work flow and raising costs. Also, screening tools have been criticized for being too expensive, too time-consuming, and too general (i.e., screening for too many different diagnoses).

Despite these problems, screening can be a valuable tool in primary care, where there is a high prevalence of psychiatric disorders. If undetected, these disorders cause emotional distress and impaired functioning. Undiagnosed mental disorders and somatization have an adverse impact on health costs, as affected patients are often high utilizers of nonpsychiatric services.[19]

The first questionnaire used for screening in primary care populations was the Cornell Medical Index, introduced in 1956. Other one-stage screening instruments borrowed from the mental health setting followed, including the General Health Questionnaire, the Beck Depression Inventory, the Zung Self-rating Depression Scale, and the Hamilton Anxiety Scale.

Newer screening tools for case finding in primary care use a two-stage screening approach. They require the administration of a short questionnaire or computer administered interview. If results are positive, more specific follow-up questions are used to query the patient. Examples of these new two-stage measures are the PRIME-MD and the Symptom-Driven Diagnostic Symptom-Primary Care (SDDS-PC). (See Chapter 13 and Appendices for more information on these screening tools.)

In recent years, older measures such as the Beck Depression Inventory have been re-examined for use in primary care screening. Another useful one-stage screening tool is the Brief Symptom Index (BSI), a revised version of the Symptom Checklist (SCL-90R). Although expensive, the 53-item BSI is multidimensional, with nine symptom subscales that include somatization, depression, anxiety, phobic anxiety, obsessive-compulsive, hostility, interpersonal sensitivity, psychosis, and paranoia. There are also three summary scales measuring overall distress. These can help the clinician assess whether somatic symptoms represent an underlying psychiatric or medical disorder.

Building Collaborative Multidisciplinary Teams

Successful management of somatization requires the development of an integrated, multidisciplinary approach. This idea was pioneered by Lipsitt, who developed the Integration Clinic at Boston's Beth Israel Hospital in the 1960s (see Chapter 1).[20] Recently there has been a resurgence of interest in integrated care, with the ac-

TABLE 3. THE MOST COMMON COMPLAINTS IN PRIMARY CARE PRACTICE

Gastrointestinal	Neurological	Autonomic	Cardiovascular	Musculoskeletal
Constipation	Dizziness	Impotence	Chest pain*	Back pain
Abdominal pain	Headache*		Edema	
Weight loss	Disturbed sleep*		Cough	
Nausea	Fatigue*		Dyspnea	
Diarrhea	Numbness			

*These symptoms tend to be least responsive to current biomedical treatments.[8]

Cultural Factors

As Western societies become more culturally diverse, healthcare providers must acquire a better understanding of the cultural significance of symptoms, especially for patients who somatize. Social scientists who study somatization find that expressing emotional distress somatically appears to be universal.[15] Patterns of expression, as well as the meaning attached to symptoms, may vary greatly with the culture. Recognizing this universality can lead to greater sensitivity on the part of clinicians.

Detecting Somatization

The intertwining of physiological and psychological features of somatization makes it difficult to detect and treat. Diagnosis and treatment are further complicated by the nature of the continuum, from normal somatization to pathological somatization disorder. For example, patients with chronic medical illnesses often seek care for concerns such as sleep or appetite disturbance, fatigue, pain, nausea, or other gastrointestinal complaints. Conversely, patients with psychiatric illnesses such as panic disorder may complain of shortness of breath, palpitations, sweating, and even chest pain.

Although understanding its role in both medical and psychiatric conditions is essential, somatization is not a diagnosis. Nevertheless, some clinicians make a "diagnosis" of somatization that can be misleading. If a patient does not meet *DSM-IV* criteria for somatization disorder, a different somatoform disorder diagnosis should be used. Another *DSM-IV* diagnosis that overlaps the phenomenology of somatization is Psychological Factors Affecting a Medical Condition. Unfortunately, lack of diagnostic precision can lead to the "diagnosis" of somatization based solely on the absence of identifiable pathophysiology. When patients are labeled as somatizers based on a diagnosis by exclusion, they often feel blamed for not producing verifiable pathology.[16]

Somatic symptoms of fluctuating or chronic medical illnesses, especially if they are susceptible to exacerbation by psychosocial stressors, may be indistinguishable from somatization in an otherwise healthy person. For example, an insulin-dependent diabetic might present with parasthesias and dizziness. These symptoms may represent either a stress-induced exacerbation of the disease, or a psychophysiological response to the stressor, reflecting increasing psychological distress.

Patient Self-Assessment

Patients with generalized anxiety disorder, panic disorder, and major depression frequently present with somatic complaints in primary care. This occurs in up to 80 percent of patients. Subsyndromal symptoms of anxiety and depression, along with somatization, are even more common.[17,18] One strategy to address this problem involves active case-finding approaches to identify such patients and triage them into appropriate behavioral, interpersonal, or pharmacologic treatments. It is not yet clear that this strategy is cost effective.

Using psychiatric screening tools in primary care is problematic. Physicians have been reluctant to use these measures, fearing discovery of new cases. Screening instruments that are too sensitive will generate extra work to evaluate newly detected "cases," impeding work flow and raising costs. Also, screening tools have been criticized for being too expensive, too time-consuming, and too general (i.e., screening for too many different diagnoses).

Despite these problems, screening can be a valuable tool in primary care, where there is a high prevalence of psychiatric disorders. If undetected, these disorders cause emotional distress and impaired functioning. Undiagnosed mental disorders and somatization have an adverse impact on health costs, as affected patients are often high utilizers of nonpsychiatric services.[19]

The first questionnaire used for screening in primary care populations was the Cornell Medical Index, introduced in 1956. Other one-stage screening instruments borrowed from the mental health setting followed, including the General Health Questionnaire, the Beck Depression Inventory, the Zung Self-rating Depression Scale, and the Hamilton Anxiety Scale.

Newer screening tools for case finding in primary care use a two-stage screening approach. They require the administration of a short questionnaire or computer administered interview. If results are positive, more specific follow-up questions are used to query the patient. Examples of these new two-stage measures are the PRIME-MD and the Symptom-Driven Diagnostic Symptom-Primary Care (SDDS-PC). (See Chapter 13 and Appendices for more information on these screening tools.)

In recent years, older measures such as the Beck Depression Inventory have been re-examined for use in primary care screening. Another useful one-stage screening tool is the Brief Symptom Index (BSI), a revised version of the Symptom Checklist (SCL-90R). Although expensive, the 53-item BSI is multidimensional, with nine symptom subscales that include somatization, depression, anxiety, phobic anxiety, obsessive-compulsive, hostility, interpersonal sensitivity, psychosis, and paranoia. There are also three summary scales measuring overall distress. These can help the clinician assess whether somatic symptoms represent an underlying psychiatric or medical disorder.

Building Collaborative Multidisciplinary Teams

Successful management of somatization requires the development of an integrated, multidisciplinary approach. This idea was pioneered by Lipsitt, who developed the Integration Clinic at Boston's Beth Israel Hospital in the 1960s (see Chapter 1).[20] Recently there has been a resurgence of interest in integrated care, with the ac-

companying belief that integration will lead to cost savings through medical cost offsets, as well as to improvement in the quality of care. This has fueled interest in population-based screening of primary care populations for symptoms of somatization, depression, and anxiety.

Prior to instituting a widespread screening program for mental disorders or subsyndromal symptoms of anxiety or depression, it is necessary to build a system for triage and referral that links primary care, behavioral medicine, and mental health clinicians. This collaborative effort is the foundation for an integrated approach, and it requires a shared vision and teamwork. First, leaders must be identified in each of the three departments to champion the process of change. Teams of three—a psychiatrist (or psychiatric clinical nurse specialist), an internist (or family physician), and a behavioral medicine specialist (a psychiatric nurse specialist, social worker, or health psychologist)—are needed for each geographically distinct clinical site. The teams may also include members of other allied health professions: nutritionists, physical therapists, occupational therapists, podiatrists, and others. A recent trend in some healthcare organizations is to extend this concept to include practitioners of alternative or complementary medicine.

Only after the details of how behavioral assessments, referrals, and care will be coordinated are determined should a case-finding plan be implemented. In large healthcare systems, the integrated approach can be piloted in one or more settings (such as health centers or large medical group practices). If an analysis of the data from the pilot sites suggests probable success, the integrated care model can be implemented throughout the system.

Von Korff and associates described four essential elements of effective co-management:

- Development of a collaborative problem definition
- A shared decision-making approach to goal setting, behavior change, and treatment planning
- Development of a continuum of self-management training and support services
- Establishment of an active and sustained follow-up program[21]

A model for collaboration between internal medicine, mental health (or psychiatry), and behavioral medicine is being developed at Harvard Pilgrim Healthcare, the largest health maintenance organization (HMO) in New England (see Chapter 9). In this model, a behavioral medicine clinician works part-time in the internal medicine clinic. This clinician is available for "curbside" consultations or to see patients at the request of the PCC. The behavioral medicine evaluation may result in advice for the PCC or for the patient, referral to a behavioral medicine group program, or referral to mental health for additional evaluation and treatment.

The behavioral medicine department at Harvard Pilgrim is particularly interested in managing the demand for general medical services by improving the detection and treatment of somatization in the primary care setting. In our culture, when people have physical symptoms, they often go to their physician to find out what is wrong. Primary care physicians are usually the first clinicians to note symptoms that suggest somatization. Because the stigma of mental illness persists, many patients will see mental health clinicians only as a last resort. Strengthening the role of the PCC as the leader of the patient care team carries an expectation that PCCs are best suited to address the issue of somatization due to their knowledge of and familiarity with the patient. This has led to a successful management approach, as follows: 1) recognize somatization; 2) have a single physician coordinate care; 3) schedule frequent, regular, brief visits; 4) limit inappropriate specialty consultations; 5) resist patient pressure to inappropriately pursue physical etiologies; and 6) after careful patient education, negotiate a reasonable plan for diagnostic evaluations as part of a shared decision-making process.[22]

In the health centers of the Harvard Pilgrim plan, somatization is treated in collaboration with the behavioral medicine department. Behavioral medicine staff are liaisons between internal medicine and mental health, to facilitate discussion of treatment options for patients who somatize. This includes availability for in-person and telephone consultations. Patients with somatization, stress-related disorders, problems coping with chronic illnesses, and subsyndromal anxiety or depression are referred to behavioral medicine, unless there are comorbid mental disorders (such as psychosis or substance abuse), suicidal risk, or severe psychosocial stressors or disability. Patients with complex problems or severe symptoms are referred to mental health.

The Personal Health Improvement Program (PHIP) was developed and coordinated by the behavioral medicine department of Harvard Pilgrim. The program is designed to treat patients with somatization, stress-related illnesses, and chronic illnesses. The goal is to reduce suffering and stress-related symptoms. Participants are given learning opportunities to observe the connections between moods and symptoms, and they learn to adopt new behaviors that can relieve their pain or discomfort. (For detailed information on this program, see Chapter 10.)

An effective clinical partnership strengthens the patient's disease management skills, enhances motivation and self-confidence, and activates and supports problem solving skills. Self-monitoring and relapse prevention techniques help maintain lifestyle changes and enhance social role functioning. Relaxation, hypnosis, biofeedback, guided imagery, and cognitive-behavioral therapy have helped alleviate pain and other distressing symptoms. Progressive exercise programs have been used to improve coping, reduce distress, and enhance self-efficacy. Structured programs for helping patients change health behaviors can reduce health risks.

Barriers to Identification and Referral

Despite these successes, there are patient, provider, and system barriers to overcome in introducing co-management programs into primary care (Table 4). Institutional barriers that impede clinicians' referral of somatizing patients include 1) inadequate knowledge about somatization, 2) lack of accessible screening and case-finding tools to identify somatizers, 3) lack of appreciation of the adverse cost impact of somatizing patients, 4) adverse impact of somatization on clinician job satisfaction, 5) lack of clinician training programs with opportunities for experiential learning, 6) lack of behavioral medicine consultative services in the primary care setting, 7) clinician inexperience or discomfort in introducing a conversation with the patient about

TABLE 4. COMMON BARRIERS TO INTEGRATION[21]

Patient Barriers
- Lifestyle changes are difficult
- Comorbid medical problems may complicate self-management
- Comorbid depression or anxiety may interfere with treatment motivation or adherence
- Illness behavior may be reinforced
- Family systems may resist change
- Inadequate social support
- Lack of information

Provider Barriers
- Historical emphasis on acute care
- Failure to take a biopsychosocial history
- Insufficient time during the clinical encounter
- Failure to provide opportunities to learn from similar patients in groups
- Inadequate follow-up plans

System Barriers
- Co-management is generally not integrated into primary care practices
- Most care is focused on office visits
- Mid-level clinicians and other allied health professionals are often underutilized
- Poor coordination of care between primary and specialty care
- Inadequate information system supports
- Financial barriers (i.e., inadequate investment in demand-management strategies and treatments)
- Poorly developed links between healthcare systems and community resources

referral, and 8) too little time during the clinical encounter. By developing new approaches to address these barriers, rates of identification and referral should increase.

Strategies to Increase Referrals

There are several strategies that can be implemented to increase clinical referrals to behavioral healthcare providers. Clinicians should be educated about somatization and the somatic manifestations of subsyndromal anxiety and depression. Presentations that highlight the cost to patients and staff—in terms of distress and dollars—may help generate the necessary commitment to developing an integrated, collaborative approach. Other strategies include 1) implementing case finding for somatization through the selection and use of screening tools; 2) providing behavioral interventions that are perceived as helpful by patients with multiple or persistent somatic complaints; 3) developing a behavioral medicine or primary care psychiatry liaison/consultation service that integrates internal medicine, behavioral health, and mental health; 4) providing educational material for patients; and 5) developing and implementing clinician training programs that provide opportunities for experiential learning. This training helps PCCs to learn in a personal and visceral way how behavioral medicine programs work to enhance somatosensory awareness and improve communication. Clinicians need to understand treatments before they feel comfortable recommending them. In addition, clinical effectiveness and cost-effectiveness should be tracked as part of the organizational quality improvement and risk management strategy.

Treatment Issues

Although many treatment-related inquiries accompany somatization, the main question is how to treat it effectively. Although somatization is a highly individualized phenomenon, some elements are common to most patients. To treat somatization, discussions of individual patient experience must be integrated with general guidelines of care. A single protocol or formula is rarely generalizable; however, there are certain general guidelines that can be used in treating most patients with somatization (Table 5).

An issue that requires sensitivity is the introduction of the idea that the patient's physical symptoms, although real, are an expression of personal distress. Educating clinicians about somatization enables them to incorporate a discussion of the normal mind-body relationship as part of routine patient encounters. Patients may then engage more openly in discussions of their symptoms from a similar perspective. They may also become less resistant to referrals.

Nevertheless, a few patients will flatly refuse to accept that any of their physical symptoms have a psychological component. A trusting alliance between these patients and their caregivers may provide a powerful tool for the PCCs who manage somatizers. This trust may elicit a willingness on the patient's part to begin the process of shifting values or adjusting beliefs. These shifts enable the PCC to introduce concepts like mind-body health and behavioral medicine (a term that is less threatening than psychiatry). Eventually, resistant patients may accept referrals to see a psychiatrist or other mental health professional.

To manage highly-resistant somatizing patients, the PCC's best allies are limit setting and consistency about the rules of care among the multidisciplinary team. For example, "doctor shopping" is discouraged. A limited number of medical visits per year should be available for treatment-resistant complaints, but the patient should be encouraged to seek either a mental health or a behavioral medicine consultation. Although setting limits may sound insensitive, colluding with these patients is detrimental to everyone. Limit setting, when combined with regular follow-up appointments and compassionate listening, enables practitioners to monitor these patients and assure that their concerns are taken seriously. In addition, this strategy prevents patients from unnecessary utilization of healthcare resources.

Outcomes Assessment

Successful implementation of an integrated approach to primary care requires the establishment of an effective feedback process. Desirable information for modifying and improving integration efforts are measures of the effectiveness of the interventions, as well as measures of customer satisfaction. Outcome measures should have demonstrated reliability and validity and should be suitable in terms of *change*. Often, patient satisfaction measures are already in use in healthcare organizations, and they

TABLE 5. GENERAL GUIDELINES FOR TREATING SOMATIZATION

1. Assess the symptoms
   - Make a careful and detailed assessment of symptoms
   - Ask patients to describe the frequency, severity, and duration of their symptoms
   - Document information that describes internal or situational factors that exacerbate these symptoms
   - Ask how these symptoms impact their lifestyle as well as the impact on family and friends

2. Discuss the desired outcome
   - Help patients identify realistic treatment goals

3. Determine the patient's psychological baseline
   - Assess patients' psychological, cognitive, and emotional perceptions about their illness
   - Explore possible secondary gain: "What would things be like if you did not have your symptoms?"
   - Rank symptoms in order of importance or order in which the symptoms seem easiest to relinquish

4. Determine the patient's psychological strengths
   - Ask patients what strengths they believe they have which help them live with their symptoms
   - Share your observations of patients' strengths
   - Discuss with patients how they think their strengths may help them relinquish their symptoms

5. Determine financial resources
   - Inquire about insurance coverage and historical use of healthcare resources
   - Involve case management as soon as possible
   - Collaborate with case management about how best to budget available financial resources

6. Determine the potential risks and benefits of diagnostic tests
   - Discuss with patients your beliefs about the need for or against certain diagnostic work-ups
   - If symptoms worsen, do not automatically repeat diagnostic tests. Instead, reevaluate items 1, 2, and 3 from above

7. Use multidisciplinary collaborative teams
   - Develop collaborative multidisciplinary teams
   - Build the interdepartmental relationships needed for a coordinated behavioral health triage and referral system
   - Research, evaluate, and improve team efficacy on a continuous basis

8. Refer to a behavioral medicine treatment program
   - Many patients, with careful consideration, can benefit from behavioral medicine programs

9. Assess for comorbid conditions
   - Rule out medical and psychiatric diagnoses
   - Consider re-testing medical work-ups if it is unclear whether the psychological processes are worsening the physical symptoms
   - Consider mental health referral if psychological baseline changes significantly or if patients' health-seeking behaviors intensify

may be redesigned to assess the success of programs in integrative care. Are PCCs satisfied that access to the behavioral interventions complements and facilitates their practice and directly benefits their patients who somatize? Is the feedback about behavioral treatment outcomes organized by individual patients (when consent is given) or provided in aggregated form? The cost benefits of clinically effective care should be calculated, with analytic support from administrators who track utilization. Furthermore, it may be possible to estimate the cost of *not* developing integrative approaches through the use of modeling techniques.

Future Directions

The terms *behavioral medicine* and *psychosomatic medicine* will become redundant modifiers in the medicine of the future. Economic forces are driving the gradual replacement of the medical model with the biopsychosocial model. The resulting transformation of medical practice should facilitate integrated approaches to managing the care of patients with somatization or those who amplify their symptoms. Patients will benefit from symptom reduction while receiving care that is more holistic. Clinicians who practice in a collaborative framework will find that practice is more satisfying.

Progress in medical information technology will lead to better methods of patient self-assessment, education, and self-care.[23,24] In turn, these methods will be more widely incorporated into primary care. Research will focus on the application of learning-based treatment models to advanced, integrated care. As security tools and protective policies evolve, automated patient assessment tools will merge with electronic personal health records. The automated patient record, vastly different from its handwritten predecessor, will be a dynamic tool for assessment, communication, education, self-care, and even treatment. Patients and clinicians will be empowered to work together in a new partnership for health.

References

1. Kroenke K, Mangelsdorff D: Common symptoms in ambulatory care: incidence, evaluation, therapy, and outcome. Am J Med 86:264, 1989.
2. Lipowski ZJ: Somatization: the concept and its clinical application. Am J Psychiatry 145:1358, 1988.
3. Bass C, Benjamin S: The management of chronic somatization. Br J Psychiatry 162:472, 1993.
4. Smith GR Jr: Toward more effective recognition and management of somatization disorder. J Fam Practice 25:551–552, 1987.
5. Kessler LG, Cleary PD, Burke Jr JD: Psychiatric disorders in primary care. Arch Gen Psychiatry 42:583–590, 1985.
6. Escobar JL, Rubio Stipec M, Canino G, Karno M: Somatic Symptom Index (SSI): a new and abridged somatization construct. J Nerv Ment Dis 177:140–146, 1989.
7. Barsky AJ, Klerman GL: Overview: hypochondriasis, bodily complaints, and somatic styles. Am J Psychiatry 140:274, 1983.
8. McCleod CC, Budd AM: Evaluation of the Personal Health Improvement Program. An innovation for the treatment of somatization in primary care. HMO Practice 11:88–94, 1997.
9. Engel GL: The need for a new medical model: a challenge for biomedicine. Science 196:129–136, 1977.
10. Dreher H: Is there a systemic way to diagnose and treat somatization disorder? Advances: The Journal of Mind-Body Health 12:50, 1996.
11. Smith Jr RG, Rost K, Kashner MT: A trial of the effect of a standardized psychiatric consultation on health outcomes and costs in somatizing patients. Arch Gen Psychiatry 52:238, 1995.
12. Barsky AJ, Borus JF: Somatization and medicalization in the era of managed care. JAMA 274:1931, 1995.
13. Lipsitt DR: Primary care of the somatizing patient: a collaborative model. Hosp Pract 31:77–88, 1996.

14. Simon G, Gater R, Kisely S, Piccinelli M: Somatic symptoms of distress: an international primary care study. Psychosom Med 58:481, 1996.
15. Kleinman A, Kleinman P: Somatization: the interconnections in Chinese society among culture, depressive experiences, and the meanings of pain. In: Culture and Depression. Edited by A Kleinman and B Good. University of California Press, Berkeley CA, 1985.
16. Wickeramasekera I: Assessment and treatment of somatization disorders: the high risk model of threat perception. In: Rhue JW, Lynn SJ, Kirsch 1: Handbook of Clinical Hypnosis. American Psychological Association, Washington DC, 1993.
17. Zung WK: Prevalence of clinically significant anxiety in a family practice. Am J Psychiatry 143:1471-1472, 1986.
18. Zung WK, Broadhead E, Roth ME: Prevalence of depressive symptoms in primary care. J Fam Practice 37:337-344, 1993.
19. Smith GR Jr: The course of somatization and its effects on utilization of health care resources. Psychosomatics 35:263-267, 1994.
20. Lipsitt DR: Medical and psychological characteristics of "crocks." Psychiatry Med 1:15-25, 1970.
21. Von Korff M, Gruman J, Schaefer J, Curry SJ, Wagner EH: Essential Elements for Collaborative Management of Chronic Illness. Center for the Advancement of Health, Washington DC, 1996.
22. Phillips S: When the body speaks its mind. Ment Med Update 4:7, 1995.
23. Miller MJ, Hammond KW, Hile MG: Mental Health Computing. Springer, New York, NY, 1996.
24. Trabin T, Freeman MA: The Computerization of Behavioral Healthcare: How to Enhance Clinical Practice, Management, and Communications. Jossey-Bass Publishers, San Francisco, CA, 1996.

Chapter 18

The Mind–Body Connection: Outcomes Research in the Real World*

Marcie Parker, Ph.D., CFLE, R. Edward Bergmark, Ph.D., and Mark Attridge, Ph.D.

"Healthcare research is an eclectic "field," not a discipline or a specialty, employs a wide range of theories and methods, and has boundaries that are vague and should remain so. Clinical epidemiology, technology assessment, critical appraisal, cost-effectiveness and cost-benefit analyses, clinical decision analysis, operations research, health systems research, [policy analysis] and health services research are all accommodated under the rubric of healthcare research."[1]

Industry leaders and corporate executives are asking challenging questions about the integration of behavioral health and primary care, the efficacy of integrated care, and its cost effectiveness. They are calling for more rigor in measuring and reporting the results of wellness and prevention programs sponsored by the workplace.[2] They want to know, for example, what are the important current measures of behavioral health service outcomes? What are the most significant improvements that need to be made?

The healthcare industry needs refined data collection, more integrated services, and an emphasis on prevention programs. Researchers need to find ways to help manage risk more effectively and to design better data systems to demonstrate that prevention is really saving money.[3] While we intuitively know that treating the person as a whole by addressing the mental and the physical needs is more effective and efficient, we need validation through research.

The research from Optum, a division of United HealthCare Corporation, seems to demonstrate a need for greater emphasis on the integration of behavioral health and primary care. This integration is reflected in our biopsychosocial model, which is a multidisciplinary health approach that recognizes the interrelated influences of biological, psychological, and social factors on the onset, course, and treatment of physical illness.

The Importance of Behavioral Healthcare

Behavioral health issues, including mental health problems, alcohol and substance abuse, stress, migraine headaches, depression, and panic disorders, are common in the United States.[4] Much recent research demonstrates the need to identify and treat depression in the primary care setting.[5-9] These issues affect Americans in every setting, with serious consequences for individuals, families, and communities. The question is why services and interventions that address behavioral health needs

*Chapter 18 ©1997 United HealthCare Corporation

do not figure more prominently in the current healthcare system. It may be due, in part, to myths about behavioral health interventions.

Two trends have converged recently in the United States—efforts to develop a national healthcare system and the need to address the national deficit. This has led to renewed efforts to identify, through outcomes research, therapies and interventions which are truly effective. The need for acute and chronic medical therapies is not usually questioned, despite a surprising lack of empirical evidence proving their efficacy. In fact, only about 12 percent of the therapeutic medical procedures in use today have been shown to be effective through systematic outcomes research.[10] On the other hand, providers, payors, and the public often question the efficacy and the need for behavioral health interventions. There is a widespread misperception that psychological services have a limited impact on the cost of medical services. In fact, extensive efforts are underway to document empirically validated therapies and their ability to reduce medical claims.[11,12]

At the same time, there is renewed interest by the general public and by public funders, planners, and policy makers in integrating behavioral health into primary care and other healthcare settings.[13] The goal is to have care flow seamlessly between the behavioral health specialist and the primary care physician (PCP) to meet the needs of the client and to lessen the perceived stigma of receiving mental health services.

Effectiveness of Behavioral Health Interventions

There have been a number of studies of the efficacy of psychological, educational, and behavioral treatments for a variety of problems. These have included a meta-analysis by Lipsey and Wilson of the findings from 302 other meta-analyses.[14] The conclusion is that well-developed psychological, educational, and behavioral treatments often produce meaningful, positive effects on the intended outcome variable. Lipsey and Wilson also report that the average statistical effect size for psychological treatments is greater than that of most successful medical treatments.

Giles, Prail, and Neims, in a review of more than 150 therapeutic outcome studies, concluded that some directive treatments (such as behavioral or cognitive behavioral treatments) were more effective than long-term psychotherapies.[15] Other reviews of the outcomes and cost effectiveness of psychotherapy and interventions have also concluded that behavioral health interventions are generally effective in improving the quality of life, well-being, and health of many clients.[16-19]

Medical cost offset studies over the past three decades have shown that medical costs for clients are reduced anywhere from 5 percent to 80 percent when clients receive psychological care. These reductions include fewer visits to the medical doctor's office as well as other kinds of healthcare utilization.[20-29] These studies provide empirical evidence of the cost effectiveness and cost offset of behavioral health interventions. Most effective are the integrated behavioral health and medical interventions.

Employee Health and Human Risk Management

In 1996 Optum conducted a national survey of benefits managers to assess their thoughts about employee health and human risk management services. The survey included detailed questions about employee concerns, in addition to the amount and effectiveness of services and training offered by the organizations. We found that managers recognize the importance of employee programs designed to improve productivity, skills, and services that help employees balance their lives between work and home. For example, working parents may be hesitant to take sick days for themselves, preferring instead to save them for days when their children are ill. By working with telephone triage nurses and their own PCPs, parents can effectively assess the severity of the child's illness and can access alternative community resources for sick-child day care.

Our research shows that employees have concerns about a diverse range of biopsychosocial issues, from physical well-being to work, family, legal, and financial issues. Figure 1 depicts high or very high at-risk responses to our employee concern survey from both the employers' as well as the employees' perspectives.

This study found that the majority of the companies surveyed provide substance abuse, mental health, family, awareness training, and health promotional services to their employees. Substance abuse/addiction was the most frequent service provided by managers (81 percent). In addition, it was also rated the highest in enhancing employee performance (88 percent) and reducing overall healthcare costs (85 percent). Over 80 percent of managers believe employee performance was improved by awareness training, family/relationship services, and mental health services provided to the employee. Over 70 percent of the managers find that pregnancy and childbirth, mental health, and health promotional services helped reduce healthcare costs.

Our survey also found that 24-hour telephone services which allowed employees to access a nurse or counselor were rated the highest by managers for optimal delivery of health and human risk services. Next highest rated were (in descending order): 24-hour

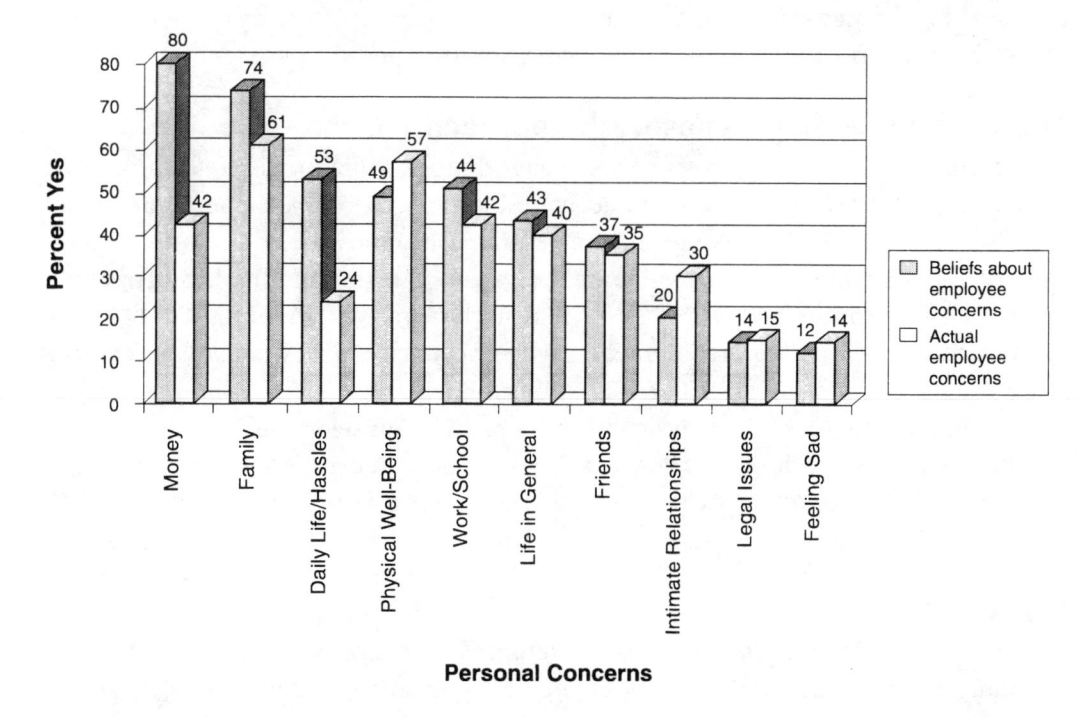

Figure 1. At-risk levels of personal concerns

access to counselors, referrals to local resources, in-person counseling sessions, on-site workshops, printed educational materials, automated telephone access, and electronic access (online, cable TV, or kiosk). Telephone medical information and counseling services also enhance the primary care system through better access to care and continuity of care.

Substance abuse programs which help supervisors carry out responsibilities in creating a drug-free workplace (45 percent) and understand workplace effects (39 percent) are more frequently offered than substance abuse programs which focus on its effects on families (23 percent). This seems to show that managers are struggling with their responsibilities and need further in-depth education. The training programs most frequently requested by managers within the upcoming year were: how to become a wise healthcare consumer, balancing work and family, achieving healthy lifestyles, and planning for retirement.

This study indicates that many benefits managers understand the value of behavioral health services, especially when integrated with primary care. Furthermore, they view the need for these services as more urgent than most employees do. This may be because benefits managers deal with many employees who are having problems and rarely interface with those who are not. Managers thus see the more global effect of problems, such as domestic abuse or substance abuse, on the entire workplace.

Many of the concerns that affect employees and morale in the workplace are complex, biopsychosocial issues. They affect all aspects of our lives—health, family, work, finances, child care, elder care, legal, and emotional. The research demonstrates that a biopsychosocial approach works, and employers and purchasers seem to agree on its value as well. The challenge is to deliver a truly integrated service and properly investigate its outcomes. Our biopsychosocial model helps callers deal with these complex, interrelated concerns, work more effectively with PCPs, develop solutions, and seek out referrals for counseling and community support groups.

The Case for a Biopsychosocial Approach

Optum® Care24 is a biopsychosocial model through which registered nurses and master's level counselors integrate triage, coordination, education, support, and advocacy by telephone. This helps prevent unwarranted healthcare use. Features include telephone integration (one number to call), systems integration (sharing of records among nurses, counselors, and PCPs), clinical integration (coordination between nurses and counselors to promote the biopsychosocial approaches to care) and report integration (quarterly and annual reports of results and caller satisfaction).

Through discussions with physicians, nurses, and counselors, as well as ongoing literature searches, we have developed a list of caller concerns that are biopsychosocial in nature and warrant close coordination among nurse, counselor, and PCP. Our most recent data (March 1997) show that the top biopsychosocial topics addressed by counselors and nurses are abdominal pain, depression, headache, chest pain, substance abuse, anxiety/panic, asthma, domestic abuse, and eating disorders. (See end of chapter for a complete list of Optum Care24 biopsychosocial conditions.)

Many of the callers were referred to their PCP, urgent care center, or emergency department. In many instances, callers also mentioned legal, financial, family, stress, marital, and sexuality issues that compounded the chief complaint. Sometimes they also mentioned work-related issues with a counselor. These concerns often centered on poor work performance, job stress, management issues, time and attendance problems, difficulties with workplace culture, and interpersonal workplace problems.

Screening Questions

To help clinicians determine when callers might want to have a Care24 consultation involving a nurse and counselor, we developed five key biopsychosocial screening questions. These questions are not used with all callers, but are used when, in the professional judgment of the counselor or nurse, they are warranted.

1. Have you had any recent life changes? (divorce, financial problems, a sick child or spouse)
2. In the past two years, have you experienced the death of a person close to you? (If yes, then as a child, did you experience the loss of someone close to you? Do you feel you had adequate support in grieving for this loss? Do you feel that you have come to a resolution of the loss? If not, what kinds of problems are you encountering as a result? Would a referral be helpful?)
3. Are you depressed?
4. Is this issue affecting other areas of your life such as work, family, relationships, other physical conditions?
5. Is your current condition affecting your ability to work or perform daily activities?

Nurses and counselors receive training jointly so they can identify either medical and/or emotional concerns which need consideration. For example, counselors are aware of the medical needs of callers and work with nurses to address these concerns. If a young woman calls with an eating disorder, the counselor confers with a nurse to assess the caller's current nutritional status. Or, an elderly woman complaining of easy bruising may be questioned about alcohol dependency and nutritional deficiency. She may be screened for possible physical abuse. If abuse is found, her living situation and social supports may need to be evaluated. Her PCP will be alerted (with her permission) to her physical abuse, her need for a safe environment, and possible coordination with community support groups and resources.

Overlap of Mental Health, Physical Health, and Work Issues

The effectiveness of the biopsychosocial approach is demonstrated in our own research, which illustrates the overlap between mental health, substance abuse, personal concerns, physical health, and work-related issues. In an analysis of 12,688 callers who phoned a counselor in the last three quarters of 1995, we looked for the overlap between mind, body, and work issues. The comorbidity data examined included:

- Work—The most commonly discussed issues were critical incident stress management following a crisis at work, sexual harassment, workplace violence, or a hostile work environment.

- Mind—Alcoholism, major depression, marital relationship problems, legal issues, a difficult adjustment related to job loss or relationship loss.
- Body—Pregnancy, childbirth, headaches, or chronic pain.

We found that 68 percent of callers have concerns in one category, 23 percent have concerns in two categories, and an astounding 9 percent have concerns in all three areas, or a trimorbidity. In addition, we noted that each category actually has many more comorbidities. For example, a person may call about a marital problem and begin discussing alcoholism, legal, and financial problems as well.

Recently, we have refined the categories considerably to provide a more detailed breakdown of callers' concerns. These categories include: individual work issues; organizational work concerns; physical issues (for the caller or those for whom they provide care); two possible categories for mental health concerns (allowing callers, for example, to indicate that they are using cocaine and are depressed); relationship issues; legal concerns; financial issues; childcare concerns; and eldercare issues. This breakdown will help us understand the sources of physical health concerns which are being seen in the primary care physician's office, the urgent care center, and the emergency department.

Severity of Caller Concerns

Each problem area is also assessed for severity, defined as how urgently the person needs professional assistance for the problem. There are four categories of severity, as reported by counselors:

Low (indefinite time period before help or educational materials are needed)
Moderate (needs help within one week)
High (needs help within 24 hours)
Crisis (needs help immediately)

Figure 2 shows the percentage of each category of severity. The majority of callers (80 percent), need educational information or assistance within a week for their concern. On the other hand, 11.5 percent of mental health, 12.8 percent of physical health, and 16.7 percent of work-related calls were high-severity calls. Additionally,

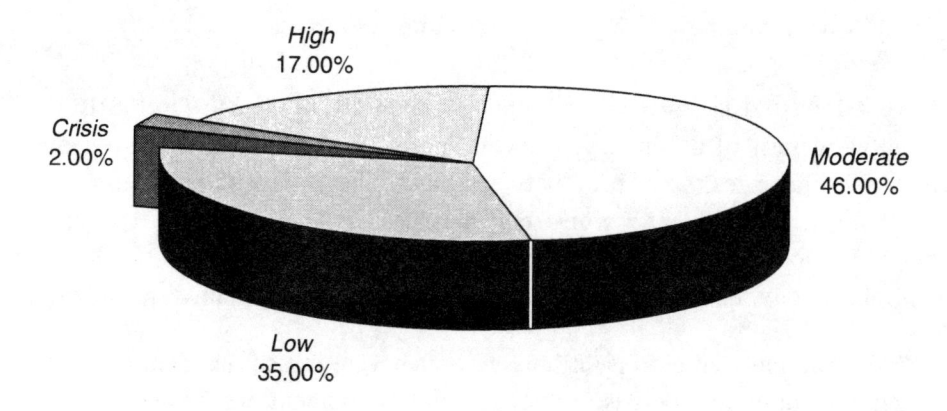

Figure 2. Assessed problem severity

1.5 percent of mental health, 1.3 percent of physical health, and 1.0 percent of work-related calls were crisis-level calls for which the callers needed immediate help to prevent injuring themselves or others.

Biopsychosocial Concerns in a Large Midwest Public Employer Group

In a separate study, we asked over 1,000 employees (randomly selected from over 75,000 employees in a large Midwest public employer group) how concerned they were about various biopsychosocial issues. These were rated on a six-point scale ranging from one (not at all concerned) to six (very high concern). The ten areas of rated concern were 1) physical well-being, 2) feeling sad (which might signal depression), 3) work/school, 4) daily life/hassles, 5) intimate relationships, 6) family, 7) friends, 8) money, 9) legal issues, and 10) life in general.

The results indicated that all areas were significantly positively correlated, ranging from $r = +0.33$ to $+0.76$. All areas of concern are interrelated, such that having greater concern in any one category indicates also having greater concern in other categories. Thus, even though a PCP may focus on a particular area of concern, such as recurrent headaches, the caller is likely to have multiple related biopsychosocial concerns as well. This lends support for an assessment based on a biopsychosocial model.

Midwestern Insurance Company Study

This study tracked medical claims costs (including mental health claims) for 246 employees, 112 spouses, and 118 of their children for a period of two years (one year before and one year after their call to Optum).

For the employees, average monthly medical claims costs before contact with Optum were $92 and, after service, $101; this represents an increase of $9 per month. However, at the family level, average medical claims per month were $295 before services were accessed and $255 after contact, a decrease of $40 per month. The family unit had reduced claim costs of 14 percent, spouses' claim costs were reduced by 32 percent, and children's claim costs were reduced by 13 percent (Table 1).

In this study, it appears that individual employee costs increased due to treatment received following contact with nurses and counselors. The primary impact of this treatment was reduced stress and medical claims for the employees' family members.

TABLE 1. MIDWESTERN INSURANCE COMPANY STUDY—CLAIMS COSTS

	Average cost per month before contact	Average cost per month after contact	Difference	Change (percent)
Employee	$92	$101	$9	+10
Spouse	$114	$77	$37	−32
Child	$89	$77	$12	−13
Family Total	$295	$255	$40	−14

Thus, the study suggests a positive effect on the health and well-being of family members when intervention is made at the individual level, and employees are assisted in addressing their biopsychosocial issues. Furthermore, this effect is significant enough to compensate for the added costs of the services which are provided to the employee.

Difficult Bosses

In 1993 we polled a nationally representative sample of more than 1,000 working Americans on the topic of difficult bosses and their impact on workers and the workplace. The actual sample size was 659 respondents: 350 men (68 percent had a male boss) and 309 women (52 percent had a male boss).

Results show the impact of behavioral health issues on healthcare and workplace productivity. Workers are more likely to get ill if they believe their boss is treating them disrespectfully. Workers who say their boss is rarely or never respectful are five to six times more likely to report physical ailments caused by the bosses' behavior than workers who say their boss is usually or always respectful. Of workers who felt they had disrespectful bosses, 25 percent of workers have left a job due to their bosses' disrespectful behavior, and one-third of the workers surveyed have considered leaving a job due to their bosses' disrespectful behavior. Also, 20 percent of workers surveyed report that their bosses' disrespectful behavior causes stress in their lives. The most common physical effects caused by bosses' disrespectful behaviors are headaches (reported by 41 percent of respondents with a bad boss, or 26.3 percent of men and 52.9 percent of women) and stomach aches (reported by 10.4 percent of respondents with a bad boss, or 8.1 percent of men and 12.3 percent of women).

After seeing the results of this survey, we also took a closer look at our assistance caller statistics. Of 88 callers who reported an interpersonal conflict with their supervisor, 54 percent also had an organizational work issue such as a merger or downsizing, 30 percent had physical problems (often headaches and backaches), and 95 percent reported problems in the mental health/substance abuse/daily living category. For these callers, early coordination with the PCP, and possibly a counselor as well, might keep physical symptoms from escalating and keep healthcare costs down.

Assistance Caller Outcomes: Results of Five Surveys

Studies were conducted to determine the kinds of outcomes experienced by callers in five problem areas: mental health issues *(Diagnostic and Statistical Manual of Mental Disorders,* Third edition, revised, or *DSM-III-R);* financial problems; substance abuse problems; work-related problems; and domestic abuse problems.

Mental Health Problems

Most callers felt they received the help they needed and were more effective in coping with their problems. Most had followed up on their recommendations, whether to a support group, counselor, behavioral health program, or other resources (Figure 3).

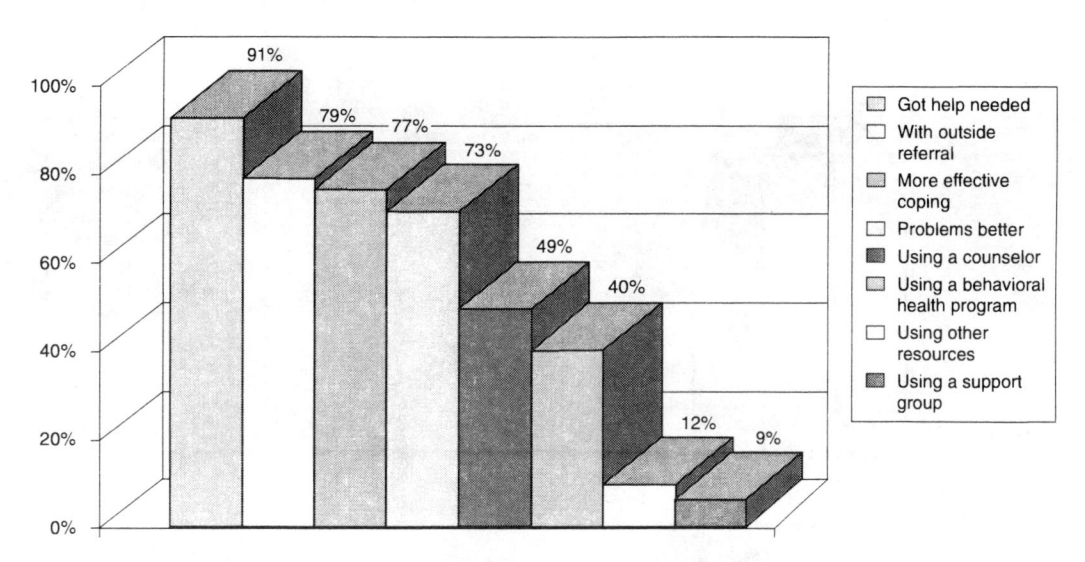

Figure 3. Survey of 330 clients with mental health issues (*DSM-III*-R)

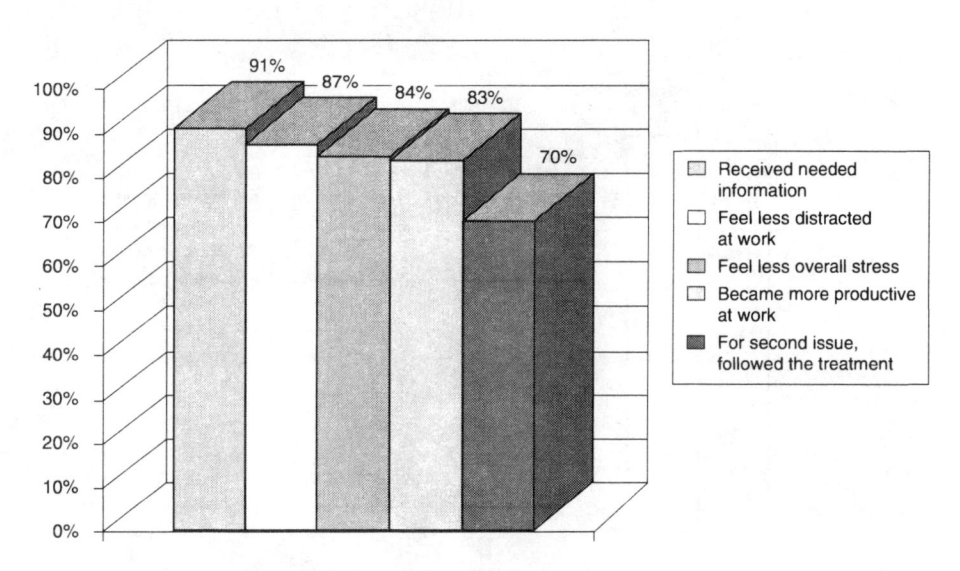

Figure 4. Survey of 109 clients with financial problems

Financial Problems

Callers in this survey said they received the information they needed from the counselor, felt less stressed in general, and could get more done at work. In addition, 70 percent of these callers with a secondary issue such as alcohol or drug abuse, depression or marital problems pursued the recommended course of treatment for the secondary issue including discussing it with their PCP (Figure 4).

Substance Abuse Problems

Most of these callers believed they were coping better after speaking with a counselor and said that their problems were improved. More than one-half had not used drugs or alcohol for four or more weeks since speaking with a counselor. Many were

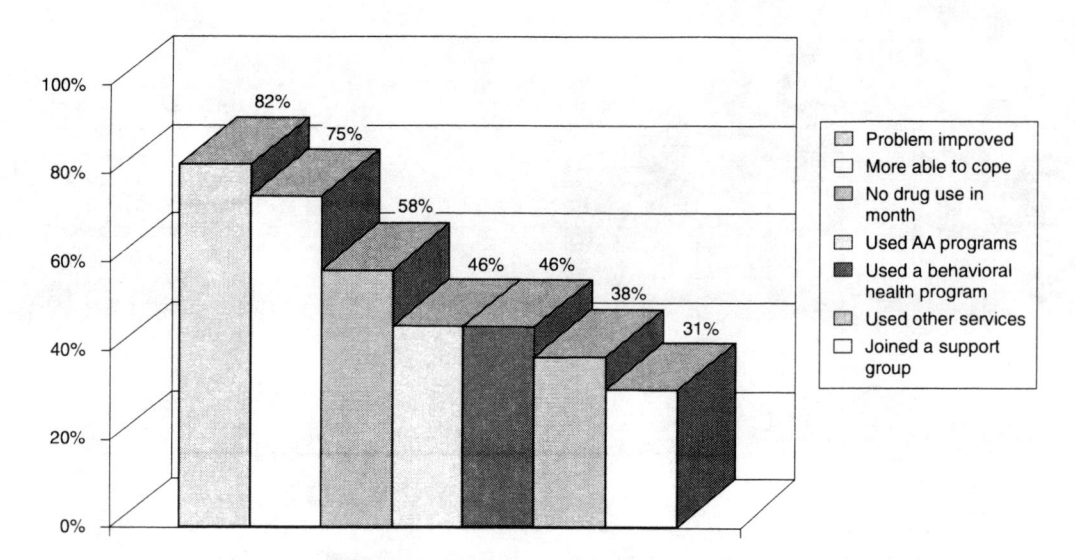

Figure 5. Survey of 83 clients with substance abuse problems

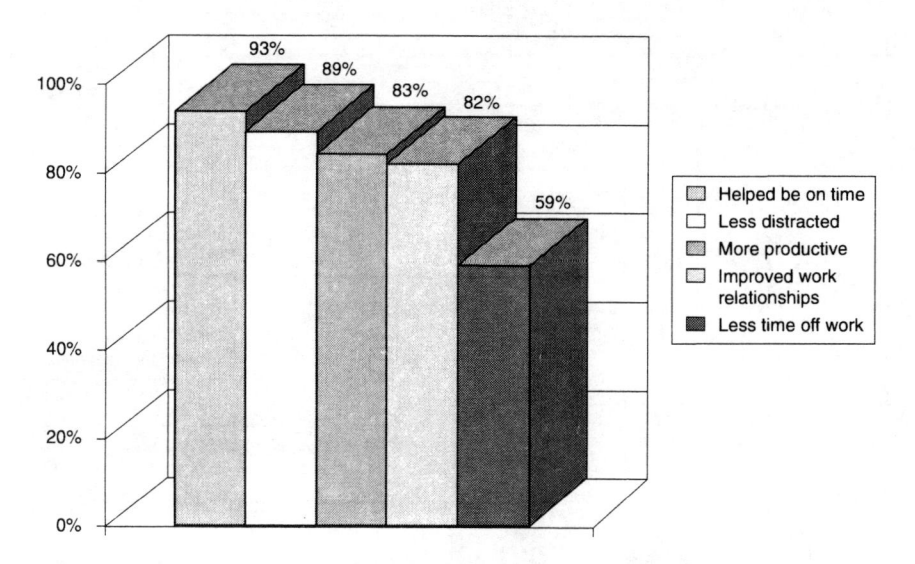

Figure 6. Survey of 66 clients with work-related problems

using a support group, behavioral health program, or Alcoholics Anonymous group (Figure 5).

Work-related Problems

The majority of Optum callers with work-related problems found that the treatment helped them become less distracted, and they felt they were more productive at work overall (Figure 6).

Domestic Abuse Problems

In another study of our abuse cases from June 1991– December 1994, we found a total of 2,627 callers with Domestic Abuse/Violent Relationship/Child Abuse as either

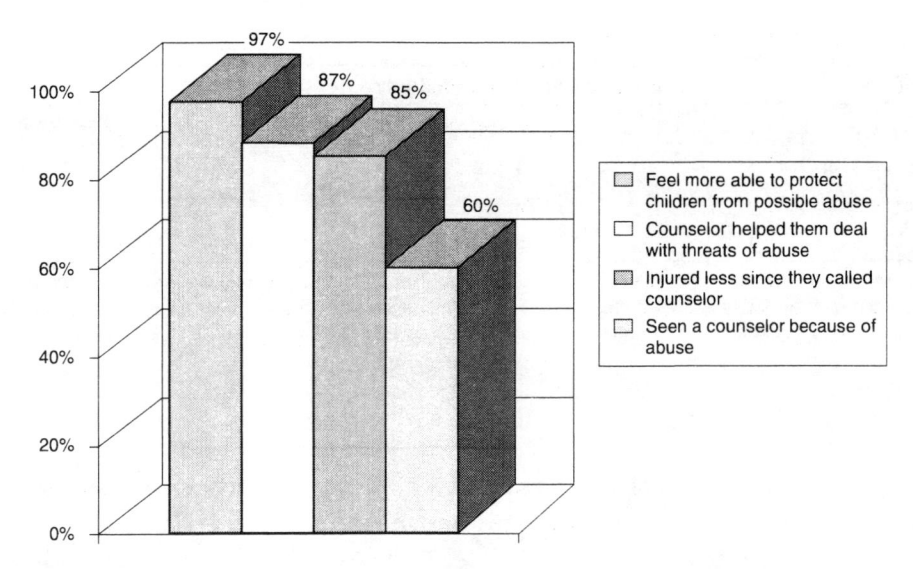

Figure 7. Survey of 49 clients with domestic abuse problems

the primary or secondary assessed problem type. This represents 3.7 percent of all new cases over this time period. Women accounted for 78 percent of abuse callers, compared to 64 percent for all callers.

The majority had been injured less frequently since calling a counselor. Most felt better able to protect themselves and their children from abuse and threats of abuse (Figure 7). Significantly, 88 percent of the callers had gone to the emergency room in the previous six months for a domestic abuse injury, and none had gone to the emergency room for domestic abuse injuries since contacting the counselor.

The results of these five surveys provide compelling evidence of the need for a biopsychosocial approach and a strong liaison with PCPs in identifying and treating these issues in a clinical setting.

Caller Satisfaction and Outcomes Surveys

Regular surveys of callers are conducted to assess utilization, satisfaction, outcomes, and clinical profiles. There is quarterly reporting of statistics which indicates how many members use services, descriptions of the reasons for calling, problem severity assessment, referral information, and satisfaction with various aspects of the service.

Results have been consistent over a number of years with our caller satisfaction survey and alternative resource study. In an analysis of the surveys of 8,013 callers in 1995 and the first half of 1996, 76 percent said their physical well-being improved after speaking with a counselor or nurse. Twenty-six percent said that if they had not called, they would have seen their PCP or had an urgent care or emergency room visit. Also, 51 percent would have taken time off from work to deal with their problem if they had not spoken with a nurse or counselor. Over 72 percent indicated that after calling, their personal relationships improved.

We also looked at healthcare visits deferred, as shown in Table 2. Currently, we are having an outside survey research firm conduct our caller satisfaction surveys.

TABLE 2. HEALTHCARE VISITS DEFERRED*

Type of visit	Number of visits deferred (percent)
Physician visits	728 (26.7)
Urgent care visits	64 (2.3)
Emergency room visits	76 (2.7)
Total	868 (32.0)

*Sample size = 2,729. Member assist calls are about 10 percent of all calls; thus, the total percentage deferred would be 29 percent. Of the 868 callers who would have gone to their physician's office, urgent care facility, or emergency room, 32 (3.7 percent) were referred to an external mental health provider (Optum Assistance data Q1–Q3, 1996).

This eliminates many possible sources of bias and may help us achieve a higher rate of response. We are also developing provider satisfaction surveys in addition to the caller surveys.

NurseLine Diversion

Data for NurseLine (our toll-free medical information line) also show diversions from the caller's original inclination. In addition to requesting information on specific health issues (80 percent of callers), many callers request direction for minor illness or injury. Registered nurses assess urgency and make recommendations for the most appropriate care setting, such as calling 911 or poison control, going to the emergency room or to urgent care, seeing the PCP now, seeing the PCP in one to two days, or trying home care or self-care.

Many times nurses validate the caller's original inclination (Figure 8). About 20 percent of the time, the nurses recommend what the caller wanted to do or reinforce the caller's original inclination. This provides the caller with reassurance and reduces caller stress. Callers are also provided with questions to ask the PCP or healthcare provider in order to make the office visit more effective and efficient.

One-fifth of the time the caller wants to take an action that is more severe than the nurse would recommend; thus, callers were recommended to a lower level of care than their original inclination. These are diversions from original inclination, often from an emergency room visit or physician visit. Savings are calculated by subtracting the cost of one from the other, so if the caller saw the physician instead of going to the emergency room, we calculate the savings as the average cost of the emergency room visit minus the average cost of the physician office visit for the region of the country from which the call originated.

Forty percent of the time the caller wants to take a less costly or less severe course of action than the nurse would recommend, and are thus recommended to a more intensive level of care. Figure 8 shows that 1 percent of callers were sent to the emergency room and 14 percent were urged to see their PCP immediately when their original inclination was to wait. In this way, we have avoided heart attacks, diabetic comas, or the effects of head trauma that might otherwise have ensued. In any given year, our nurses recommend that 60,000 callers to go to the emergency room or to see their physician immediately.

THE MIND-BODY CONNECTION: OUTCOMES RESEARCH

What the Caller Wanted to Do for Problem*

		Do Nothing	Home Care	Call MD	See MD	UR	ER	911
		13.42%	24.67%	38.91%	9.83%	2.58%	10.54%	0.03%
What the Nurse Recommended	Home Care	5.24%	5.78%	8.25%	1.01%	0.09%	0.58%	0.00%
	MD Follow-Up 1–2 Days	3.21%	5.69%	9.40%	3.73%	0.47%	1.14%	0.01%
	Call MD Now	2.95%	7.97%	13.94%	2.45%	0.55%	2.18%	0.01%
	See MD Now	1.89%	4.96%	6.88%	2.57%	1.46%	6.19%	0.00%
	911-Emergency	0.14%	0.27%	0.44%	0.07%	0.02%	0.46%	0.02%

*Based on 16,079 NurseLine Clinical Calls in Fall of 1995

☐ Lighter shaded area represents the **40%** of callers who were recommended to a more **intensive** level of care.
▓ Darker shaded area represents the **20%** of callers who were recommended to a more **appropriate** level of care.

Figure 8. NurseLine recommendations versus caller inclinations

In a study of whether or not callers actually followed through on the nurses' recommendations, we called 10 percent of the callers one week after their original call. We found that 90 percent had followed the suggested course of action.

In some instances, callers who initially access nurses via NurseLine actually require both nursing and mental health consultation. These are often substance abusers, alcoholics, or persons with depressive illness who "test out" the line and make sure they will receive respectful and nonjudgmental acceptance. Once they feel comfortable, they will call a counselor or allow themselves to be transferred from the nurse to the counselor in the same call.

In 2 percent to 10 percent of calls, the nurse determines that the caller also needs to speak with a counselor and makes the referral with the caller's permission. Sometimes, callers do not understand the mental health component of their physical symptoms, and the nurse can educate and refer them to their PCP or to a counselor. Alternatively, callers may be comfortable seeking help for physical concerns but are not willing to seek help for mental health issues. Nurses can provide invaluable education and support, enabling the caller to make the transition to the PCP and, ultimately, a counselor.

Results of this research show that demand-side management should be for the purpose of optimizing the use of healthcare resources, not denying access to care. We believe that quality managed care does not lead to blanket denial of access to care, but rather to providing the right care, at the right time, and in the most appropriate setting.

Medical Cost Offset

We joined with the Wisconsin Education Association Insurance Group (WEA) and William Mercer, Inc. in a three-way partnership to assess a demand-side management program on outpatient medical utilization and associated costs. This medical cost offset study examined the two-year impact of a medical information service (NurseLine) on outpatient utilization among approximately 48,000 active employees insured by WEA. Use of a 24-hour telephone-based medical information service, self-care book, monthly wellness newsletter, and maternity education program was tested to assess cost-effectiveness in reducing medical services utilization. Preliminary findings indicate up to a 4.5 to 1 return on investment for program participants.

The study was designed to assess the impact of the medical information service on outpatient utilization and associated claims expenses. The null hypothesis of "no difference" was tested to assess whether a group offered the program would show lowered utilization of specific outpatient medical services over a two-year period when compared to a similar control group. It was anticipated that the reduction in outpatient services utilization, measured as savings in claims dollars, would exceed program costs.

The study compared the claims experience of the experimental group versus the control group for a specified set of medical services. Outpatient utilization rates, measured as services per 1,000 enrollees, were obtained for physician office visits, emergency room admittance, hospital outpatient services, and outpatient physician and medical facility surgical services.

The utilization rate was approximately 8 percent. Use of combined outpatient services showed an increasing trend for both groups over the two experimental periods. However, the experimental group showed a 19 percent lower rate of increase compared to the control group. Lower utilization of outpatient services over the two-year period for this particular homogeneous group generated a savings-to-cost ratio of 4.5 to 1.

The results provide encouraging indications that the service, as evaluated in this study, may be associated with reductions in the use of medical services. Furthermore, these reductions were observed over a two-year period, generating savings which exceeded program costs by a considerable margin. While the self-care book and newsletter may be helpful, access to a registered nurse 24 hours a day was the single most important component of the program. The study needs to be replicated with diverse populations throughout the United States to determine whether these savings apply more broadly.

Disease State Management

Many companies are leveraging the research presented to develop disease state management programs. *Disease management* involves a set of interventions applied to the care of persons with targeted chronic diseases in order to improve the course and outcome of their disease, prevent acute exacerbation, and improve the quality of their lives.

Three common goals of disease management are 1) improving the quality of care and reducing the cost of care for those with the targeted chronic disease; 2) focusing on high-cost conditions of moderate to high prevalence with national guidelines and standards for treatment; and 3) supporting Health Plan Employer Data and Information Set (HEDIS) initiatives from the National Committee for Quality Assurance (NCQA) for improved health plan performance in the management of chronic conditions.

Disease state management combines several research methods into a powerful clinical intervention program. Medical claims data are first analyzed to identify potential program participants with disease-specific claims in the past year. Participants are then interviewed with a survey profile to categorize them into mild, moderate, or severe levels. Survey data also assess the reaction of participants to written educational materials sent to the home and to clinical intervention. At 6 months and at 12 months from the introduction of the disease management program, participants are profiled to assess changes in clinical outcomes, medical utilization, knowledge and understanding of the disease, and satisfaction with care. A longitudinal follow-up of claims history at the one-year point is used to validate the self-report survey information. Thus, our disease management process combines claims data, survey data, and risk profiling to target individuals who may need an advanced level of case management and preventive intervention coordinated through their PCP.

The clinical objectives of disease state management are to educate participants to self-manage their illness, in order to achieve desired clinical, financial, and quality of life outcomes. These objectives are achieved through improved relationships with the PCP, the care manager, the family, and the managed care organization.

In the first stage of disease management, the focus is on primary prevention (health promotion and disease prevention). Stage two is the actual disease management, and stage three focuses on long-term care. Program deliverables include participant identification and profiling, telephone education, disease-specific educational materials, physician-oriented interventions, specialty partners to manage high-level interventions, 24-hour telephone access to registered nurses, and outcomes research, measurement, and reporting.

Current disease management programs include congestive heart failure, low back pain, diabetes (Type I and Type II), and asthma (pediatric and adult). A program for depression is under development. We are now in the first year of collecting data to measure return on investment for disease state management, and we hope to have these results in the near future.

Conclusion

Our research demonstrates the need for healthcare providers to understand and accept the indivisible nature of physical health and behavioral health and to incorporate this concept into their daily practice. Primary care physicians who do not routinely screen for depression may be providing sporadic, symptomatic relief for a variety of physical symptoms while delaying resolution of an underlying problem.

Behavioral health professionals should be aware of the medical "mimics" of mental disorders and how to spot them.[30] A behavioral health provider, counseling a participant with drug or alcohol dependency, needs to recognize the physical damage that results from substance abuse. The counselor can then provide more effective support and encouragement as the caller seeks medical evaluation with a PCP.

Most people intuitively understand the interrelationship between physical and mental health needs. Providers must begin to pay more attention to this important interplay as well. A collaborative, supportive, respectful working relationship among counselors, nurses, and PCPs can significantly enhance the quality of care and reduce medical claims costs.

We continue to develop the biopsychosocial approach through the ongoing training of our counselors and nurses, efforts to include communication with primary care providers, and development of standards and guidelines for services that integrate all the concerns of daily living. Managed care organizations have an opportunity to encourage the re-integration of the mind and body through outcomes research that shows the value of the biopsychosocial model and through incentives in the service delivery system that encourage integration.

References

1. White KL: Healthcare research: old wine in new bottles. The Pharos (Summer):12–16, 1993.
2. Burns J: The need for more rigor when measuring and reporting results (Editor's Memo). Business and Health, January:8, 1995.
3. Peck RL: Employers look at behavioral healthcare. Behav Health Management November/December:10–11, 1996.
4. Bergmark RE, Dell P, Attridge M, Parker, MK: Creating an integrated Healthcare System: the health and human risk management model. Managed Care Q 4:36–42, 1996.

5. Rush JA, Golden WE, Walton Hall G, et al: Guideline overview: Depression in primary care. In: The Medical Outcomes and Guidelines Sourcebook. Agency for Healthcare Policy and Research (5):200, 1993.
6. Valente SM: Recognizing depression in elderly patients. Am J Nurs December:19, 1994.
7. Sturm R, Jackson CA, Meredith LS, et al: Mental healthcare utilization in prepaid and fee-for-service plans among depressed patients in the medical outcomes study. Health Services Res 30:319–340, 1995.
8. Wells KB, Hays RD, Burnam MA, et al: Detection of depressive disorder for patients receiving prepaid or fee-for-service care. JAMA 262:3298, 1989.
9. Baer L, Jacobs DG, Cukor P, O'Laughlen J, Coyle JT, Magruder, KM: Automated telephone screening survey for depression. JAMA 273:1943, 1995.
10. Zalta E: "Outcomes and Quality Care: An Overview." Presentation to the 1995 National Managed Healthcare Congress, Washington DC, April 1995.
11. Chambless DL, Sanderson WC, Shoham V, et al: An update on empirically validated therapies. Clin Psychol 49:5–22, 1996.
12. Goldberg RJ: Integrating Behavioral Health Services with General Medical Care. Manisses Communications Group, Providence RI, 1996.
13. Clay RA: Making the next move into primary care. APA Monitor, January:34, 1997.
14. Lipsey MW, Wilson DB: The efficacy of psychological, educational, and behavioral treatment. Am Psychol 48:1181–1209, 1993.
15. Giles TR, Prail EM, Neims DM: Evaluating psychotherapies: a comparison of effectiveness. Intl J Mental Health 22:43–65, 1993.
16. VandenBos GR: Outcome assessment of psychotherapy. Am Psychol 51:1005–1006, 1996.
17. Hollon S: The efficacy and effectiveness of psychotherapy relative to medications. Am Psychol 51:1025–1030, 1996.
18. Tengs TO, Adams ME, Pliskin JS, et al: Five-hundred life saving interventions and their cost-effectiveness. Risk Analysis. 15:369–389, 1995.
19. Jacobson NS, Christensen A: Studying the effectiveness of psychotherapy. Am Psychol 51:1031–1039, 1996.
20. Turkington C: Help for the worried well: psychological interventions cut medical hospital costs and help people feel better. Psychol Today August:44–48, 1987.
21. Cummings NA: The successful application of medical offset in program planning and in clinical delivery. Managed Care Q 2:1–6, 1994.
22. Jones KR, Vischi TR: Impact of alcohol, drug abuse and mental health treatment of medical care utilization: a review of the literature. Med Care 17(suppl 2):1–82, 1979.
23. Mumford E, et al: A new look at evidence about reduced cost of medical utilization following mental health treatment. Am J Psychol 141:1145–1158, 1984.
24. Lobeck F, Traxler WT, Bobinet DD: The cost-effectiveness of a clinical pharmacy service in an outpatient mental health clinic. Hosp Community Psychiatr 40:643–645, 1989.
25. Jacobs DF: Cost-effectiveness of specialized psychological programs for reducing hospital stays and outpatient visits. J Clin Psychol 43:729–735, 1987.
26. Smith GR, Miller LM, Monson RA: Consultation liaison intervention in somatization disorder. Hosp Community Psychiatr 37:1207–1210, 1986.
27. Cooper CL, Sadri G: The impact of stress counseling at work. J Soc Behav Pers 6:411–423, 1991.
28. Aivazyan TA, Zaitsev VP, Yurenev AP: Autogenic training in treatment and secondary prevention of essential hypertension: five-year follow-up. Health Psychol 7(suppl):201–208, 1988.
29. Shi L: Health promotion, medical care use, and costs in a sample of worksite employees. Evaluation Rev 17:475–487, 1993.
30. Hedaya RJ: Understanding Biological Psychiatry. WW Norton & Company Inc., New York NY, 1996.

Appendix A
Optum® Care24 Biopsychosocial Conditions

Definition: Biopsychosocial care is a multidisciplinary health approach that recognizes the interrelated influences of biological, psychological, and social factors on the onset, course, and treatment of physical illness.

*1. Abdominal pain (adults)
2. Alzheimer's disease
3. Angina (see cardiac conditions)
4. Anorexia nervosa (general information)
*5. Asthma (adult/pediatric)
6. Bipolar disorder
7. Breast cancer surgery
8. Bulimia (general information)
9. Cardiac conditions
*10. Cardiac/tachycardia (adult/pediatric)
*11. Chest pain
12. Chronic chemical dependency
13. Chronic fatigue syndrome
*14. Chronic headache
15. Chronic illness
16. Chronic pain management
17. Communicable disease/AIDS
18. Communicable disease/STDs
19. Domestic abuse
*20. Dysmenorrhea
21. Eczema
22. Fibromyalgia
23. Gyn/Breast cancer risk factors
24. Gyn/Breast implant support groups
25. Gyn/Hysterectomy (general information)
26. Gyn/Menopause
27. Gyn/Menstrual cycle/ovulation
28. Gyn/Ovarian cancer
29. Gyn/Sterilization
*30. Headache
31. Herniated disk
32. Hypertension
33. Hypoglycemia
34. Infertility (Male/Female)
35. Irritable bowel (general information)

36. Lupus (discoid or systemic)
*37. Male/Painful intercourse
38. Male/Vasectomy
*39. Medical reference protocol
*40. Medical overdose
41. Multiple sclerosis
42. Neurodermatitis
43. Nicotine patch
44. Obesity
*45. Ortho/Amputation–traumatic
46. Parkinson's disease
47. Peds/Bedwetting/Enuresis
48. Peds/Day care
49. PG/Chronic health problems
50. PG/Diabetes/Gestational
*51. PG/Ectopic pregnancy
52. PG/Genetics and counseling
*53. PG/Miscarriage (general information)
54. PG/Post abortion instruction
55. PG/Smoking and pregnancy
56. PG/Stress
57. PG/Uterine Anomalies
58. Postpartum depression
59. Premenstrual syndrome
60. Psych/Anxiety and panic
61. Psych/Depression
62. Sciatica
63. Sleep disorder/Insomnia
64. Substance-related disorders
65. Alcohol withdrawal
66. Nicotine withdrawal
67. Opioid withdrawal
68. Sedative, hypnotic, or anxiolytic withdrawal
69. Temporomandibular joint syndrome (TMJ)
70. Ulcer/Peptic disease

*Symptom-based conditions

PG=Pregnancy-related

Part V.
THE FUTURE OF BEHAVIORAL HEALTH AND PRIMARY CARE INTEGRATION

Chapter 19

Training for Interdisciplinary Practice: Trends in Clinical Psychology and Family Medicine

Thomas M. DiLorenzo, Ph.D. and Harold A. Williamson, M.D., M.S.P.H.

The integration of primary care and behavioral health is too new an area for there to be trained leaders yet. Current use of the term *interdisciplinary* usually connotes care or education conducted by two specialties within the same general field. However, enough knowledge has been gained in this rapidly changing and growing area that educators must begin to think about how a training component can be added to traditionally narrow parochial fields.

While there are many other behavioral health (e.g., social work, psychiatric nursing) and primary care (e.g., internal medicine, pediatrics) disciplines in which integration can occur, this chapter will focus on the integration of clinical psychology and family medicine training. Because of unique training requirements in family medicine residencies, psychologists and family physicians have already often worked together in clinical and training settings.[1] Clinical psychology and family medicine have their own unique histories and training models. These will be discussed separately, and integrated training models will also be described.

Historical Perspectives

Clinical Psychology

Clinical psychology's contemporary roots lie in the assessment of mental processes.[2] Work in the area of interventions was taking place in the early 1900s, and this area exploded when the need developed to treat men returning from World War II with emotional difficulties. Many of the standard therapies were developed in the decades from the 1950s through the 1970s. Psychoanalysis was developed first, followed by Gestalt therapy, existential therapy, family therapy, and transactional analysis. In the late 1960s and early 1970s, the cognitive-behavioral revolution was occurring.[2] Interestingly, cognitive-behavioral therapy is popular today in the managed care arena because of the following attributes: 1) emphasis on short-term therapy; 2) grounding in empiricism; 3) use of outcome variables; and 4) reliance on empirically validated treatments (similar to the movement in medicine called evidence-based medicine).

Graduate Education. In 1949, the first conference on graduate education in clinical psychology was held in Boulder, Colorado. The scientist-practitioner model (or Boulder model) of graduate training was defined during this conference. The model asserts that:

- Clinical psychologists shall pursue their training in university departments.
- They shall be trained as psychologists first and clinicians second.

- They shall be required to serve a clinical internship.
- They shall achieve competence in diagnosis, psychotherapy, and research.
- The culmination of their training shall be the Ph.D. degree, which involves an original research contribution to the field.[2]

Late in the 1960s, critics of the scientist-practitioner model began to develop a different model based more on clinical training than on scientific training. These programs or "schools of professional psychology" were considered practice-based, while the Ph.D. programs were considered research-based. However, the difference is less a dichotomy than a continuum. Peterson noted in 1986 that "at least 10 kinds of organizations are in operation, all training people for careers in professional psychology." In addition to the departmentally based Ph.D. programs, there are practitioner programs within university psychology departments and/or psychiatry departments of medical colleges, university-based professional schools, free-standing professional schools, departments of professional psychology, schools of general psychology, psychiatry departments of medical colleges, schools of professional psychology within theological institutions, consortia arrangements involving several institutions of higher education, and external degree programs.[3]

There are now over 175 doctoral programs in clinical psychology accredited by the American Psychological Association (APA). Unfortunately, there is no formal, global method currently available to change any aspect of graduate education, except possibly with accreditation or licensing requirements. In general, little curricular time is currently spent on training in the interface of primary care and behavioral health. The exceptions to this are the health psychology programs or tracks that have been developed in traditional departments of psychology or in medical schools over the past 15 years. Graduate students in these programs are more likely to receive additional education in the physiological aspects of health and disease.

Internship/Residency. All clinical psychology programs require an internship or residency (these terms are used interchangeably in psychology). Most internships require a one-year commitment and are considered to be the capstone of applied experience for training in clinical psychology. In the early years, graduate students had little clinical experience prior to the internship year. However, a significant amount of clinical experience before internship (through clerkships) is now the rule rather than the exception.

Post-Doctoral Fellowships. As with many other disciplines, training in psychology has become more specialized. Graduate-level training is still widely considered to be generalist, while training in the internship and post-doctoral years is considered to be specialized. Other requirements come into play as well, as one considers a professional career in clinical psychology. All states now require one to two years of post-doctoral supervised training before a person is eligible to take the licensure exam. Some of these post-doctoral training programs in professional psychology are organized, but many have been established in a post hoc fashion. With more planning and foresight, this training experience could also include a component of the primary care/behavioral health interface.

Family Medicine

The term *graduate education* might be applied to the four years of medical school that occur after a student earns a bachelor's degree. Within the field of medicine, however, graduate medical education generally refers to residency, which is a three- to five-year clinical training period after the completion of medical school.

Medical School. Before 1910, medical education in the United States largely took place through clinical apprenticeships. Basic science and clinical courses, usually conducted in large lecture formats, were followed by a sort of indentured apprenticeship with an experienced clinician. In the early 1900s, a report by Abraham Flexner criticized medical education as haphazard, unstructured, and not tied to particular educational theories or to an institutional infrastructure. Following this report, medical education underwent radical changes, including a reduction in the number of institutions for training physicians and a standardized curriculum. This curriculum usually consisted of two years of basic science education, largely lecture and laboratory, and two years of clinical training, usually supervised patient care in large city hospitals accompanied by clinical lectures. With some variation, this format continues to be the basic underpinning of American medical education.

More recently, innovations in medical education have included early clinical experiences, based on the premise that basic science teaching must be understood in a clinical context. Education in community and outpatient settings resurfaced in the 1970s and 1980s and continues to be a prominent theme. Medical education has become somewhat more interactive, with lectures giving way to problem-based learning in small groups.

Internship/Residency. Historically, after completing medical school, students entered a one-year rotating internship. This internship was hospital-based and included rotations in a number of different specialties. The goal was to develop a broad base of knowledge and skills. Large hospital wards were the most convenient, and in many ways believed to be the best environment for internships. During the first half of the 20th century, advances in the biological understanding of disease and technology and the shift of patient care and diagnostic technology to hospitals encouraged subspecialization within medicine. Specialized residency training, from three to seven years in duration, rapidly supplanted the rotating internship. Subspecialty training consisted of a two-year clinical or research fellowship after the completion of the standard three-year residency. By the late 1960s, the number of generalists in training had plummeted. Reports from several government agencies and private foundations raised concerns about the lack of organized training in primary care and advocated a return to generality.

Three-year residencies in family medicine were subsequently encouraged by organized medicine, grant funding, and government agencies. These residencies aimed to develop the knowledge, attitude, and skills necessary for a particular kind of primary care practice. Older models taught students and residents what the faculty knew, and what was needed to care for sick patients in tertiary care hospitals. For the first time, a significant portion of training moved to the outpatient setting, where residents cared for panels of "their own" patients, under close supervision of faculty physicians. Residents still spend about half their time in the inpatient setting, learning basic skills and principles of patient care. Accreditation requirements for family medicine residencies ensured that the training experience would closely approximate both inpatient and outpatient practice experience.

The designers of these residencies recognized that primary care practitioners required knowledge and skills in social and behavioral medicine. The legislation and competitive grant funding that allowed these residencies to proliferate actually required that a "behaviorist" (usually a psychologist) be a part of the faculty.[4] In general, the amount of behavioral science training in family medicine residencies is considerably greater than that provided in internal medicine or pediatrics.[5] Over the past 20 years, many general internal medicine programs, general pediatric programs, and combined general medicine/pediatrics programs have been developed. These programs have focused on outpatient care and a broader range of generalist skills.

Current Models of Training

Clinical Psychology

Undergraduate. Most academicians believe that undergraduate study in psychology provides a broad exposure to many areas of psychology. However, there are certainly important ways for the undergraduate to find out about and prepare for a career in clinical psychology at the primary care interface.

Graduate. There are several standard models of training at the graduate level. The degree of science woven into each of these programs varies. However, basic to each program is a core curriculum, practical experience, and the need for research production. Most graduate curricula encompass core areas of psychology, including basic clinical psychology. Often, a program will have a variety of tracks (e.g., child, adult, health) that are represented by various courses. Appendix A shows how a traditional clinical psychology curriculum could be changed to include more course work at the interface of primary care and behavioral health.

In graduate school, practical experience is often obtained through job placements called clerkships. These clerkships have been developed by clinical graduate programs to provide students with valuable clinical training before internship. Usually, these clerkships are in traditional mental health settings such as community mental health centers and outpatient clinics. Clerkships may be one place where training can occur in primary care/behavioral health settings. Finally, with most Ph.D. programs in psychology, graduate students are required to make an original research contribution to the field. A dissertation and/or master's thesis and other research projects are completed by students in their graduate years.

Internships. In addition to Veterans Administration internships, many locations are now accredited to offer the internship experience, including counseling centers, medical schools, community mental health centers, and private behavioral health centers. Although specific internships may be narrowly focused, most often an intern will have the opportunity to gain experience with adults and children, with inpatients and outpatients, and with a myriad of diagnoses and problems. Rotations are often three, four, or six months in duration, and the intern has the opportunity to work with other behavioral health professionals during each rotation.

Post-Doctoral Fellows. There are few good models of post-doctoral education for entering the practice of professional psychology. Upon completion of the internship, individuals usually find supervised training in the job environment so that the post-doctoral requirements for licensure are fulfilled.

Influence of Managed Care. While there is no question that managed care has influenced the practice of psychology, it has not had a major effect on graduate psychology training programs. Unlike family medicine, there are few federal training dollars involved in graduate education. Therefore, the federal government has little impact in making systematic changes in the field of psychology.

As managed care affects the practice of professional psychology, there will be a decrease in the number of students entering graduate training in professional psychology. The skills that need to be developed in graduate education will change as well. There will be a greater focus on problem-oriented, solution-focused, time-effective treatments and empirically validated treatments.[2,6] Since primary care physicians (PCPs) are often the gatekeepers in a managed care world, future professionals must be able to apply preventive strategies in the PCP's office. Students should receive training in early diagnosis, symptom relief, and in a developmentally focused behavioral health care orientation, especially in common disorders such as depression and anxiety.[7] Finally, students need more training in the areas of consultation, supervision, and in the use of a myriad of management techniques in the organizational setting.[8]

Potential Changes in Training. Although we believe that undergraduate training in psychology should remain general, there are several changes that could be made to the curriculum to make students more aware of the primary care/behavioral health interface. These changes could bring this interface and work-related learning (service learning) components into the course content. A new type of certification as a health service provider (nondoctoral-level clinician) could be created.

Many courses could be offered to undergraduate students to help them consider the interface with primary care. For example, an undergraduate course in health psychology with family medicine physicians as lecturers would provide behavior/disease connections. Other basic courses should include psychophysiology and drugs and behavior. For the first time, the University of Missouri is offering a course to undergraduates on clinical psychology with medical populations, which is designed to sensitize undergraduate students to patients with medical problems.

A new concept in undergraduate education is service learning. As part of a standard course, students are required to work in some applied setting to understand the theoretical concepts in a practical way. We already have a service learning component to a community psychology class, in which undergraduate students spend a semester working (for course credit) in a state hospital under the direct supervision of a psychologist.

Finally, as health dollars continue to shrink, we should be open to nondoctoral-level clinicians performing the bulk of what we now call psychotherapy. Recently, several members of the University of Missouri psychology department met with the deputy director of the state department of mental health to discuss the possibility of the university developing an undergraduate track in mental health services, possibly leading to a new type of certification. These types of opportunities will increase in the future.

The real socialization process of selling primary care/behavioral health integration will begin in graduate studies. Three ways that this interface could be introduced into graduate education include changes in the curriculum, enhancement of clerkship/practicum placements, and innovative faculty involvement (e.g., serving as mentors/fellows of students from other departments or being involved in collaborative research projects).

Making curricular changes in a program is a relatively easy way to introduce the concepts behind primary care/behavioral health integration at the graduate level. A course is now being taught in the clinical psychology program—Psychotherapy, Managed Care, and Empirically Validated Treatments—which will replace older courses. Rather than a traditional survey of psychotherapies, the instructor has incorporated important aspects of managed care and empirically validated treatments into the conduct of psychotherapy. Important aspects of the PCP's practice are described as well as how they relate to treatment (especially the treatment of depression). The area of health psychology is a perfect example of psychology's relevance to the future of healthcare.[7] A collaborative effort could also be developed for family physician faculty members to serve as instructors in some of the health-oriented courses.

For some time, we have been considering the possibility that our clinical graduate students could be trained in nontraditional settings to enhance their integration skills. We developed a practicum site in the department of psychiatry last year and are pursuing a clerkship/practicum in one of the satellite clinics of the family and community medicine department. This site is really the essence of training in the primary care/behavioral health interface.

At present, collaboration that takes place between the faculties of psychology and family medicine at the University of Missouri mostly occurs at the research level. Both groups have expressed the desire to integrate more fully at the training level: graduate student training for psychology, and fellowship training for family medicine. In this way, faculty from each department will serve as mentors for students and/or actually hire the students/fellows to be integrally involved in various grant activities.

In the last few years, internships have been developed that include rotations in primary care. The prime force behind this has been the realization that interns can serve important roles in the primary care setting. However, a more focused effort is needed to create a better internship experience. Broskowski details what is needed.

> "Internships must be redesigned to maximize the experience of working across a range of mental health and medical care settings, including large, multispecialty group practices, health maintenance organizations (HMOs), general hospitals, and specialized units for the treatment of specific medical conditions (e.g., physical rehabilitation, cardiac care, respiratory diseases). Behavioral interventions will be valued in general clinical settings as the evidence for their impact on reduced medical costs, improved health status, and member satisfaction increases."[7]

Graham and Fox also make a cogent argument for the need for systematic, formalized post-doctoral education for psychological practice. Unfortunately, although this need has been noted repeatedly over the years, the "exact nature and content of such training" has yet to be determined.[9]

Medical Education/Family Practice

The educational path leading to an M.D. degree, with a few exceptions, has not changed substantially since the adoption of standardized curricula. Following the undergraduate degree there are four years of medical school, which train students in the basic and clinical sciences relevant to medical practice. In general, there are at least two years of clinical sciences training, consisting of a combination of in-hospital and outpatient settings. Here the medical student learns to take histories, conduct physical examinations, develop a differential diagnosis and evaluation, and outline a treatment plan. Students assume progressive responsibility, but are always under the close supervision of a resident and/or faculty physician.

In the first two years of medical school, students typically have lecture and/or small group sessions devoted to principles of behavioral science. This usually includes human development, human sexuality, domestic violence, addictive behaviors, and sometimes psychopathology. Students also typically spend two months in a psychiatry rotation structured around inpatient care.

Following medical school, students choose a specialty in which to complete a residency. Using a national computer process, students are assigned to residency programs. Residencies in primary care fields are usually three years; others are three to five years in duration. During residency the new physician will assume progressive responsibility for patient care, further honing skills learned during medical school. The resident should be and usually is under the supervision of an attending faculty physician who assumes professional, legal, and financial responsibility for the patient's care. Traditionally, residency programs were completed in large, inner city hospitals, whose patients were often indigent. Residency training is now supported by a number of private hospitals and healthcare organizations.

Medical student and residency education is often uni-disciplinary. With the exception of family medicine residencies, there is usually little formal interaction between physicians-in-training and other health-related trainees. The content of residency programs is determined by a residency review committee composed of representatives of the American Association of Medical Colleges, the American Medical Association, the specific specialty professional organization, the specialty-specific academic organization, and the certifying board for the specialty. Each of the primary care disciplines has different requirements regarding mental health and behavioral issues (see Appendix B).

The residency review committee for family medicine requires that "Knowledge and skills in this area should be acquired through a program in which behavioral science and psychiatry are integrated with all disciplines throughout the resident's total educational experience. Training should be accomplished primarily in an outpatient setting through a combination of longitudinal experiences and didactic sessions. Intensive short-term experiences in the facilities devoted to the care of chronically ill patients should be limited. Instruction must be provided by faculty who have the training and experience necessary to apply modern behavioral and psychiatric principles to the care of the undifferentiated patient. Family physicians, psychiatrists, and behavioral scientists should be involved in teaching this curricular component."[10]

Most family practice residencies use psychologists, psychiatrists, and/or social workers as teachers and providers of services. The behavioral health curriculum in family medicine residencies may be in "block" form (a two-month rotation of inpatient and outpatient mental health services) or longitudinal (seeing a panel of patients once a month with a supervising psychologist). In addition, lectures and seminars on the use of psychotropic medication, appropriate referrals, and the interface between medical and psychological illnesses are a major portion of the curriculum.[5]

Medical education has, in general, moved toward 1) earlier clinical experiences for medical students; 2) an increased focus on interactive, small group, and collaborative learning exemplified in problem-based learning; and 3) education in community settings. At the residency level, family medicine has continued to focus on innovations in outpatient practice. Innovations have included a move toward a longitudinal curriculum (as opposed to monthly rotations), community-oriented primary care projects aimed at blending clinical practice with public health, a curriculum in total quality improvement (TQI), and innovative curricula to help residents function better in managed care settings.

Influence of Managed Care. Managed care has influenced medical education in many ways.[11,12] The academic health centers that typically comprise the infrastructure for medical education have been threatened by managed care plans. Many have not been able to respond to the increasing focus on primary care and the reduction in reimbursement for medical services. Managed care organizations have generally been unwilling to allow resident physicians to act as gatekeepers in their managed care plans. This has been a dilemma for primary care programs, because one of their major educational tenets is to allow continuity of care experiences in managing health and illness. On the other hand, managed care has heightened the visibility of PCPs and influenced an ever-increasing number of students to pursue careers in primary care. In 1995 it became clear that these market forces would "trickle down" to influence medical student decisions. There was a rapid rise in interest in primary care residencies.[13]

Recent studies suggest that primary care residencies have had varying experiences with managed care health plans, ranging from highly successful adaptations to serious reductions in patient numbers available for teaching practices.[14] It is important for those in health and health-related professions to think beyond managed care. This is especially true of educators, who must understand that managed care is the messenger, not the message. The message is that healthcare must be coordinated, personalized, accountable, cost-effective, evidence-based, and understood and delivered in the context of populations, not individuals. It is the responsibility of educators to understand this message and ensure that future health professionals respond to it.

Potential Changes in Training. Medical education institutions are continuing to move greater portions of their training programs out of hospitals and into communities. Fewer patients will spend fewer days in teaching hospitals across the nation. Training will take place "at the point of need." It is also likely that medical education will be much more responsive to market needs in the future. Organized medicine has increased its focus on the oversupply of physicians and the maldistribution by specialty and geography. Current recommendations to reduce the overall output of physicians and redistribute the specialty choices of graduates will meet considerable resistance. Nonetheless, organized medicine in the United States is determined to avoid an oversupply. Changes in the funding of medical education through the Health

Care Financing Administration and state legislatures are likely to become the driving forces that move physician workforce trends.[15,16]

The Pew Health Professions Commission has identified six strategies to prepare medical professionals for the future:

- Ensure that medicine's vision of professional accountability includes the prevention of disease and the preservation and enhancement of the health of individuals and of the collective community.
- Educate physicians who possess the general skills, attitudes, and knowledge needed by all physicians regardless of career path.
- Develop community-based educational programs that balance the tertiary care experience for medical students, residents in areas of general care, and other health professionals, while providing educational outreach to the community.
- Encourage medical faculty to develop competencies needed to fulfill the Pew Commission's vision of medicine and to demonstrate the role of physicians with individual patients and within the community.
- Expand the research orientation of the academic health center to include the problems identified within the population and resulting from an assessment of community needs.
- Emphasize lifelong learning, inquiry-based education, and student-centered learning in medical education.[17]

Some institutions will probably continue to use an interdisciplinary model, particularly in rural and urban underserved areas. Social service agencies are beginning to recognize that human service professionals are not well trained to work collaboratively. As resources are shrinking in an era of welfare reform, there is a need for professionals skilled in collaborative work relationships. This trend will also be present within medical education, where managed care organizations and "vertically-integrated networks" will seek individuals with demonstrated collaborative skills.

The inexorable rise in managed care will lead to the requirement that trainees understand TQI, peer review, case management, disease management, community-oriented primary care, electronic medical records, interactive televideo, and electronic information systems. These last tools will allow long-distance learning and consultations, as well as improved communication among healthcare providers.

Less likely, but possible, is the emergence of a single-discipline PCP. Many educators agree that, were we to invent the concept of primary care anew, we would probably not create three separate specialties (family practice, internal medicine, and pediatrics). Combined residencies have been proposed, and a few are in pilot phases. Whether the years of traditional separation of these specialties will yield to a more rational single primary care provider is unclear.

Future Trends

Uni-disciplinary implies education and care conceived and delivered without regard for the role of other health-related professionals. *Multi-disciplinary* refers to education and service delivery in which there is a recognition of the contribution of others, but not necessarily communication or integration. *Interdisciplinary*, both within educational and service delivery contexts, implies a relationship in which various disciplines communicate, coordinate, and work together. *Trans-disciplinary* is a mostly theoretical concept in which disciplines assume one another's traditional roles. We advocate a training perspective that encourages students to move along this continuum as quickly as possible.

Curriculum

There has always been an interest in joint curricula within different disciplines. Such a curriculum could be delivered in lecture format, in which trainees at various levels would receive similar information about the roles and competencies of various professionals and the value of collaborative practice, communication skills, community needs assessment skills, and community leadership. Although such a format makes sense, there are barriers to its implementation including scheduling difficulties and student disinterest. Small group seminars, built around existing curricular requirements for several disciplines, seem more likely to be successful.

At the University of Missouri-Columbia and the University of New Mexico, a problem-based learning format has been a highly successful technique for interdisciplinary education. In these settings, students in medicine, nursing, occupational and physical therapy (and soon psychology and social work) use a case-based method called problem-based learning to "solve" problems presented by a real-life "patient," whose history is presented in an unfolding fashion. Carefully selected cases reveal the scope of work of other disciplines and the need for inter-professional communications skills. These "real-life" cases have created spirited interchange and a true sense of teamwork. Creating the appropriate cases requires special pedagogical skills and is time consuming, but the result is a highly efficient method in which to achieve interdisciplinary goals.

Practicum Experiences

When interdisciplinary goals require a more intensive interaction between trainees, a joint clinical practicum offers a closer collaboration between professionals. This method seems most appropriate for psychology trainees who will choose a practice affiliated with a primary care group. These collaborative models already exist, and research suggests that they can be quite successful.[18-21] When establishing such experiences, we recommend that students at similar levels of training be paired with each other. A psychology graduate student's first clinical experience, for example, should probably not be with a senior family medicine resident.

Working in a primary care outpatient office, the psychology trainee and his/her psychology supervisor would receive referrals from the medical practice. The number of cases required by psychology trainees for their practicum can easily be obtained from a family medicine teaching practice. Formal and informal discussion among the trainees regarding their mutual patients/clients can be facilitated by trainee supervisors, who have numerous opportunities to model successful professional interactions. An advanced psychology trainee can provide curriculum for medical students or family practice residents through leadership in lectures and seminars.

Joint research and publication by faculty also help to create an interdisciplinary milieu. In this training context, it is important to recognize the possibility of the psychology trainee's sense of isolation and uniqueness.[1] One could minimize these feelings by setting up teams of psychology faculty, family medicine faculty, family medicine residents, interns from each discipline, psychology graduate students, and medical students.

Biopsychosocial Models of Education/Training. Traditional medical training has often erred in supporting the dualism in mind and body. Medical philosophers and medical educators have often struggled with the concept. It has been easier for medical training to focus on biomedical issues that have been strongly reinforced by scientific discoveries and the use of medical technology. However, over the past decade there has been continued interest in the biopsychosocial model in primary care training.[21] This model has found particular favor in family medicine settings, in which experienced clinicians find the traditional biomedical model lacking as they attempt to assist their patients. In this context, medical sociologists, anthropologists, and health-related psychologists have found much common ground with family medicine educational philosophies.

Integration of Healthcare Training. The rapid development of medical care organizations and "vertically-integrated networks" provide a substantial opportunity for joint educational experiences. It seems reasonable for large HMOs, for example, to support the joint training of PCPs and psychologists, so that such trainees could fit comfortably within these integrated care models. With the exception of a few old and well-established HMOs, however, these delivery structures have not yet shown substantial interest in supporting medical education, much less interdisciplinary education.[11,12]

Policy Issues. A number of policy issues surface regarding the integration of service and care. What is the proper training of a psychologist to work in a primary care setting? Should PCPs be responsible for recognizing behavioral health problems and then referring to mental health professionals, or should they provide almost all mental health services? How many primary care/behavioral health specialists are needed? What is a minimum joint interdisciplinary curriculum?

When physicians and psychologists train and practice in a joint setting, several problems remain. When a patient is jointly cared for by a mental health specialist and a physician in the same practice, who is responsible? This has professional, ethical, financial, and legal ramifications. Is the psychologist a "partner" in a financial sense or an "employee" of a practice? In some interdisciplinary practices, both disciplines use the same method of documentation (i.e., the patient's chart). This raises certain ethical questions for mental health specialists and occasionally causes problems with insurers who request copies of medical records. However, it also results in a fundamentally important form of communication between these two professions.

Cost Offset in Training Models: Using Faculty in Innovative Ways. Creative financing for medical education is increasingly the norm in the current era of cost restraint. We must be equally creative in funding interdisciplinary education. About one-third of a family medicine resident's estimated educational costs are reimbursed through billings from services provided, one-third comes from the Health Care

Financing Administration directly and indirectly, and another third must come from other sources. In the last decade, those other sources have frequently been the billings of faculty physicians. In this way, the difference between an "academic physician" and a "private practice physician" has become progressively blurred. The increased reliance on clinical income has given academic medical centers the potential for fiscal autonomy and has required academic physicians to have a more realistic financial understanding of medical practice. However, these advantages have been offset by the decreased time and energy of faculty for teaching and research.

On the other hand, psychology faculty in traditional departments are often on "hard money," and flexibility exists in their workloads. Traditional content courses, supervision of practicum experiences of graduate students, and the administrative costs of running programs are often covered by a base salary, which means that psychology faculty are somewhat "protected" for the time being.

Conclusion

In this chapter we have provided descriptions of psychology and family medicine training, including suggestions for more integrated models of training. Although the focus is on the integration of psychology and family medicine, the concepts apply to other behavioral health and medical disciplines as well. We believe that integrated training of professionals will lead to improved quality of care and outcomes.

References

1. Shapiro J, Schiermer DC: Clinical training of psychologists in family practice settings: an examination of special issues. Family Med 25:443–446, 1993.
2. Phares JE, Troull TJ: Clinical Psychology, Fifth Edition. Brooks/Cole Publishing, Pacific Grove, California, 1997.
3. Peterson DR: Organizational dilemmas in the education of professional psychologists. In: Quality in Professional Psychology Training: A National Conference and Self Study, Callan, JE, Peterson DR, Stricker, G, (eds). National Council of School Professional Psychology, San Diego, California, 1986.
4. Ransom DC: Yes, there is a future for behavioral scientists in academic family medicine. Family Systems Med 10:305–315, 1992.
5. Strain JJ, Pincus HA, Gise LH, Houpt J: Mental health education in three primary care specialties. J Med Educ 61:958–966, 1986.
6. Cummings NA: Impact of managed care on employment and training: a primer for survival. Prof Psychol Res Pract 26:10–15, 1995.
7. Broskowski AT: The evolution of health care: implications for the training and careers of psychologists. Prof Psychol Res Pract 26:156–162, 1995.
8. Clements CB: Training in human service management for future practitioner-managers. Prof Psychol Res Pract 23:146–150, 1992.
9. Graham SR, Fox RE: Postdoctoral education for professional practice. Am Psychol 14:1033–1035, 1991.
10. American Academy of Family Physicians: American Academy of Family Physicians Recommended Core Educational Guidelines for Family Practice Residents: Human Behavior and Mental Health. Am Fam Phys 51:1599–1603, 1995.
11. Blumenthal D: Managed care and medical education: the new fundamentals. JAMA 276:725–727, 1996.
12. Veloski J, Barzansky B, Nash DB, Bastacky S, Stevens DP: Medical student education in managed care settings: beyond HMOs. JAMA 276:667–671, 1996.

13. Dunn MR, Miller RS: The shifting sands of graduate medical education. JAMA 276:710-713, 1996.
14. Stiffman MN, LeFevre ML: Are resident physicians serving as primary care providers for managed care patients? Family Med 29:94-98, 1997.
15. Council on Graduate Medical Education: Improving Access to Health Care through Physician Workforce Reform: Directions for the 21st Century. Third report to Congress and the Department of Health and Human Services, October 1992.
16. Council on Graduate Medical Education: Recommendations to Improve Access to Health Care through Physician Workforce Reform. Fourth report to Congress and the Department of Health and Human Services, January 1994.
17. Pew Health Professions Commission: Health Professions Education for the Future: Schools in Service to the Nation. San Francisco CA, 1993.
18. Belar CD: Collaboration in capitated care: challenges for psychology. Prof Psychol Res Pract 26:139-146, 1995.
19. Bray JH, Rogers JC: Linking psychologists and family physicians for collaborative practice. Prof Psychol Res Pract 26:132-138, 1995.
20. Drotar D: Influences on collaborative activities among psychologists and pediatricians: implications for practice, training, and research. J Pediatr Psychol 18:159-172, 1993.
21. McDaniel SH: Collaboration between psychologists and family physicians: implementing the biopsychosocial model. Prof Psychol Res Pract 26:117-122, 1995.

Appendix A
Traditional versus integrated curricula for clinical psychology.

Example of current curriculum in a clinical psychology program.	Example of a curriculum that integrates primary care/behavioral health with traditional clinical training.
FIRST YEAR *Fall* Core area—Social Psychology Orientation to Psychotherapy Statistics—ANOVA Thesis Prep *Winter* Core area—Developmental Psychometrics Statistics—Multiple Regression Thesis	**FIRST YEAR** *Fall* Core areas—Social/Developmental Clinical Block (DSM, Interviewing, Child Assessment/ Treatment) Statistics—ANOVA Thesis Prep *Winter* Core areas—Biological/Cognitive Clinical Block (Adult Assessment and Treatment, Ethics, Paperwork) Statistics—Multiple Regression Thesis
SECOND YEAR *Fall* Core—Biological Experimental Psychopathology Statistics—MANOVA Thesis *Winter* Core—Cognitive Orientations to Psychotherapy II Intellectual Assessment Thesis Completion	**SECOND YEAR** *Fall* Practicum in a Primary Care Setting Psychopathology in PCP Office Diagnosis and treatment as related to critical pathways and practice guidelines Statistics—MANOVA Thesis *Winter* Practicum in a Primary Care Setting Managed Care and Empirically Validated Treatments Consultation Thesis Completion
THIRD YEAR *Fall* Practicum in a State Hospital Personality Testing Clinical Research Methods Comprehensive Exams *Winter* Practicum in a State Hospital Neuropsychological Assessment Personality Disorders Comprehensive Exams	**THIRD YEAR** *Fall* Practicum in a Primary Care Setting Supervision Management Techniques Comprehensive Exams *Winter* Practicum in a Primary Care Setting Health Psychology Community Psychology Comprehensive Exams

FOURTH YEAR
Fall
Practicum in a Mental Health Setting
Dissertation

Winter
Practicum in a Mental Health Setting
Dissertation

FIFTH YEAR
Internship/Residency

FOURTH YEAR
Fall
Practicum in a Behavioral Health Center
Dissertation

Winter
Practicum in a Behavioral Health Center
Dissertation

FIFTH YEAR
Internship/Residency

Appendix B
Sample Curriculum for Family Medicine Residents

FIRST-YEAR ROTATIONS

Introduction to Family Practice – 1 month

Emergency Medicine – 1 month

Inpatient Pediatrics – 2 months

Obstetrics – 2 months

Internal Medicine – 2 months

Well Baby Nursery – 1 week

Family Practice Inpatient Block – 3 months

Vacation – 3 weeks

Family Practice Clinics – 2 per week

SECOND-YEAR ROTATIONS

Newborn Intensive Care Unit – 1 month

Behavioral Science – 1 month

Geriatrics – 1 month

Orthopedics – 1 month

Ophthalmology – 2 weeks

Surgery – 1 month

Rural Satellite Practice – 1 month

Medical Intensive Care Unit – 1 month

Cardiology/CCU – 1 month

Obstetrics or Electives – 1 month

Other Electives – 1.5 months

Vacation – 1 month

Family Practice Clinics – 3 or 4 per week

THIRD-YEAR ROTATIONS

Family Practice Inpatient Block (Supervising Resident) – 2 months

Community Medicine/Pediatrics – 1 month

Rural Satellite Practice – 1 month

Rural Surgery – 1 month

Urology/ENT – 1.5 months

Dermatology – 1 month

Gynecology – 1 month

Obstetrics or Elective – 1 month

Other Elective – 1.5 months

Vacation – 1 month

Family Practice Clinics – 3 or 4 per week

Chapter 20

Computerized Technology: Integrative Treatment Outcome Technology in Primary Care Practice

Len Sperry, M.D., Ph.D., and Peter Brill, M.D.

Providing cost-effective diagnosis and treatment of behavioral health conditions in primary care patients is problematic and presents a challenge to both providers and administrators. The basic issue is not *whether* to integrate primary care with behavioral health services, but rather *how* to integrate them. From a practical standpoint, primary care physicians (PCPs) have limited face-to-face time with patients in need of behavioral health services, as well as limited time to interact with behavioral health providers. Specifically, the challenge involves the following three components:

- Information identification—how to quickly and accurately diagnose the need for services
- Information utilization—how the treatment provided can be easily and appropriately measured and monitored
- Information transfer—how data on patient need and treatment outcome is shared between different providers and administrators

The ideal primary care practice would comfortably blend humanistic treatment with integrative information technology. Fortunately, such technology is now becoming available. The basic challenge can be addressed with an integrative outcome system that can screen for behavioral health conditions, suggest treatment intervention options, predict the likelihood of treatment success, and monitor the results over the course of treatment. The system should also provide useful management information such as cost-efficacy, provider profiling, and clinic profiling. The "high tech" system would facilitate "high touch" clinical and administrative relations with patients, and would assist clinicians in providing a seamless continuum of treatment between PCPs and behavioral health providers.[1]

Focused, effective information technology can greatly facilitate the integration of primary care and behavioral health services. Specifically, computerized treatment outcome systems can effectively assist with diagnosis, measurement, and monitoring of behavioral health treatments. In addition, these systems can provide useful management data about patient treatment outcomes and provider efficacy.

Factors That Hinder and Facilitate Integration

Integration of primary care and behavioral health services has only been partially accomplished, due to various professional and practice issues. One important barrier has been physician reluctance to diagnose and treat behavioral health disorders in medical settings. This reluctance was based on factors such as adequacy of training, perceived competency in diagnosis and treatment, inadequate reimbursement for cognitive services, and physician discomfort with patients' emotional problems. Another factor is the common belief that patients feel uncomfortable discussing psychological problems with physicians.

For example, PCPs' perceptions that their patients did not want to discuss their depression accounted for one-third of the variance in physician belief of whether depression is an important clinical problem. This perception was strongly associated with the clinicians' discomfort about exploring depression.[2] In a national survey of family physicians, two-thirds reported that patient resistance to psychiatric diagnosis and treatment was an obstacle in providing service or referral.[3]

There is little or no empirical evidence for this belief. Rather, data suggest that patients are more satisfied with their care if their physician addresses psychosocial matters, and that patients wish to discuss these concerns with their PCP. However, because behavioral health issues are among the most ambiguous of patient concerns, physicians tend to minimize or ignore them.

Problems with referring patients and communicating with behavioral health providers has also hindered integration. Additionally, the adequacy and validity of efforts to diagnose behavioral health issues and monitor the effect of behavioral health treatment have been barriers. System considerations, such as whether behavioral health services are "carved in" or "carved out," can either complicate or facilitate the process.

Fortunately, recent technological advances can help remove some of these barriers to integration. Screening tools, outcomes measurements, and computerized outcomes monitoring and management systems can greatly reduce physician discomfort. Outcomes measurement instruments and behavioral health screening tools are essentially "behavioral lab tests." The reports generated from these instruments resemble laboratory test reports that physicians are familiar with reviewing.

In medicine, lab tests are used to confirm the physician's clinical formulation. For this reason, behavioral health screening tools and outcomes measures appeal to PCPs. These measures—and the information management systems of which they are a part—give physicians more control over behavioral health issues because of their objective measurement capability. In clinically ambiguous presentations, screening instruments and outcomes measures add even more value.

Similarly, screening tools and outcomes measures have appeal and add value from the patient's perspective. Patients may feel more comfortable disclosing personal problems on a paper-and-pencil measure than face to face with their physician. A clinical practice that uses screening instruments and serial outcomes measures communicates to patients that the data is important in their treatment. Patients are already familiar with lab tests, and if the screening tools and outcomes measures are presented to them as behavioral lab tests, their cooperation may be higher.

Technological Support for Integrated Services

Three computerized outcomes systems useful in integrating primary care and behavioral health services are Compass-PC, Outcome for Windows, and the Outcome Questionnaire-45 (OQ-45). Behavioral health screening tools are often used in conjunction with these outcomes systems, usually preceding the utilization of an outcomes measure. (See Chapter 15 for a discussion of some common behavioral health screening instruments.)

Compass-PC

This scale measures treatment progress based on both the patient's and the clinician's perspective. The scales are designed to be completed at various intervals throughout the course of treatment, so that a patient's progress can be monitored in relation to a database of similar patients. This system measures treatment outcomes as well as assessing treatment quality. Three patient self-report scales—Subjective Well-Being, Current Symptoms, and Current Life Functioning—are combined into a Mental Health Index. Additional patient scales include assessments of presenting problems and the patient's perceptions of the therapeutic relationship. Clinicians' ratings on the Global Assessment Scale and the Life Functioning Scales are combined to form the Clinical Assessment Index. Higher scores represent more healthy individuals, and cutoff scores for the Mental Health Index and Clinical Assessment Index indicate when the patient has returned to normal functioning. Two related instruments are the Compass-OP and Compass-INT for outpatient and inpatient mental health treatment.[4]

Compass-PC is usually administered to a patient if a behavioral health screen suggests that significant psychiatric symptomology or distress is present. Or, it may be reserved for situations when psychiatric symptoms are reported or observed, at which time the patient and practitioner would complete the instrument. An appropriate psychosocial or psychopharmacologic treatment plan might entail direct treatment by the PCP or referral to a behavioral health provider. The instrument would be completed periodically throughout the course of treatment.

A unique feature of Compass-PC is the self-description subscale, which assesses personality style factors with considerable clinical relevance in the primary care setting. This feature is valuable in predicting resistance to treatment, as well as medication adherence. Patient profiling helps the PCP identify and deal with difficult patients.

Outcome for Windows

This program is an outcomes management system developed specifically for medical treatment.[5] The software documents clinical, functional, and financial outcomes, as well as patient descriptors, quality of life, and patient satisfaction. It can provide predictors for costs, length of stay/number of sessions, and patient improvement. The current software program is generic, with a common set of database variables that can be added to or modified to meet user needs.

Outcome for Windows is designed to determine how a treatment plan for a given patient compares—in duration, cost, and outcomes—to successful treatment plans for other patients with similar presentations. After entering the diagnostic code and pertinent patient characteristics, the software draws all similar cases from the database and creates an outcome report with predictive information. It addresses predictive issues such as the number of treatment sessions required to decrease symptoms and achieve functional improvement, the average cost of treatment for similar patients, the most effective treatment protocol for the diagnosis, global assessment of functioning, quality of life rating, and pain rating after treatment as compared to similar patients. Furthermore, Outcome provides information on other factors, including decrease in medication use following treatment and patient satisfaction with treatment.

Outcome Questionnaire-45

The OQ-45 is a patient self-report instrument designed for repeated measurement of patient progress through the course of therapy and at termination. The instrument consists of 45 items and takes approximately seven minutes to complete. It is written at a sixth-grade reading level. The OQ-45 attempts to measure positive feelings and satisfactions as well as symptoms. It is designed to address less dysfunctional populations, such as Employee Assistance Program (EAP) participants. Typically, the instrument is completed at each treatment session.

The OQ-45 is based on the premise that outcomes assessment should evaluate patient functioning in three domains: 1) symptomatic distress, 2) interpersonal problems, and 3) social role adjustment.[6] The instrument is divided into three subscales that correspond to these domains. The Symptom Distress scale emphasizes symptoms from the most frequently diagnosed mental disorders, including depression, anxiety, and substance abuse. The Interpersonal Relations scale includes items that assess problems with friendships, family life, and marriage. The Social Role Performance scale includes items that assess patient levels of dissatisfaction, conflict, or distress in employment, family roles, and leisure.

Because a significant percentage of patients with untreated yet diagnosable mental illness present in the primary care setting, a variant of the Outcomes Questionnaire-45 was developed, the OQ-10. This 10-item screening tool has been used to identify patients who present for treatment of a medical condition but who resemble patients more typically found in inpatient and outpatient mental health populations. Such patients may have concurrent psychiatric disorders that are not being treated, or they may have a psychiatric disorder rather than a physical illness. The OQ-10 can alert the PCP to the need for further psychological evaluation, to determine the appropriateness of mental health treatment. Use of the OQ-10 can facilitate integrated medical and behavioral health services.

Illustrations of Outcomes System Use in Primary Care

How would an outcomes system be used in primary care? The following clinical case examples illustrate how this information technology can serve as a vital link in the integration of primary care with behavioral health services. Detailed, computerized feedback information involving diagnosis, treatment interventions, outcomes, and follow-up of two primary care patients are described.

Case 1

Terri R. is a 39-year-old married white female who has been followed for diabetes mellitus (type I) in this clinic for approximately 14 years. Her diabetes has been well controlled on Ultralente. At a recent appointment, she complained of insomnia, palpitations, a four-pound weight loss, and lightheadedness. She admitted that she was experiencing considerable family stress because her daughter had left for college, leaving the patient and her husband alone for the first time since the daughter was born.

Physical examination and laboratory tests were within normal ranges. A behavioral health screen indicated that anxiety symptoms were pronounced.

She was prescribed Zoloft for her anxiety, and the drug information sheet was reviewed with her. She was directed to complete Compass-PC, after which a follow-up appointment was scheduled in two weeks. At the next appointment, she noted that while her sleep was better, she was still quite anxious and worried. A review of the Compass-PC treatment progress report indicated that her Mental Health Index was low, but her Anxiety and Depression scale scores were high. Both Family and Intimacy functioning were low, and one critical sign involving alcohol/drug use was reported. Laboratory tests showed slight glycosuria and urine ketones. Her Zoloft dosage was increased, and the patient was counseled about the interaction of alcohol and diabetes. The second Compass-PC was completed, and the patient was scheduled to return in three weeks.

The patient reported minimal improvement at the next appointment. A review of the Compass-PC treatment progress report showed that, although the Mental Health Index had improved slightly, Family and Intimacy functioning were still low. When these low rankings were pointed out to the patient, she disclosed that significant marital problems existed and that her husband wanted a trial separation. Medication was continued at the same level, and a referral for individual and couples counseling by the clinic's social worker was made. Another Compass-PC was scheduled following six weeks of counseling; medical follow-up was scheduled for eight weeks.

Terri appeared much less anxious at the next appointment. She had attended three individual sessions with the social worker and three joint sessions that included her husband. A review of the treatment progress report showed Mental Health Index in the normal range, as were anxiety and depression ratings. Intimacy and Family functioning levels had increased moderately. Zoloft was continued at the same dosage, and she and her husband would continue for two more counseling sessions and then as needed after the last session. Medical follow-up was scheduled in three months.

Case 2

A young woman presented with depression, abdominal pain, tension headaches, peptic ulcer disease, and insomnia. She met the criteria for the *Diagnostic and Statistical Manual,* Fourth edition *(DSM-IV)* Adjustment Disorder with Mixed Anxiety and Depressed Mood. Her score on the Global Assessment of Function scale (GAF) was 61, with her highest GAF during the past year being 90. Medical evaluation was positive for a duodenal ulcer, for which Zantac was prescribed. A complete psychological evaluation was undertaken and analyzed by Outcome for Windows, and two protocols were compared. Protocol I included visits with a family physician and medication management. Protocol II used a combined approach that included physician, medication, psychological counseling, and biofeedback treatment.

It appeared that overall improvement was much greater with protocol II, as noted by a higher quality of life rating, lower pain rating, cessation of medication use, and a higher GAF following treatment. The cost of protocol II was $2,035 more than protocol I, but the overall effects were greater for all variables measured. Furthermore, only 3 percent of patients treated with protocol II returned for treatment of the same symptoms within the following 12 months, compared to 27 percent with protocol I.

Compared to the cost associated with protocol II treatment, it appeared that the patient's outcome was excellent, with improvement across all areas and a projected cost savings of $577 over treatment with protocol I. She no longer needed medication and her physical symptoms and GAF ratings returned to premorbid levels. By using outcomes data in this way, the provider is able to plan treatment and predict long-term outcomes, total costs, and the number of sessions needed to maximize treatment outcomes. This data is useful not only in planning treatment but also in supporting treatment decisions to patients, case managers, other providers, and third-party payers.

Conclusion

Outcomes measures and their related outcomes management systems will continue to facilitate the integration of primary care and behavioral health services. Technological advances permit assessment and diagnosis of psychological factors that mimic or complicate medical treatment. Such systems allow a seamless continuum of care between general medical providers and behavioral health specialists, as well as removing many obstacles that have hindered the integration of services—most significantly, the PCP's discomfort with patient behavioral health issues. Behavioral data gathered from health screening tools and outcomes measures provide the physician with a "behavioral lab test" to facilitate and monitor treatment. It can also provide management data about clinical practice patterns.

References

1. Pollin I, DeLeon P: Integrated health delivery systems: psychology's potential role. Prof Psychol 27:107–108, 1996.
2. Main DS, Lutz LJ, Barrett JE, Matthew J, Miller RS: The role of primary care clinician attitudes, beliefs, and training in the diagnosis and management of depression: a report from the Ambulatory Sentinal Practice Network Inc. Arch Fam Med 2:1061–1066, 1993.
3. Orleans CT, George LK, Houpt JL, Brodie H: How primary care physicians treat psychiatric disorders: a national survey of family practitioners. Am J Psychiatry 142:52–57, 1985.
4. Sperry L, Brill P, Howard K, Grissom G: Treatment Outcomes in Psychotherapy and Psychiatric Interventions. Brunner/Mazel, New York NY, 1996.
5. Keatley M, Lemmon J, Miller T, Miller M: Using 'normative' data for outcomes comparisons. Behav Health Manage 15:20–21, 1995.
6. Wells M, Burlingame G, Lambert M, Hoag M, Hope C: Conceptualization and measurement of patient change during psychotherapy: development of the outcome questionnaire and youth outcome questionnaire. Psychother 33:275–283, 1996.

Suggested Reading

Lyons J, Howard K, O'Mahoney M, Lish J. The Measurement and Management of Clinical Outcomes in Mental Health. John Wiley and Sons, New York NY, 1997.

Sederer L, Dickey B (eds). Outcomes Assessment in Clinical Practice. Williams & Willkins, Baltimore MD, 1996.

Sperry L, Brill P, Howard K, Grissom G. Treatment Outcomes in Psychotherapy and Psychiatric Interventions. Brunner/Mazel, New York NY, 1996.

Sperry L, Fink P (eds). Special issue: treatment outcomes in clinical practice. Psychiatr Ann 27:95-134, 1997.

Vibbert S, Young M (eds). The 1997 Behavioral Outcomes and Guidelines Sourcebook. Faulkner & Gray, New York NY, 1996.

Resource Information

Outcome for Windows
Evaluation Systems International, Inc.
777 29th Street, Suite 400
Boulder CO 80303
(303) 443-2200

OQ-45 and OQ-10
Algorithms for Behavioral Care, Inc.
44 Roseville Road
Westport CT 06880
(800) 357-1200

Chapter 21

The Future of Primary Care/Behavioral Health Integration: Questions... and Some Answers?

Grant E. Mitchell, M.D. and Joel D. Haber, Ph.D.

It has become increasingly difficult in healthcare today to implement changes that improve the quality of care, decrease medical costs, and increase patient and provider satisfaction. Integration of behavioral health and primary care is one such change that can produce these results. Research data convincingly and consistently support the integration of behavioral health and primary care.

Primary care practice is the ideal place for closer collaboration with the behavioral health sector. Carve-out mental health programs once considered state of the art are no longer accepted with such fervor. A growing awareness of the significance of unrecognized mental health problems in primary care, medical cost offset data, and quality of care issues support the biopsychosocial model of care. Before such integration takes place, however, a number of problems must be carefully considered. These include recognition of mental disorders, barriers to appropriate management, screening issues, treatment, and training of primary care practitioners.

Recognition

As stated elsewhere in this volume, about half of all mental healthcare is delivered in the primary care system. Approximately 25 percent of medical outpatients and 30 to 60 percent of medical inpatients suffer from behavioral health disorders.[1-4] Further, 90 percent of the most common complaints presented in primary care have no clear organic basis. These include chest pain, fatigue, dizziness, headache, edema, back pain, dyspnea, insomnia, abdominal pain, and numbness.[5]

The problem however, is not only the extent of behavioral health problems in primary care, but the difficulty many primary care clinicians have in recognizing these disorders. Studies suggest that many of these patients with mental disorders are not properly diagnosed or treated, leading to significant comorbidity, patient dissatisfaction with treatment, provider frustration, and excess costs.

Models presented in this book delineate successful collaborative efforts aimed at improving the recognition and treatment of mental disorders in the primary care setting. Depression, one of the most common disorders, has been extensively researched and studied in the primary care sector and thus has been the target of improved screening and recognition efforts. Patients with anxiety disorders, substance abuse, and somatization also frequently present in primary care and are receiving increased attention by researchers and clinicians. A small subset of these populations are considered high utilizers of medical services in that they disproportionately consume healthcare dollars. Many of these patients are believed to be suffering from undiagnosed or inadequately treated mental illnesses. It has been difficult to identify the cause of their high utilization and problematic to manage them in primary care settings.

Solutions

Logic and experience dictate that screenings for behavioral health problems should take place in primary care. There is usually an established relationship between the primary care provider and the patient. Also, the stigma of addressing behavioral health issues in this setting appears to be reduced. The practice of undergoing an annual physical examination provides an additional opportunity to perform a behavioral health screening.

Yearly physical exams should be replaced by a "personal health evaluation," which includes both physical and emotional screenings. The evaluation would include a brief behavioral health screening questionnaire and follow-up by the primary care physician (PCP) if problems are identified. These screenings would further reduce stigma if their use becomes standard practice. This would help patients understand that both emotional and physical health issues are important.

For truly successful integration, screening and recognition efforts should be offered at sites other than the PCP's office. The workplace is another important location for integrated primary care health teams to perform personal health evaluations. These efforts could focus on screening for work-related stress and disability. Supervisors should also be trained by these teams to recognize common behavioral health disorders that may contribute to disability. Earlier identification of such problems might reduce the millions of dollars in disability claims, where physical problems may have little correlation to the actual degree of disability.

Primary care practitioners in training should be taught to recognize behavioral health problems, particularly through the use of simple, validated screening measures. Such training should ideally be provided by multidisciplinary teams whose members emphasize the mind-body connection. These teams can encompass a variety of behavioral health professionals based on the needs of the setting and population. An opportunity exists for mental health practitioners to join PCPs already in practice by providing them with training on behavioral health disorders. This could be accomplished through on-site informal lunch meetings, newsletters, or even through casual discussion. Collaborative relationships introduce the process of integration in already established practices and may lead to further initiatives being implemented.

Other efforts should target patients with subsyndromal conditions, in addition to those with disorders that meet the *Diagnostic and Statistical Manual for Mental Disorders*, Fourth edition *(DSM-IV)* criteria. Subsyndromal anxiety and depression may account for more of the behavioral health disorders than those with actual *DSM-IV* conditions (see Chapter 15). Tools that assist in the recognition of these subsyndromal conditions will prove valuable in future integrated delivery systems because detection will enable us to determine the impact such conditions have on functioning and how best to treat them.

Barriers

The stigma of mental illness, the culture of primary care medicine, and the lack of reimbursement for addressing behavioral health problems in primary care all present significant barriers to integration. Additionally, patients often express emotional issues through physical complaints to primary care providers, either because they are unaware of the emotional issue, or they believe that physical symptoms are expected and necessary to gain entry into the office. Some PCPs are uncomfortable with interpreting these complaints as emotional for fear the patient will become angry and leave the practice. Many also feel unprepared to manage behavioral issues even when they are diagnosed.

In many insurance plans, a primary care visit is less costly for the patient than a visit with a mental health provider, due to lower copayments. Higher copayments for mental health actually reduce the use of services by those who would benefit most from treatment. While this barrier to access may reduce utilization in the mental health specialty setting, evidence is increasing that these patients use significantly more medical resources.[6]

Solutions

A greater number of conferences, published articles, and lectures on the identification and treatment of mental health problems in primary care have begun to increase awareness of these barriers. For example, The National Depression Screening Program has helped reduce the stigma of depression by facilitating a more open dialogue regarding this condition. The availability of patient education materials that describe behavioral health disorders have contributed to their being viewed as important health issues instead of personality problems or signs of weakness. The introduction of selective serotonin reuptake inhibitors (SSRIs), with their ease of use and lower incidence of side effects, have also made the treatment of depression more acceptable to both patients and PCPs.

Financial incentives designed to enhance the recognition and treatment of mental disorders will improve the quality of life for patients and may decrease overall medical costs. Insurance companies should create parity with regard to copayments for mental health conditions and should reimburse PCPs for performing a personal health evaluation at a higher rate than for a physical examination. This is necessary to compensate for the increased time involved in addressing behavioral health issues. If an uncomplicated mental health problem is detected, it can be treated by the appropriately trained PCP; alternatively, further evaluation by a mental health practitioner may be needed.

Integrating medical/surgical and behavioral health services under one payment system can reduce the likelihood of cost shifting from one specialty to another. Scripps Health Systems in California recently announced a new healthcare delivery system which not only integrates behavioral health, but will create parity between medical/surgical and mental health benefits.[7]

Screening

Screening instruments to identify patients with mental disorders in primary care settings have been validated and are now widely available. They have been developed to provide a simple, standardized screening method for PCPs to use in their offices. PRIME-MD and SDDS-PC are examples of these instruments. Patients fill out a brief questionnaire, the results of which direct a more detailed interview conducted by the PCP, nurse, or mental health professional (see Appendices 3 and 4).

These screening tools have not gained widespread acceptance among primary care providers. Although the measures are brief, many clinicians find them to be too time-consuming. False negatives and false positives have contributed to reluctance to use these screening tools. Even when symptoms are detected, some PCPs are unsure of the course of treatment to follow. This is particularly true when patients report some symptoms but not enough to meet criteria for a *DSM-IV* mental disorder (i.e., subsyndromal conditions).

Solutions

Researchers should concentrate on developing new screening instruments that require less time for administration and scoring, provide accurate diagnoses, and most important, reveal information that has clinical relevance to their treatment of the patient. A new screening tool, known as the Patient Problem Questionnaire (PPQ), has been designed to respond to some of these concerns (see Appendix 5).

Advances in computer technology provide new opportunities to perform mental health screenings. Current tools are now being modified to include Computer Assisted Telephone Interview (CATI) versions. These enable patients to call a toll-free number and be interviewed by a computer, which queries them and records their responses. A report of the results is then sent or faxed to the PCP. Other options include screening via the Internet. All of these methods reduce the administrative burden on the primary care practitioners and their staff members.

Resistance to improving the screening and recognition of behavioral health disorders has been partly due to the fear of significant costs associated with the treatment of large numbers of patients with a variety of mental health symptoms and partly to the difficulty that primary care practitioners experience in determining the clinical relevance of these symptoms. While we advocate the screening of every new patient through use of the personal health evaluation, we are not suggesting that every identified mental health symptom requires treatment. Instead, if the screening reveals a potentially significant mental health problem, an integrated team would assist the PCP in determining the extent to which the symptoms interfere with social and occupational functioning, and thus require treatment. Once this determination is made, treatment must be targeted to the symptoms causing the dysfunction. Such medically necessary treatment should be reimbursed by the health plan.

Treatment

It is estimated that 50 percent of mental healthcare is delivered by primary care practitioners. However, many PCPs find that treatment of behavioral health disorders in primary care is difficult due to time constraints, lack of knowledge and comfort with treatment options, and difficulty of reimbursement for these services. Since behavioral health disorders are often successfully treated, assisting primary care practitioners in the management of these disorders will lead to healthier patients and more confident clinicians.

Solutions

Several chapters in this book have described the treatment of the more common behavioral health disorders seen in primary care. The treatment programs have many components, some of which include disease management, telephone triage, joint case management, patient education, and prevention initiatives.

Many primary care clinicians avoid the treatment of behavioral health disorders because they believe such disorders involve long-term therapy and consume excessive time. However, Katon et al found that interventions limited to patient education, prescription medication, and four to six sessions of cognitive-behavioral therapy (provided by a mental health practitioner) led to a significant reduction in depressive symptoms.[8]

Because patient education materials are so important, they should be available in a variety of formats. Education programs on specific mental disorders, stress management programs, support groups for individuals and families, pamphlets, and audio/video tapes are particularly useful aids. The creation of a national data bank for these resources would further increase awareness and enhance their use.

Standardized treatment guidelines and algorithms that have been developed by the American Psychiatric Association and others should be adapted, if necessary, for use in primary care. Employing these protocols can decrease the fear of treating mental disorders and help PCPs determine when a patient should be referred to a behavioral health specialist. Software is already available for the primary care practitioner that includes linked screening, diagnosis, and treatment algorithms.

A related and growing area of interest is the inclusion of alternative health treatments in traditional settings. While conventional medicine has been mostly successful in addressing acute illnesses and injuries, alternative therapies in conjunction with conventional therapies are intended to produce better treatment outcomes in chronic illness and facilitate lifestyle changes.

Holistic therapies may be considered truly integrated therapies. These treatments embrace the biopsychosocial approach and allow patients to participate more fully in the healing process. Some of these include Chinese medicine, acupuncture, herbal medicine, homeopathy, massage, yoga, biofeedback, and imagery.

Physicians can work with nonphysician alternative practitioners in many ways. At Columbia-Presbyterian Complementary Care Center, imagery and healing are used to promote patient recovery prior to cardiac surgery, as an alternative to standard cardiac treatment.[9] Behavioral and relaxation techniques such as hypnosis, imagery, biofeedback, and meditation have been used successfully for conditions such as chronic pain and insomnia.[10] These alternative treatments delivered in primary care settings must continue to undergo analysis that focuses on outcomes, patient satisfaction, and cost effectiveness. Medical schools have increasingly been incorporating the study of alternative medicine into their curricula. The establishment of the Office of Alternative Medicine at the National Institutes of Health has further legitimized the study and validation of these alternative techniques.

While much of the discussion involving integration has focused on integrating behavioral health into primary care, it is also important to consider the potential benefits of incorporating primary care into behavioral health. For many seriously mentally ill individuals, the only contact with the healthcare system may be through their mental health professional. This setting could provide an important opportunity to address their physical health needs by having a primary care provider on site or by providing additional training to behavioral health practitioners in the screening and treatment of physical illnesses.

Finally, it is important to remember that mental health information that is recorded in the medical record must have certain protections; releasing this information can stigmatize patients and prevent them from obtaining insurance, employment, and loans. Computerized systems have been developed to address this concern. Access to the medical record can be controlled by incorporating graded security systems into the software.

Training

Previous chapters in this book have highlighted the paucity of behavioral health training in many primary care residency programs. The average internal medicine residency program devotes less than two hours per year to behavioral health training.[11] The difficulty that many PCPs have in recognizing mental disorders is not only due to a lack of knowledge but is also due to the lack of training in interviewing and communication skills. While behavioral health training programs usually teach these basic skills, they often fail to adequately prepare trainees to adapt these skills to the primary care environment.

Solutions

Behavioral health should be further integrated into the medical school curriculum simultaneously with physical disease states. This can best be accomplished not by adding material to the program, but instead by reorganizing the teaching of behavioral health concepts. Such "educational integration" would avoid establishing the separation of mind and body fostered by the current system.

Clearly, education in interview techniques and communication skills must be expanded in primary care training programs if PCPs are to feel comfortable and confident with these issues (see Appendix 6). Interviewing tools such as the BATHE technique (see Chapter 13), if utilized by PCPs, would provide both relationship building and a brief system of screening.[12] This clinical model for interviewing patients helps the PCP deal with psychosocial issues that may otherwise be difficult to address.

Residency programs that offer multiple board certification should also be expanded. For example, a physician with training in pediatrics and child psychiatry would indeed be a valuable member of an integrated team. Because a portion of residency education is often funded through patient care revenue, PCPs in residency programs should be reimbursed for addressing uncomplicated behavioral health issues. There is also a deficiency in behavioral health programs that teach the biopsychosocial model but do not adequately teach trainees how to work in the primary care environment. Overcoming this will require an increased emphasis on the evolving role of the behavioral health practitioner from an independent specialist to an on-site, collaborative consultant.

Models of Integration

For many years, our healthcare system has been fragmented. Care has traditionally been provided by specialists who often focus on their area of expertise. Payment systems often carve out mental health benefits. Recently, PCPs have been given more responsibility for coordinating clinical care and have been encouraged to manage a patient's total health before referring to a specialist. Accomplishing this goal will require increased cooperation with specialists. Different levels of collaboration can exist between the primary care practitioner and behavioral healthcare provider. Doherty, McDaniel, and Brady have formulated a general conceptual framework that describes five levels of collaboration that can exist in integrated systems (see Appendix 2).[13]

Level I

"Minimal Collaboration" refers to a distinct separation between mental health and medical/surgical services in which little collaboration occurs. This is the model that describes most private practices.

Level II

This can be considered "Basic Collaboration from a Distance." At this level, practitioners operate in different settings but have occasional telephonic or written communication about patients. An example might be a medical group that refers their mental health patients to outside behavioral health practitioners but shares basic information with each other.

Level III

"Basic Collaboration on Site" describes the type of integration where mental health practitioners and PCPs are co-located and do communicate. However, the interaction between practitioners is not coordinated in any systematic way. An example might be a consultation-liaison service in a hospital.

Level IV

In "Close Collaboration in a Partly Integrated System," practitioners are co-located and work together as a team, but some operational and financial aspects of the system remain distinct. A brain-injury rehabilitation program might operate with this level of integration.

Level V

This level refers to "Close Collaboration in a Fully Integrated System." All healthcare personnel function as a unit with members having distinct but equivalent roles in the system. Scripps Health Systems in California may represent this ultimate level of collaboration.

Doherty and colleagues point out that higher levels of integration are required to adequately address complex biopsychosocial problems. Because most primary care providers still practice in systems that only minimally collaborate with mental health practitioners, their treatment of mental disorders should probably be limited to uncomplicated cases. A goal for these practices should be to move along this continuum to a higher level of collaboration in order to provide better care to patients with more complex mental health disorders.

Conclusion

The changing roles of the behavioral health practitioner and the primary care provider have already been extensively discussed. However, the most important member of the integrated healthcare team is the patient. The term *patient* is defined as an individual who is receiving care or treatment.[13] This definition highlights the more passive role that patients have traditionally played in the doctor-patient relationship. Patients should instead be active members of the integrated team, with their own rights and responsibilities in the management of their health.

The abbreviation *PCP* should also stand for the *primary care partnership* that includes the patient, the primary care practitioner, and other healthcare providers. When patients are more involved in their care, treatment is more likely to be successful due to the increased sense of self-control and mastery. Patients should thus be encouraged to assume as much responsibility as they can manage. Although educating patients will require additional resources, ultimately it will improve their health and reduce the burden on primary care providers.

The primary care partnership can be viewed as a fluid system. The relative activity of the members changes, depending on the health needs of the patient. For example, the PCP might assume a more prominent role in directing the care of an individual who has suffered an acute myocardial infarction (MI). After the acute event is stabilized, the behavioral health provider might become the more active partner by assisting the PCP and the patient in managing the behavioral sequelae of the MI. Later, the patient might assume the more active role by instituting lifestyle changes to maintain and improve his or her health.

We must strive to maintain reasonable expectations of the PCP's role. It is unfair to expect PCPs to be experts in all areas. However, as coordinators of the primary care partnership, a wide variety of health issues could be more successfully managed, in terms of quality of care, patient satisfaction, cost effectiveness, and physician time.

It is likely that some PCPs will not embrace these ideas. This may be especially true for those already in practice. One method to aid in gaining acceptance might be to identify a subgroup of PCPs who have an interest in behavioral health disorders and encourage them to receive additional training. For example, in a primary care group these individuals could assist in screening and treating those with uncomplicated mental disorders. While this would represent a significant improvement for many primary care practices, an important goal would be to eventually incorporate behavioral health professionals into the practice to assist in the assessment and treatment of more complex cases.

A review of the chapters in this volume convincingly shows that integration is not a new idea, nor is it to be easily accomplished. A number of challenges exist that must be carefully researched and thoughtfully implemented. Some of these are listed below, corresponding to the chapter order of this book. Other challenges will no doubt arise as integration efforts proceed.

- *Barriers*. When patients with behavioral health disorders are jointly cared for in an integrated system, who is primarily responsible for their mental healthcare? Are there increased legal risks for PCPs managing these behavioral health problems?

- *Models.* How will integrated models address the risk of increased utilization of mental health services that results from case finding?
- *Recognition.* Will the increased recognition of behavioral health symptoms result in improved health outcomes?
- *Screening.* Should screening instruments focus less on *DSM-IV* diagnoses and more on identifying patients with clinically significant pathology who are likely to benefit from treatment?
- *Treatment.* How do integrated systems address the issue of treatment variability among practitioners?
- *Training.* How will integrated training programs be funded as managed care continues to grow?

Finally, while the cost and potential savings associated with integration have been extensively discussed, we should not feel compelled to justify the expense of behavioral health treatment solely through the medical cost offset. The most critical potential outcome of integration systems is the improvement of personal health and quality of life for patients.

References

1. Spitzer RL, Williams JB, Kroenke K, et al: Utility of a new procedure for diagnosing mental disorders in primary care: the PRIME-MD 1000 study. JAMA 272:1749-1756, 1994.
2. Ormel J, Von Korff M, Ustun TB, et al: Common mental disorders and disabilities across cultures: results from the WHO collaborative study on psychological problems in general health care. JAMA 272:1741-1748, 1994.
3. Cavanaugh VS: The prevalence of emotional and cognitive dysfunction in a general medical population: using the MMSE, GHQ, and BDI. Gen Hosp Psychiatry 5:15-24, 1983.
4. Moore RD, Bone LR, Geller G, et al: Prevalence, detection and treatment of alcoholism in hospitalized patients. JAMA 261:403-407, 1989.
5. Kroenke K, Mangelsdorff AD: Common symptoms in ambulatory care: incidence, evaluation, therapy, and outcomes. Am J Med 86:262-265, 1989.
6. Cole SA, Raju M: Overcoming barriers to integration of primary care and behavioral healthcare: focus on knowledge and skills. Behavioral Healthcare Tomorrow 5:31-37, 1996.
7. Grinfield MJ: Physician, hospital accord to reinvent managed care. Psychiatric Times 14(5):1-3, 1997.
8. Katon W, Robinson P, Von Korff M, et al: A multifaceted intervention to improve treatment of depression in primary care. Arch Gen Psychiatry 53:924-932, 1996.
9. Moore NG: The Columbia-Presbyterian Complementary Care Center: comprehensive care of the mind, body, and spirit. Alternative Ther 3:30-32, 1997.
10. Chilton M: Panel recommends integrating behavioral and relaxation approaches into medical treatment of chronic pain, insomnia. Alternative Ther 2:19-28, 1996.
11. Lipkin M: Can primary care physicians deliver quality mental healthcare? Behavioral Healthcare Tomorrow 5:48-53, 1996.
12. Lieberman JA: BATHE: an approach to the interview process in the primary care setting. J Clin Psychiatry 58:3-6, 1997.
13. Doherty WJ, McDaniel SH, Baird MA: Five levels of primary care/behavioral healthcare collaboration. Behavioral Healthcare Tomorrow 5:25-27, 1996.

Annotated Bibliography

Treatment of Mental Disorders in Primary Care and Specialty Settings: Utilization, Recognition, Treatment Delivery, Outcome, and Quality of Care

Marcia Kaplan, M.D.

Utilization

1. Olfson M, Pincus HA: Outpatient psychotherapy in the United States, I: volume, costs and user characteristics. Am J Psychiatry 151:1281–1288, 1994.

   Psychotherapy accounts for 8% of outpatient medical costs. Users of psychotherapy reported poorer general health, higher medical costs, and more functional impairment than non-users. Not all mental health care is psychotherapy, although mental health specialists commonly provide psychotherapy.

2. Olfson M, Pincus HA: Outpatient psychotherapy in the United States, II: patterns of utilization. Am J Psychiatry 151:1289–1294, 1994.

   Long-term psychotherapy accounted for 16% of psychotherapy users and 63% of psychotherapy expenditures. Medication use and psychiatric hospitalization were more common among long-term users. Long-term and short-term psychotherapy tend to be provided by different healthcare professionals for different kinds of conditions. Research is needed to define conditions under which long-term psychotherapy achieves benefits that equal or surpass those of other procedures.

3. Simon GE, VonKorff M, Durham ML: Predictors of outpatient mental health utilization by primary care patients in a health maintenance organization. Am J Psychiatry 151:908–913, 1994.

   Utilization of mental health services increased with poorer general health and decreased with higher out-of-pocket cost for mental health visits. Use of mental health services was high, and increasing copayments reduced use of services without respect to severity of illness.

4. Simon GE, Grothaus L, Durham ML, et al: Impact of visit copayments on outpatient mental health utilization by members of a health maintenance organization. Am J Psychiatry 153:331–338, 1996.

   In a staff model HMO, institution of a $20 copayment was associated with a 16% decrease in likelihood of service use, but no decrease in number of visits per year among users. An increase to $30/visit did not further decrease likelihood of use, but did decrease number of visits per year by 9%. Higher copayments restricted access regardless of clinical need.

5. Landerman LR, Burns BJ, Swartz MS, et al: Relationship between insurance coverage and psychiatric disorder in predicting use of mental health services. Am J Psychiatry 151:1785–1790, 1994.

   Using data from the second wave of the ECA project, authors found that insurance coverage was strongly associated with care, whether or not patient had a psychiatric diagnosis. The association between coverage and probability of care was strongest among those with a psychiatric disorder. These findings are not consistent with the claim that failing to provide insurance will reduce discretionary but not necessary mental health utilization.

6. Olfson M, Pincus HA: Outpatient mental healthcare in nonhospital settings: distribution of patients across provider groups. Am J Psychiatry 153:1353–1356, 1996.

Data from the 1987 National Medical Expenditure Survey showed that 4% of noninstitutionalized Americans, or 9 million people, made 84 million outpatient mental health visits. Psychiatrists provided more treatment than psychologists for schizophrenia, bipolar illness, substance abuse, and depression, but provided less treatment for anxiety disorders. General medical physicians provided the most treatment for adjustment disorders and substance abuse. Mental health professionals provided most treatment for childhood mental disorders and mental retardation.

7. Henk HJ, Katzelnick DJ, Kobak KA, Greist JH, Jefferson JW: Medical costs attributed to depression among patients with a history of high medical expenses in a health maintenance organization. Arch Gen Psychiatry 533:899–904, 1996.

High utilizers with depression used $1500 more than nondepressed patients in healthcare costs. Costs of treatment of depression accounted for only a small portion of total medical costs for depressed high utilizers.

8. McFarland BH, Johnson RE, Hornbrook MC: Enrollment duration, services use and costs of care for severely mentally ill members of a health maintenance organization. Arch Gen Psychiatry 53:928–944, 1996.

Severely mentally ill members of an HMO were enrolled for longer duration than controls with no chronic disease, but not as long as controls with diabetes. Costs of mental health treatment for the severely mentally ill were higher than for controls, but outpatient general medical usage was not higher. Inpatient medical/surgical utilization for the severely mentally ill was equal to usage of pharmacy controls (anyone using outpatient pharmacy services during a given period of time). There was no evidence for disenrollment or refusal to offer services to severely mentally ill patients despite contract limiting services to short-term acute conditions. The integrated delivery system provided by the HMO may be particularly valuable for the severely mentally ill, more so than "carved out" mental health services.

9. Dickey B, Normand ST, Norton EC, et al: Managing the care of schizophrenia. Arch Gen Psychiatry 53:945–952, 1996.

Review of the Massachusetts statewide managed care plan for all Medicaid beneficiaries between 1992 and 1994 shows that per-patient expenditure for schizophrenic patients dropped slightly and inpatient days dropped slightly. There was a small increase in readmission within 30 days for this group. Most patterns of care remained the same.

Recognition, Treatment Delivery, and Outcome

10. Wells KB, Golding JM, Burnam MA: Psychiatric disorder in a sample of the general population with and without chronic medical conditions. Am J Psychiatry 145:976–981, 1988.

The prevalence of any psychiatric disorder in the past six months was 25% for patients with one or more chronic medical conditions, compared to 18% for those without chronic medical illness. Forty-two percent of the chronically ill had a lifetime psychiatric disorder, compared with 33% of those without chronic medical illness. Persons with chronic medical conditions were more likely to have lifetime substance abuse and recent affective and anxiety disorders. Arthritis, cancer, lung disease, heart disease, neurologic disorder, and physical handicap were associated with psychiatric disorder, but hypertension and diabetes were not.

11. Tiemens BG, Ormel J, Simon GE: Occurrence, recognition and outcome of psychological disorders in primary care. Am J Psychiatry 153:636–644, 1996.

Recognition of psychological disorders was not associated with better outcome. Increasing recognition will lead to improved outcomes only if primary care providers have the skills and resources to deliver adequate care.

12. Sherbourne CD, Wells KB, Hays RD, et al: Subthreshold depression and depressive disorder: clinical characteristics of general medical and mental health specialty outpatients. Am J Psychiatry 151:1777-1784, 1994.

Patients with a subthreshold depressive disorder had rates of positive family history that were almost as high as patients with major depression. Patients with depression had a higher rate of comorbid anxiety disorder. Treatment rates for patients with subthreshold depressive disorder were considerably lower than for patients with depression in the general medical sector but not in the mental health sector.

13. Brown C, Schulberg HC, Madonia MJ, Shear MK, Houck PR: Treatment outcomes for primary care patients with major depression and lifetime anxiety disorders. Am J Psychiatry 153:1293-1300, 1996.

Depressed patients with comorbid anxiety disorders presented with significantly more psychopathology and tended to terminate prematurely more often than patients with major depression alone. Medication and psychotherapy are effective treatments for both types of patient, but there is poorer response in those with anxiety disorders. It is important to identify the presence of an anxiety disorder in depressed patients.

14. Ormel J, Oldehinkel T, Briman E, Brink W: Outcome of depression and anxiety in primary care. Arch Gen Psychiatry 50:759-766, 1993.

Long-term outcome of patients with psychiatric symptoms was evaluated at 1- and 3-year follow-up. Partial remission rather than full recovery was the rule, and was associated with residual disability. Depression had better outcome than mixed depression and anxiety. Authors suggest a different model for following patients with residual symptoms and disability.

15. Wells KB, Katon W, Rogers B, Camp P: Use of minor tranquilizers and antidepressant medications by depressed outpatients: results from the Medical Outcomes study. Am J Psychiatry 151:694-700, 1994.

Depressed outpatients' use of medication was followed: 23% had used an antidepressant and 30% had used a minor tranquilizer. Psychiatrists' patients were most likely to have used medication. The more severely depressed patients were more likely to take antidepressants. Patients in prepaid plans were twice as likely as those in fee-for-service plans to use minor tranquilizers.

16. Olfson M, Broadhead WE, Weissman MM, et al: Subthreshold psychiatric symptoms in a primary care group practice. Arch Gen Psychiatry 53:880-886, 1996.

Subthreshold symptoms were as or more common than Axis I diagnoses, and many patients also had other Axis I diagnoses. Depressive and anxiety symptoms were associated with impairment. Authors suggest that patients with subthreshold symptoms of depression or anxiety have a broad psychiatric assessment.

17. Sherbourne CD, Wells KB, Meredith LS, Jackson CA, Camp P: Comorbid anxiety disorder and the functioning and well-being of chronically ill patients of general medical providers. Arch Gen Psychiatry 53:889-895, 1996.

Patients with hypertension, diabetes, and heart disease, with and without comorbid anxiety disorders had significantly lower health-related quality of life. Patients with comorbid anxiety had lower levels of functioning than those without, and anxious hypertensive or diabetic patients were as debilitated as those with heart disease or depression. Anxiety disorders in the chronically ill should be identified and treated in primary care settings.

18. Meredith LS, Wells, KB, Kaplan SH, Mazel RM: Counseling typically provided for depression. Arch Gen Psychiatry 53:905-912, 1996.

Less than one-half of patients with depression received at least three minutes of counseling from primary care physicians, while almost all depressed patients received counseling from mental health specialists. Counseling rates were lower in prepaid than fee-for-service general medical practices. Psychiatrists and psychologists provided longer sessions and more formal psychotherapeutic technique than did general medical practitioners.

19. Schulberg HC, Block MR, Madonia MJ, et al: Treating major depression in primary care practice. Arch Gen Psychiatry 53:913–919, 1996.

Seventy percent of patients given psychotherapy or pharmacotherapy versus 20% of patients assigned to physician's usual care were recovered from depression at 8 months after diagnosis, because usual care patients were not communicating with their doctors about their symptoms.

20. Katon W, Robinson P, von Korff M, et al: A multifaceted intervention to improve treatment of depression in primary care. Arch Gen Psychiatry 53:924–932, 1996.

Depressed patients were randomized to intervention (behavioral treatment and counseling to improve compliance with medication) versus usual care. At 4-month follow-up, intervention patients were more compliant, more satisfied with their care, and less depressed than usual care patients. Intervention patients with subsyndromal depression had less improvement in depression severity.

21. Judd LL, Paulus MP, Wells KB, Rapoport MH: Socioeconomic burden of subsyndromal depressive symptoms and major depression in a sample of the general population. Am J Psychiatry 53:1411–1417, 1996.

Using responses from the NIMH ECA program, subjects were divided into three groups: no depression, major depression, and subsyndromal depressive symptoms. There was significantly greater impairment of job and physical functioning, health status, and financial status in those with major depression and subsyndromal symptoms compared with no disorder. Subsyndromal depression is a clinical and public health problem that needs further study.

22. Lieberman JA: Compliance issues in primary care. J Clin Psychiatry 57(suppl 7):76–82, 1996.

Mental health problems are not adequately diagnosed and treated by primary care practitioners, which leads to inappropriate medications being prescribed, and to noncompliance. Doctors leave the medical education process with a predisposition to view problems from a biomedical perspective and do not recognize their considerable ability, within the doctor-patient relationship, to intervene in psychosocial problems and thereby improve compliance. Specific techniques for counseling patients are described.

23. Krupnick JL, et al: The role of therapeutic alliance in psychotherapy and pharmacotherapy outcome: findings in the National Institute of Mental Health Treatment of Depression Collaborative Research Program. J Consult Clin Psychol 64:532–539, 1996.

This study examines the relative importance of treatment type (cognitive, interpersonal, imipramine, or placebo plus clinical management) and therapeutic alliance in the outcome of 225 depressed outpatients rated by Hamilton and Beck scores. Therapeutic alliance was similar for all treatment types and accounted for more of the variance in outcome than treatment method. Alliance was just as important for drug treatment as for psychotherapy. The patient's contribution to the alliance, rather than the therapist's, was the important factor in outcome. It is possible that alliance measured some other factor of patients (such as readiness to change). These results help explain the poorer outcome of depressed patients in primary care settings where medication may be offered without attention to the treatment alliance. More delineation is necessary as to whether the alliance can be fostered or is a preexisting characteristic of the patient.

24. Miller MD, Schulz R, Paradis C, et al: Changes in perceived health status of depressed elderly patients treated until remission. Am J Psychiatry 153:1350–1352, 1996.

Elderly depressed patients who did not respond to treatment rated their health as poorer than those who did respond. Patients who initially rated their health as fair to poor were less likely to recover from depression. Self-rating of health improved with resolution of depression.

25. Norquist G, Wells KB, Rogers WH, et al: Quality of care for depressed elderly patients hospitalized in the specialty psychiatric units or general medical wards. Arch Gen Psychiatry 52:695–701, 1996.

A higher percentage of admissions to psychiatric units were considered appropriate, overall psychological assessment was better on psychiatric units and patients were more likely to receive psychological services in psychiatric units. There were more medical complications on psychiatric units, and medical care was better on medical wards, but clinical status on discharge was better for those in psychiatric units compared to general medical wards.

26. Chacko RC, Harper RG, Gotto J, Young J: Psychiatric interview and psychometric predictors of cardiac transplant survival. Am J Psychiatry 153: 1607-1612, 1996.

Prospective study of heart transplant patients who were assessed pre-transplant for psychiatric diagnosis, coping skills, and social support. Measures of coping and social support based on patient self-assessment were the best predictors of survival. Interview determined ratings of social support and pre-transplant compliance were potential predictors. Axis I diagnoses were associated with post-transplant hospital utilization and axis II disorders were associated with post-transplant health behavior.

Quality of Care

27. Brook RH, Cleary PD. Quality of health care, part 2: measuring quality of care. New Eng J Med 335:966-970, 1996.

28. Chassin M: Quality of health care, part 3: improving the quality of care. New Eng J Med 335:1060-1063, 1996.

29. Blumenthal D: Quality of health care, part 4: the origins of the quality-of-care debated. New Eng J Med 335:1146-1149, 1996.

30. Berwick DM: Quality of health care, part 5: payment by capitation and the quality of care. New Eng J Med 335:1227-1231, 1996.

31. Blumenthal D, Epstein AM: Quality of health care, part 6: the role of the physicians in the future of quality management. New Eng J Med 335:1328-1331, 1996.

This six-part series offers an excellent, clearly stated overview of the issues involved in maintaining quality in the face of ongoing changes in financing and delivery of healthcare.

Part VI.
APPENDICES

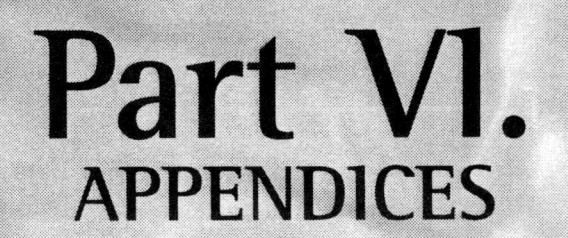

Appendix 1

Mental Disorders in General Medical Practice: Adding Value to Healthcare Through Consultation-Liaison Psychiatry

This appendix contains the ... slide show and accompanying lecture notes developed by the Academy of Psychosomatic Medicine. It presents statistics that reveal the impact of behavioral illness on general medical practice, and illustrates why an integrated system may be crucial to effective diagnosis and treatment. The data presented here focus on the high number of behavioral disorder sufferers who get lost in the general healthcare system.

Founded in 1954, the Academy of Psychosomatic Medicine serves as an arena for collaboration and exchange of ideas in psychiatric medicine and consultation-liaison psychiatry. The Academy is an international organization with over 1000 members whose mission is to aid "patients with comorbid medical and psychiatric illness and the interaction between them. This focus entails clinical work, research, and teaching as well as leadership in the provision of consultation-liaison services."

Copyright © 1996 Behavioral Healthcare Tomorrow. All rights reserved. No part of this publication may be reproduced, stored in a retrieval system, or transmitted in any form or by any means, electronic, mechanical, photocopying, or otherwise, without prior written permission of the copyright owner.

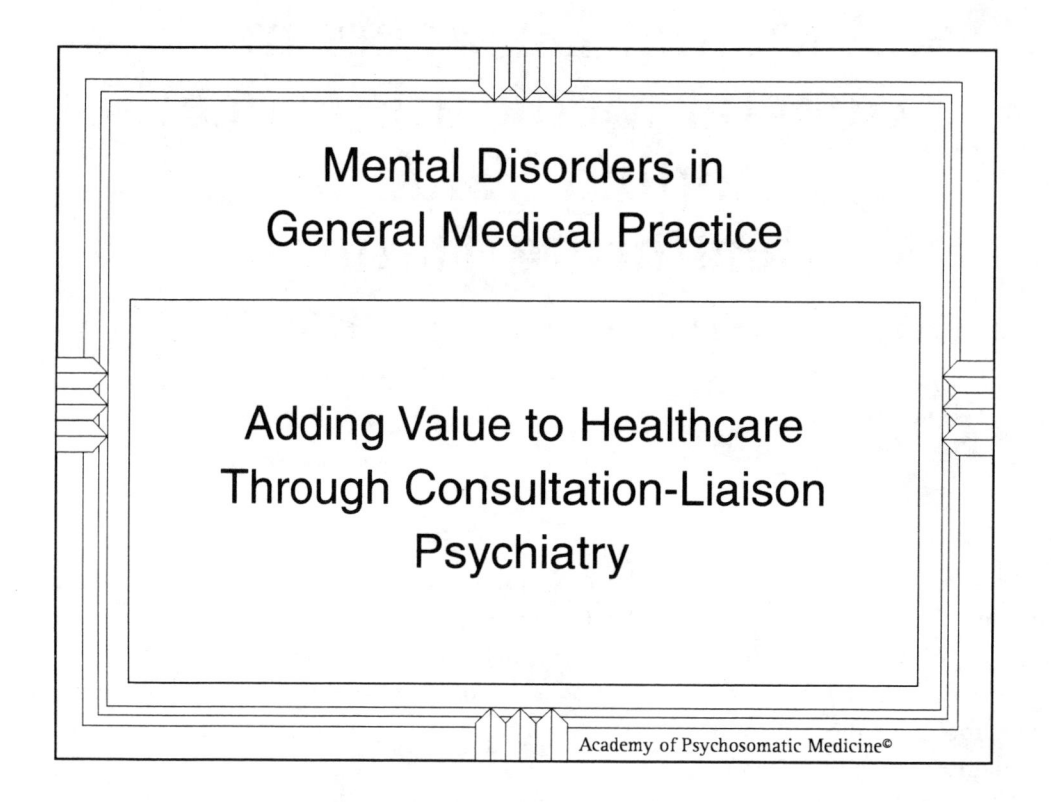

> # Mental Disorders in
> # General Medical Practice
>
> ## Adding Value to Healthcare Through Consultation-Liaison Psychiatry
>
> *Academy of Psychosomatic Medicine©*

SLIDE 1 Mental Disorders in General Medical Practice: Adding Value to Healthcare Through Consultation-Liaison Psychiatry

This slide presentation reviews the impact of mental disorders in patients receiving care in the general medical sector. Mental disorders in medical patients are common, poorly recognized and treated, and are responsible for excessive utilization and costs of general medical services. For the primary care provider, such patients tend to require a disproportionately large amount of time and attention.

Integration of mental health services with general medical services has been documented in numerous studies to improve functioning and outcome of medical patients and to decrease costs. The data support the cost-efficacy of integrating a behavioral healthcare team into all systems of healthcare. The clinical leadership of this team should be provided by a psychiatrist with expertise in the assessment and management of mental disorders in medical patients. Psychiatrists with consultation-liaison training have the experience, knowledge and skill to serve as clinical leaders of this behavioral team.

This integrated approach can help improve physicians' efficiency and efficacy in the emerging healthcare environment.

Copyright © 1996 by the Academy of Psychosomatic Medicine. All rights reserved. No part of this publication may be reproduced, stored in a retrieval system, or transmitted in any form or by any means, electronic, mechanical, photocopying, recording, or otherwise, without prior written permission of the copyright owner.

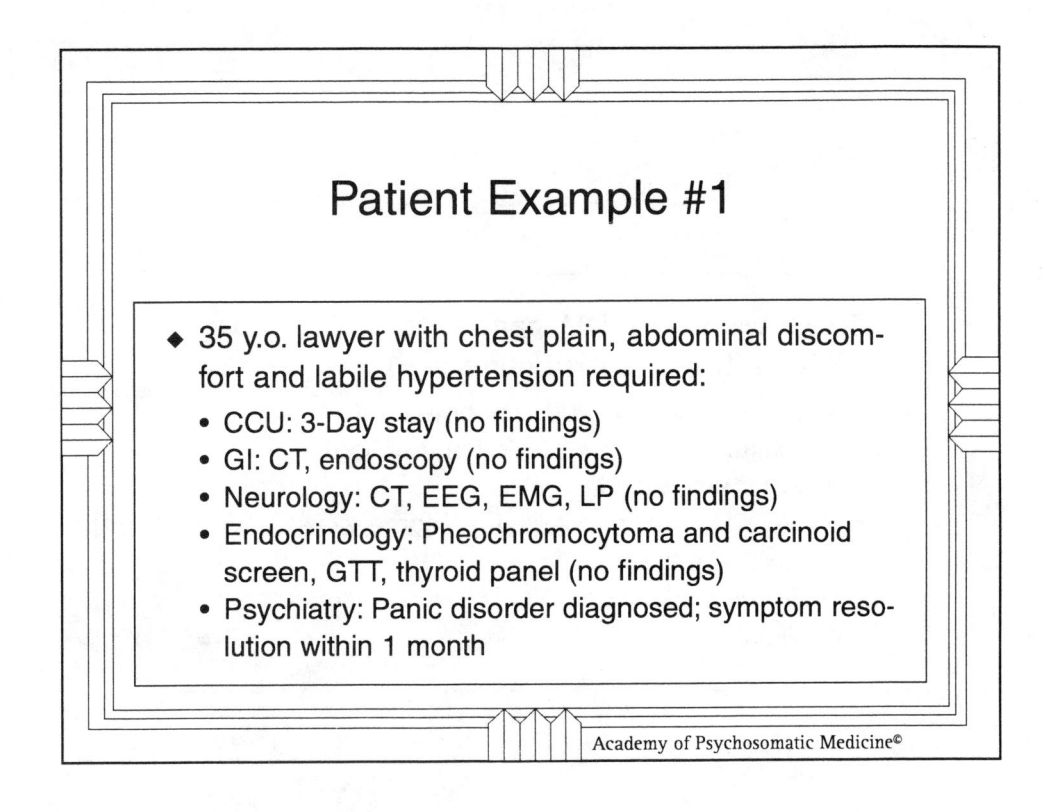

> ## Patient Example #1
>
> - 35 y.o. lawyer with chest plain, abdominal discomfort and labile hypertension required:
>   - CCU: 3-Day stay (no findings)
>   - GI: CT, endoscopy (no findings)
>   - Neurology: CT, EEG, EMG, LP (no findings)
>   - Endocrinology: Pheochromocytoma and carcinoid screen, GTT, thyroid panel (no findings)
>   - Psychiatry: Panic disorder diagnosed; symptom resolution within 1 month
>
> Academy of Psychosomatic Medicine©

SLIDE 2 Patient Example #1

This is the first of two case histories typical of the kinds of high-cost patients in current systems of care whose psychiatric symptoms may confound proper management (Katon and Roy-Byrne 1989).

A 35-year-old lawyer with chest pain, abdominal discomfort and a history of labile hypertension was admitted to the cardiac care unit for three days. During that time he underwent extensive cardiac testing, including laboratory tests, echocardiogram, and stress tests. All proved negative. He also underwent a GI workup that included a CT scan and an endoscopy, which were negative. A neurologic workup that included a CT scan, EEG, EMG and LP also proved negative as did an endocrine workup to rule out pheochromocytoma, carcinoid syndrome, thyroid disorders and diabetes. Finally, a consult from a consultation-liaison psychiatrist was obtained. Panic disorder was diagnosed and treated with an antidepressant. One-month later the patient had resumed full activities and was without significant symptoms.

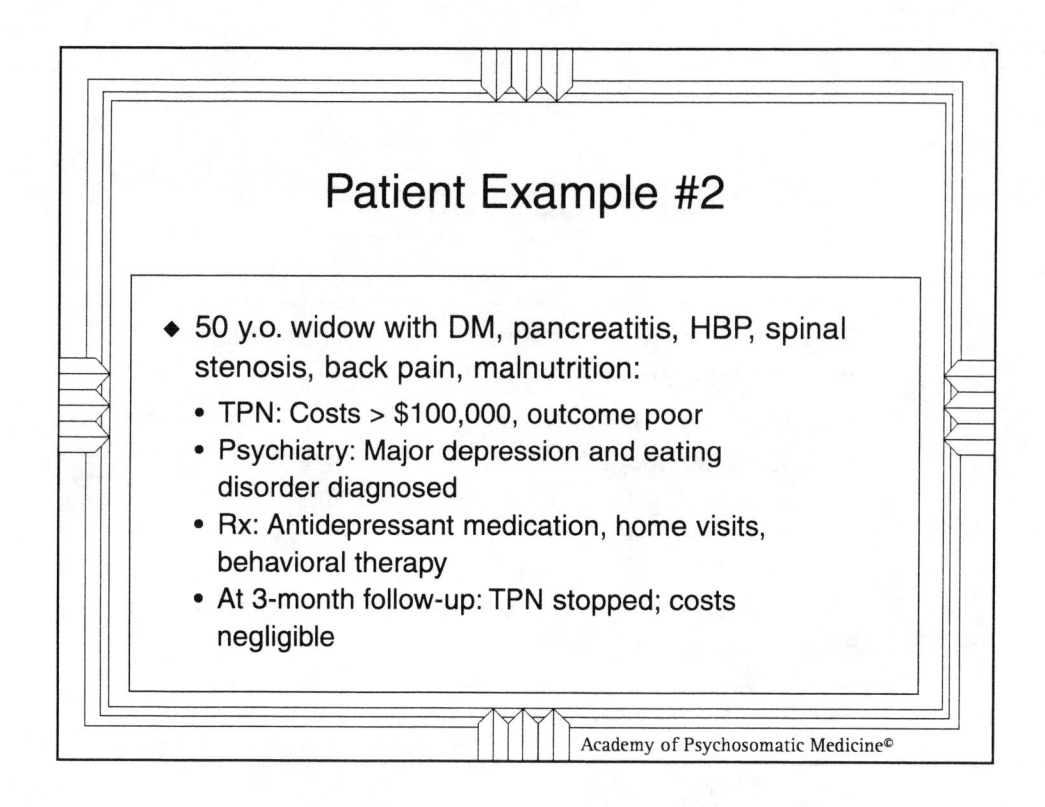

> # Patient Example #2
>
> ◆ 50 y.o. widow with DM, pancreatitis, HBP, spinal stenosis, back pain, malnutrition:
>   - TPN: Costs > $100,000, outcome poor
>   - Psychiatry: Major depression and eating disorder diagnosed
>   - Rx: Antidepressant medication, home visits, behavioral therapy
>   - At 3-month follow-up: TPN stopped; costs negligible
>
> Academy of Psychosomatic Medicine©

SLIDE 3 Patient Example #2

A 50 year-old widow enrolled in a large midwestern HMO had multiple problems: diabetes mellitus, pancreatitis, high blood pressure, spinal stenosis, back pain and malnutrition (Baird 1996).* The HMO incurred very high costs in caring for this patient, much of which could have been avoided. Prolonged TPN alone cost $100,000. Despite this, her condition remained poor. Finally, a psychiatric consultation was obtained. The patient was diagnosed with major depression and an eating disorder. Antidepressant medication, visits by a home health psychiatric nurse, and behavioral therapy directed at the eating disorder were all promptly initiated. An assessment made at three months post-treatment found her condition greatly improved. TPN had been discontinued and the continuing treatment costs were modest, consisting only of the cost of the antidepressant and occasional home visits.

TPN = total parenteral nutrition

*Baird M: Personal communication. Case presentation at the "Primary Care/Behavioral Healthcare Summit," San Diego, March 1996.

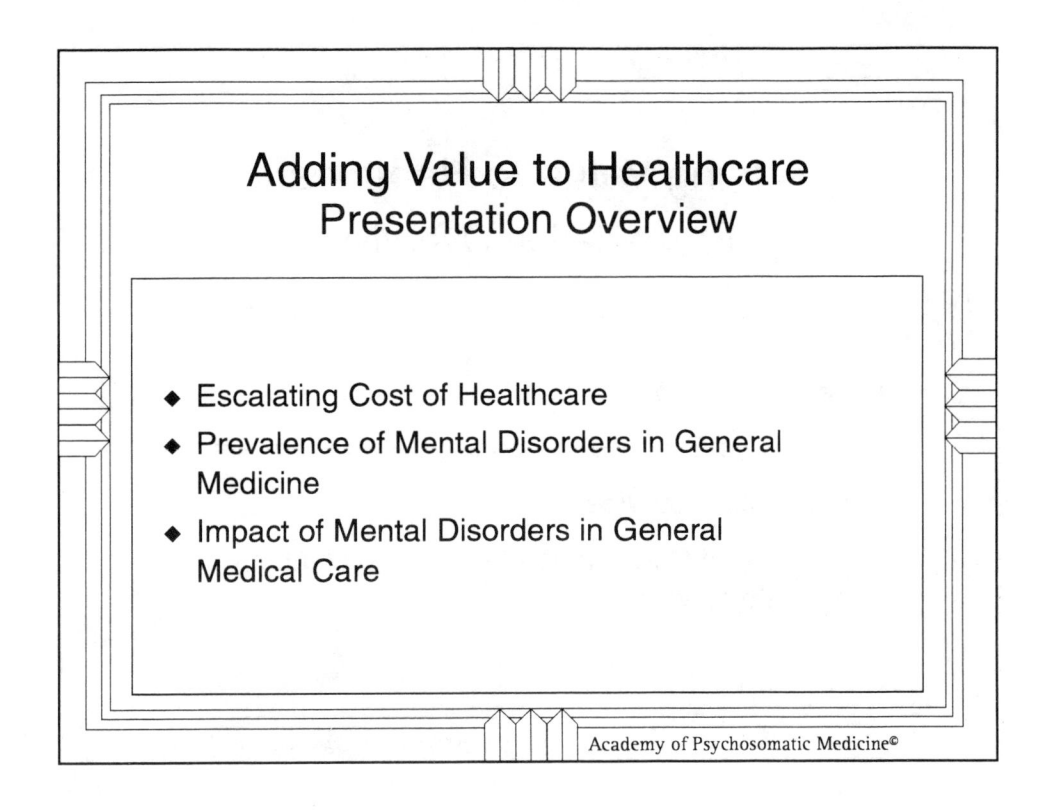

> **Adding Value to Healthcare**
> **Presentation Overview**
>
> - Escalating Cost of Healthcare
> - Prevalence of Mental Disorders in General Medicine
> - Impact of Mental Disorders in General Medical Care
>
> Academy of Psychosomatic Medicine©

SLIDE 4   Adding Value to Healthcare
Presentation Overview

These two case histories illustrate the insidious effects that mental disorders can have on the cost-effectiveness of healthcare and on patient functioning and well-being. Not least, mental disorders also create considerable frustration for providers.

During the course of this presentation, we will demonstrate that the escalating cost of healthcare is at least partly due to the high prevalence of unrecognized or inadequately treated mental disorders in the general medical sector. We'll also show that the presence of unrecognized or inadequately treated psychiatric comorbidity increases healthcare costs and utilization and compromises patient functioning, over and above the subjective distress caused to the patient.

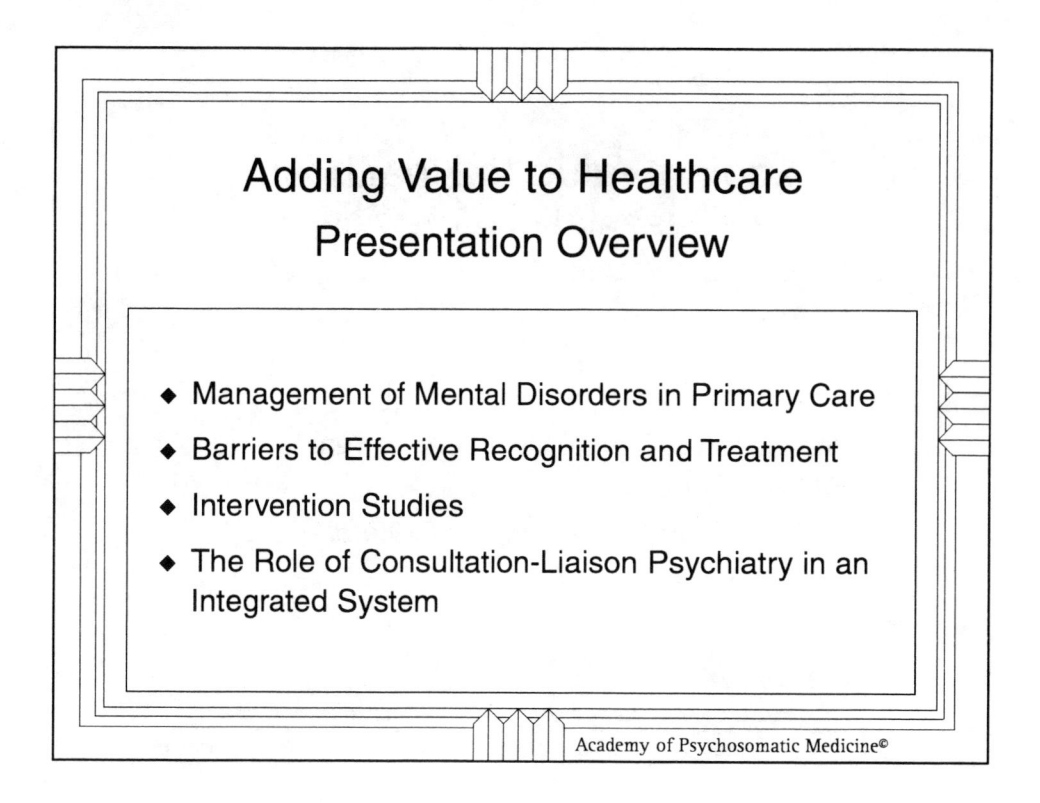

Adding Value to Healthcare
Presentation Overview

- Management of Mental Disorders in Primary Care
- Barriers to Effective Recognition and Treatment
- Intervention Studies
- The Role of Consultation-Liaison Psychiatry in an Integrated System

Academy of Psychosomatic Medicine©

SLIDE 5 Adding Value to Healthcare
Presentation Overview

In this slide presentation, we will discuss problems in the management of mental disorders in the general medical sector, describe barriers to better care and propose solutions. Studies documenting the clinical and cost-efficacy of psychiatric interventions demonstrate the unique role that C-L psychiatry can play in a behavioral healthcare team that is integrated with general medical care.

Escalating Costs of Healthcare

Per Capita ($)

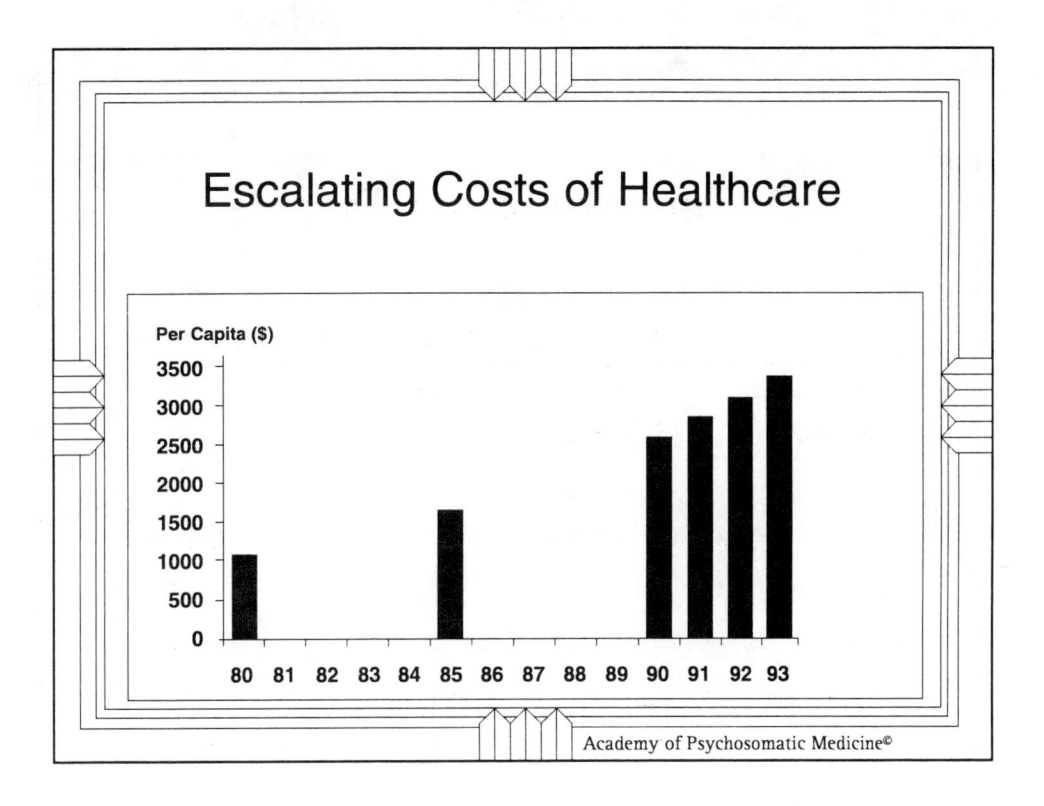

Academy of Psychosomatic Medicine©

SLIDE 6 Escalating Costs of Healthcare

As this chart indicates, national healthcare costs over the past 15 years have consumed an ever increasing portion of the resources of the United States. Per capita annual healthcare costs were $1068 in 1980; by 1993 the figure was $3299 (US Department of Commerce 1994). The need to contain these costs while maintaining quality of care has led to the rapid adoption of the managed care concept in our healthcare system.

Managed care has undoubtedly slowed the escalation of overall healthcare costs. Direct costs for treating mental disorders have dropped from almost 15% of general healthcare expenses in some settings to about 4% in intensively managed healthcare systems. Additional significant savings could be made if the hidden costs of unrecognized or untreated mental disorders in the general healthcare system could be reduced. This presentation asserts that the integration of behavioral healthcare services into general medical care can decrease costs, while improving clinical outcomes at the same time.

Prevalence of Mental Disorders

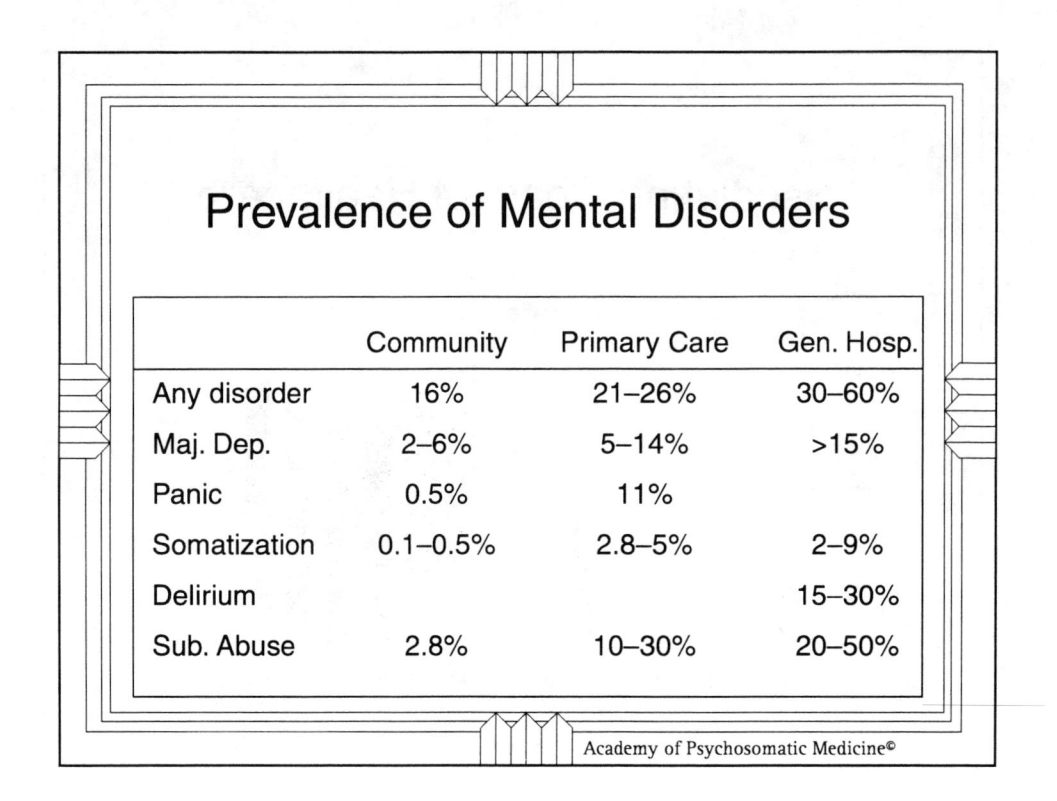

	Community	Primary Care	Gen. Hosp.
Any disorder	16%	21–26%	30–60%
Maj. Dep.	2–6%	5–14%	>15%
Panic	0.5%	11%	
Somatization	0.1–0.5%	2.8–5%	2–9%
Delirium			15–30%
Sub. Abuse	2.8%	10–30%	20–50%

Academy of Psychosomatic Medicine©

SLIDE 7 Prevalence of Mental Disorders

As this table shows, psychiatric disorders are common in the community and much more common in general medical outpatient and inpatient populations.

One-month and point prevalence studies demonstrate that 16% of community samples suffer from psychiatric disorders (Regier et al 1988, Regier et al 1993), while at least 21-26% of medical outpatients and 30-60% of medical inpatients meet criteria for significant mental disorders (Spitzer et al 1994, Ormel et al 1994, Cavenaugh et al 1983, Cohen-Cole et al 1993, Moore et al 1989).

[An additional 13% or more of medical outpatients also have subthreshold mental disorders, which are associated with significant morbidity and impairment in quality of life (Spitzer et al 1994, 1995).]

Looking at the most frequently seen disorders, major depression is 2-3 times more common in medical patients than in the community (Regier et al 1993, Rush et al 1993, Coyne et al 1994, Kessler et al 1987); panic and somatization disorders occur 10-20 times more frequently in medical patients (Smith 1994, Katon and Roy-Byrne 1989) and substance abuse disorders are 3-5 times more common (Regier 1993, US Department of HHS 1990, Moore et al 1989). While delirium occurs very infrequently in the community, it is present in 15-30% of medically ill hospitalized patients (Francis et al 1992).

Prevalence of Mental Disorders in Chronic Physical Illness

Condition	Prevalence (%)
All Conditions	24.7
Well	17.5
Neurologic Disorder	37.5
Heart Disease	34.6
Chronic Lung Disorder	30.9
Cancer	30.3
Arthritis	25.3
Diabetes	22.7
Hypertension	22.4

Academy of Psychosomatic Medicine©

SLIDE 8 Prevalence of Mental Disorders in Chronic Physical Illness

The prevalence of coexisting mental and chronic medical disorders was studied in a community sample of 2,554 persons (Wells et al 1988). The age- and sex-adjusted prevalence of any mental disorder in the preceding 6 months was 24.7% for those with a chronic medical condition and 17.5% for those with no medical condition.

[The prevalence of a lifetime mental disorder was 42.2% for those with a chronic medical condition and 33% for those without a chronic condition.]

Arthritis, cancer, lung disease, neurologic disorder, and heart disease were especially strongly associated with mental disorders.

[Persons with chronic medical conditions were more likely to have lifetime substance use disorders and recent affective and anxiety disorders.]

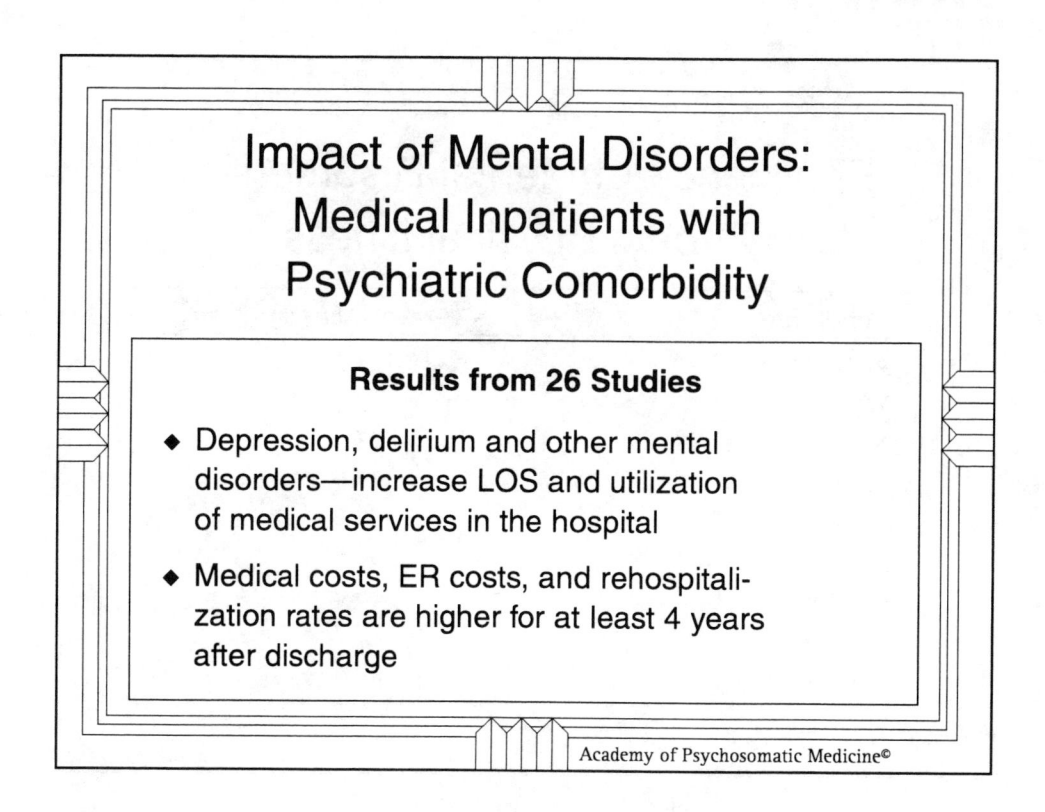

> **Impact of Mental Disorders:**
> **Medical Inpatients with**
> **Psychiatric Comorbidity**
>
> **Results from 26 Studies**
>
> ◆ Depression, delirium and other mental disorders—increase LOS and utilization of medical services in the hospital
>
> ◆ Medical costs, ER costs, and rehospitalization rates are higher for at least 4 years after discharge
>
> Academy of Psychosomatic Medicine©

SLIDE 9   Impact of Mental Disorders:
Utilization by Medical Inpatients with Psychiatric Comorbidity

Mental disorders in medical inpatients are associated with increased length of stay and increased costs. In a review of 26 international and American outcome studies, Saravay and Lavin (1994) found that 89% of all studies with sample sizes greater than 110 patients showed a significant association between psychiatric comorbidity and length of hospital stay. The authors also found that psychiatric comorbidity increased post-discharge costs, including emergency room visits and rehospitalizations, and that these costs persisted for at least four years after the initial discharge (Saravay and Lavin 1994; Saravay 1996).

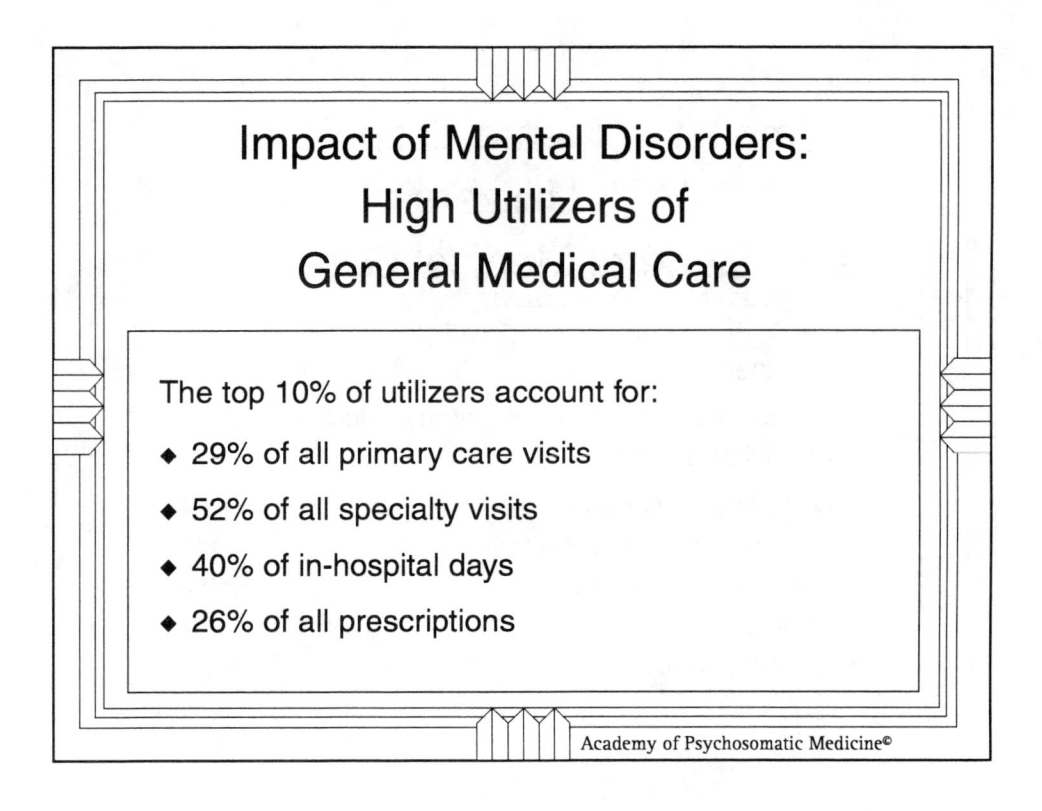

Impact of Mental Disorders: High Utilizers of General Medical Care

The top 10% of utilizers account for:

- 29% of all primary care visits
- 52% of all specialty visits
- 40% of in-hospital days
- 26% of all prescriptions

Academy of Psychosomatic Medicine©

SLIDE 10 Impact of Mental Disorders: High Utilizers of General Medical Care

The prevalence of psychiatric comorbidity is especially high among patients who use the most general medical care.

A study from the University of Washington in Seattle found that 767 patients identified as the top 10% of utilizers of healthcare in a large Northwestern HMO were responsible for 29% of all primary care visits; 52% of all specialty visits; 40% of in-hospital days; and 26% of all prescriptions (Katon et al, 1990).

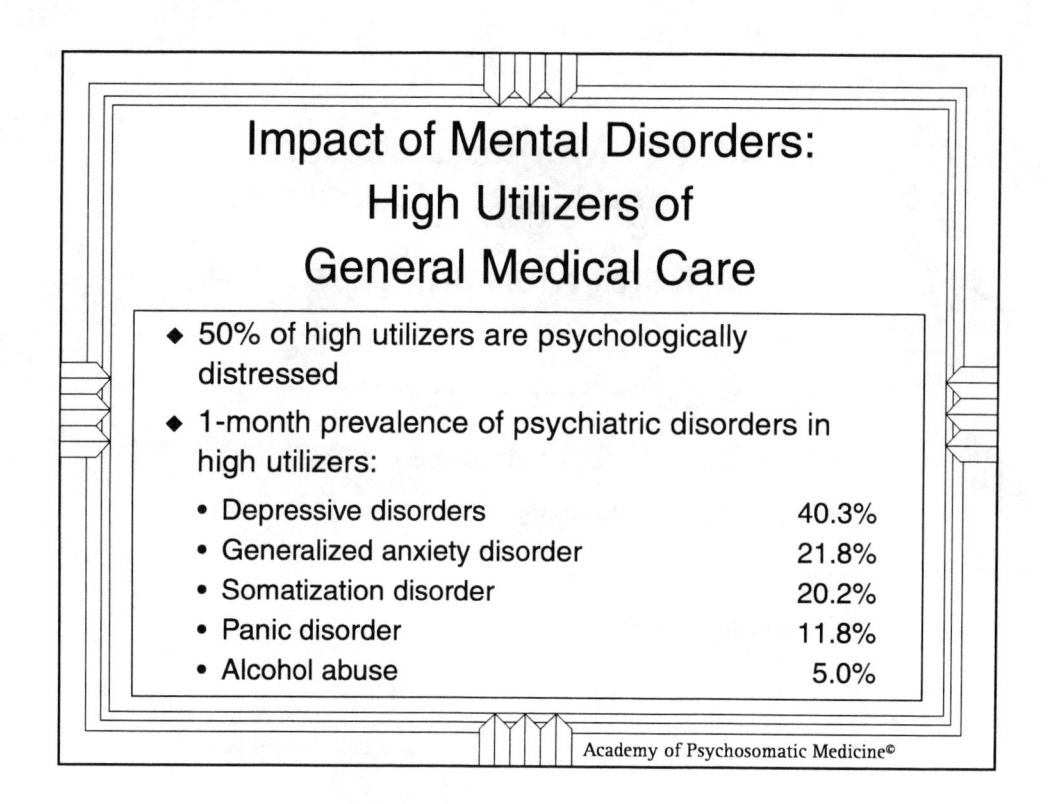

> **Impact of Mental Disorders: High Utilizers of General Medical Care**
>
> - 50% of high utilizers are psychologically distressed
> - 1-month prevalence of psychiatric disorders in high utilizers:
>
> | | |
> |---|---|
> | Depressive disorders | 40.3% |
> | Generalized anxiety disorder | 21.8% |
> | Somatization disorder | 20.2% |
> | Panic disorder | 11.8% |
> | Alcohol abuse | 5.0% |
>
> Academy of Psychosomatic Medicine©

SLIDE 11 Impact of Mental Disorders: High Utilizers of General Medical Care

Among those high utilizers of healthcare, 50% overall were psychologically distressed: 40% were found to have major depression or dysthymia; 21.8% were diagnosed with generalized anxiety disorder; 20.2% suffered with somatization disorder; 11.8% were identified as having panic disorder; and 5% were found to have an alcohol abuse/dependence disorder. These statistics reflected one-month prevalence rates (Katon et al 1990).

The next four slides review the general healthcare utilization patterns of patients with somatization disorder, depression, anxiety, and alcoholism.

> **Impact of Mental Disorders:**
> **Utilization in**
> **Somatization Disorder**
>
> - Use 9 times the healthcare services of the general population
>
> - Spend an average of 7 days/month in bed
>
> Academy of Psychosomatic Medicine©

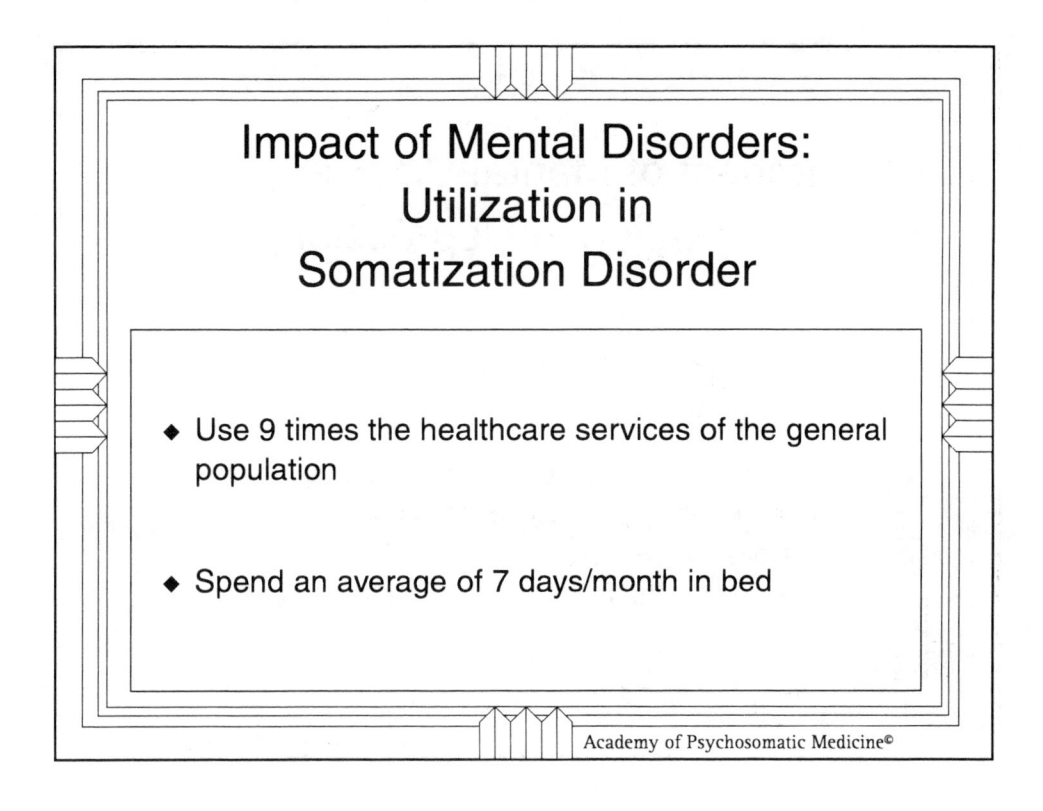

SLIDE 12 Impact of Mental Disorders: Utilization in Somatization Disorder

Among patients with mental disorders, those with somatization disorder can be especially difficult to diagnose accurately and are strikingly high users of healthcare services, much of which is unnecessary once the condition is recognized. In a review of the literature, Smith reported that patients with somatization disorder use nine times the healthcare services of the general population and spend an average of seven days a month in bed (Smith 1994).

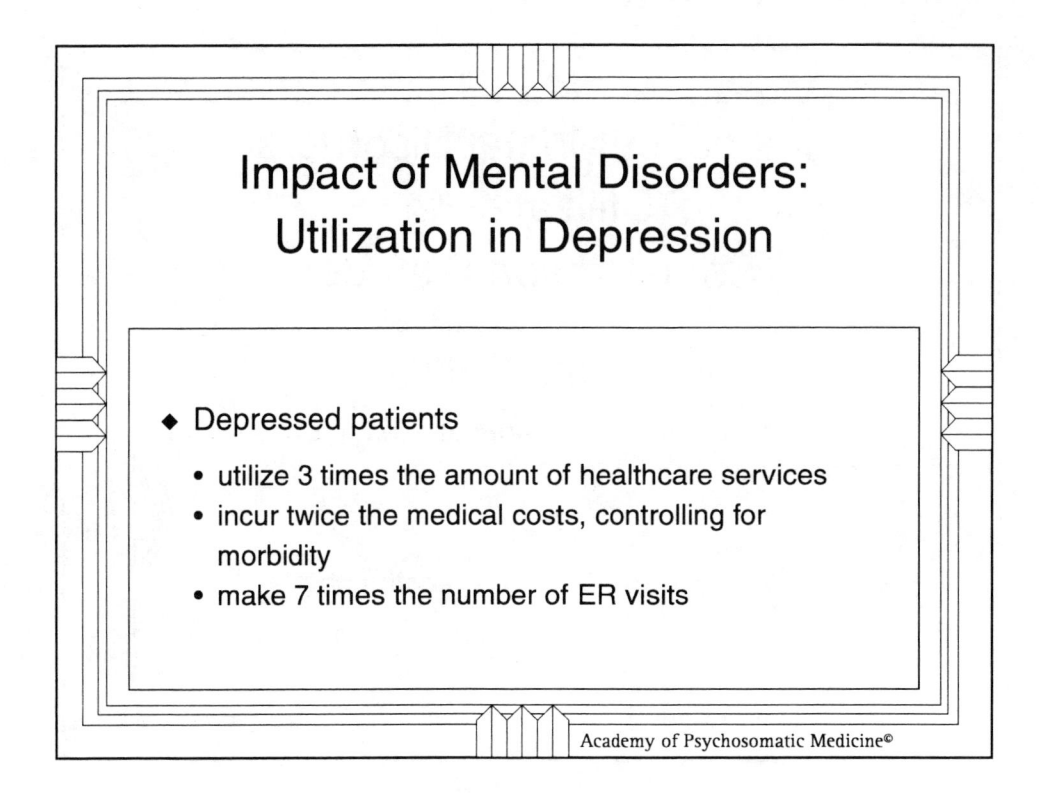

> **Impact of Mental Disorders:
> Utilization in Depression**
>
> ♦ Depressed patients
>   - utilize 3 times the amount of healthcare services
>   - incur twice the medical costs, controlling for morbidity
>   - make 7 times the number of ER visits
>
> Academy of Psychosomatic Medicine©

SLIDE 13 Impact of Mental Disorders: Utilization in Depression

Patients with depression often present to primary care physicians with somatic complaints, and tend to be high utilizers of services. Studies show that depressed patients use healthcare services three times more often than nondepressed patients (Katon and Schulberg 1992). Their medical costs, even after controlling for severity of general medical comorbidity, are twice as high as costs for nondepressed patients (Simon et al 1995a, Simon et al 1995b). They also make seven times more visits to the emergency room than nondepressed patients (Johnson et al 1992).

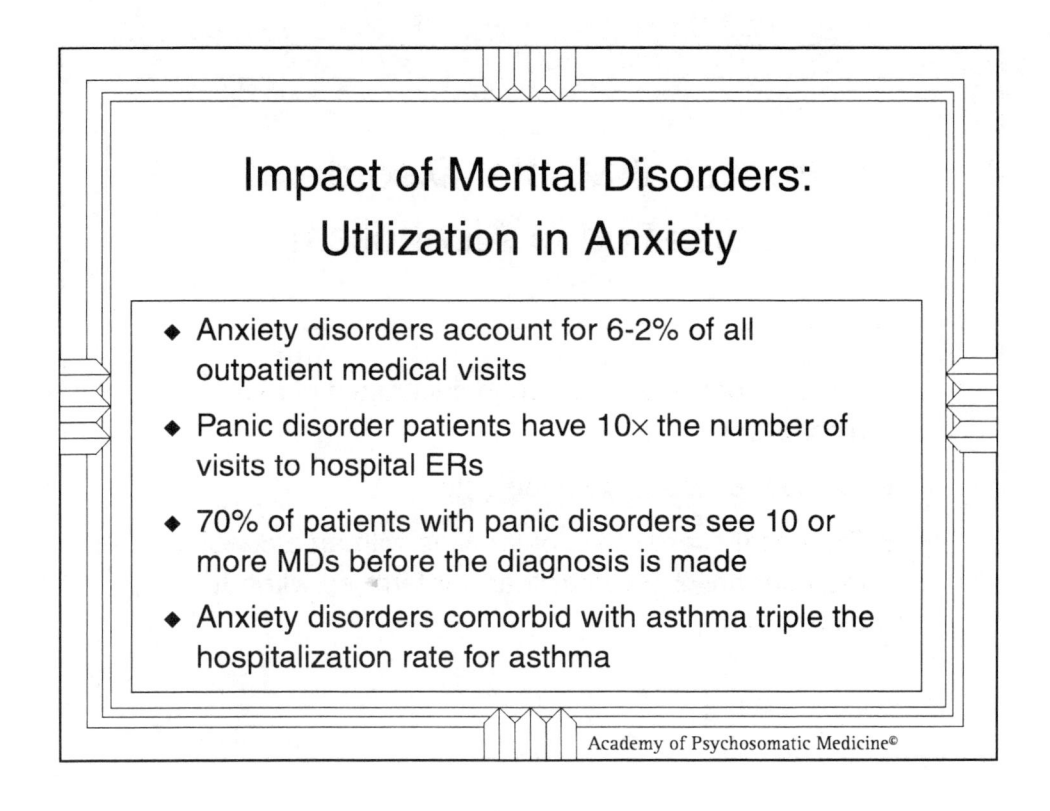

> **Impact of Mental Disorders:
> Utilization in Anxiety**
>
> - Anxiety disorders account for 6-2% of all outpatient medical visits
> - Panic disorder patients have 10× the number of visits to hospital ERs
> - 70% of patients with panic disorders see 10 or more MDs before the diagnosis is made
> - Anxiety disorders comorbid with asthma triple the hospitalization rate for asthma
>
> Academy of Psychosomatic Medicine©

SLIDE 14   Impact of Mental Disorders: Utilization in Asthma

Anxiety disorders also account for excessive utilization of healthcare resources.

In primary care practice, 6-12% of all patients suffer from anxiety disorders (Katon and Roy-Byrne 1989). Patients with panic disorder make ten times more visits to the emergency room than non-anxious patients. Seventy percent of patients with panic attacks will see ten or more physicians before the diagnosis is made (Ballenger 1987).

When anxiety attacks coexist with medical disorders such as asthma, the hospitalization rate can triple (Katon and Roy-Byrne 1989).

[The Epidemiologic Catchment Area study, which has studied the risks and rates of psychiatric disorders in a sampling of over 18,000 patients in five cities, found that panic disorder is associated with pervasive social and health consequences similar to or greater than those associated with major depression (Markowitz et al 1989).]

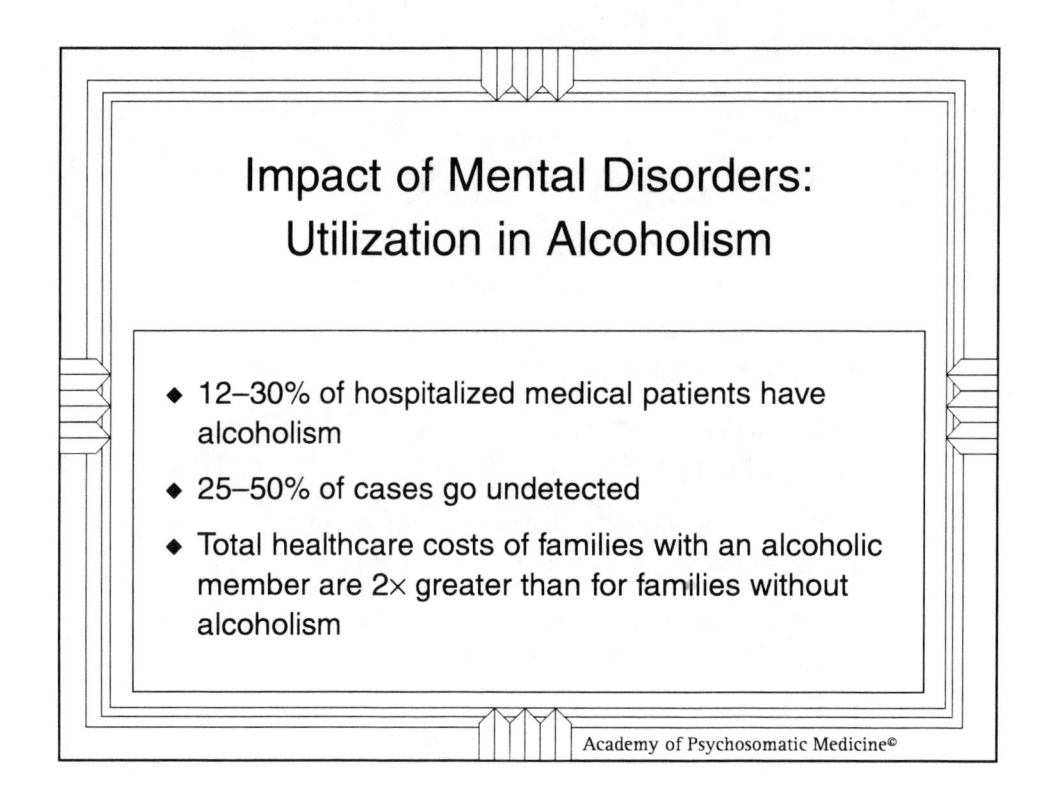

Impact of Mental Disorders: Utilization in Alcoholism

- 12–30% of hospitalized medical patients have alcoholism
- 25–50% of cases go undetected
- Total healthcare costs of families with an alcoholic member are 2× greater than for families without alcoholism

Academy of Psychosomatic Medicine©

SLIDE 15 Impact of Mental Disorders: Utilization in Alcoholism

Current estimates indicate that approximately 10 million adult Americans, or 7% of those 18 years of age or older, have an alcohol abuse or dependency disorder (US Department of HHS 1990). A study conducted at Johns Hopkins University found 12–30% of their hospitalized patients screened positive for alcoholism but one-fourth to one-half of cases were unrecognized. Physicians were less likely to identify alcoholic patients with higher incomes, higher educational levels, those with private insurance, women, and those who denied heavy alcohol intake (Moore et al 1989).

Another study, a four-year longitudinal analysis of insurance claims filed by federal employees, found that families with alcoholic members had twice the total healthcare costs as families without alcoholic members (Holder et al 1986).

The next five slides review the impact of mental disorders on the costs of healthcare, on functioning and disability, and on general medical morbidity and mortality.

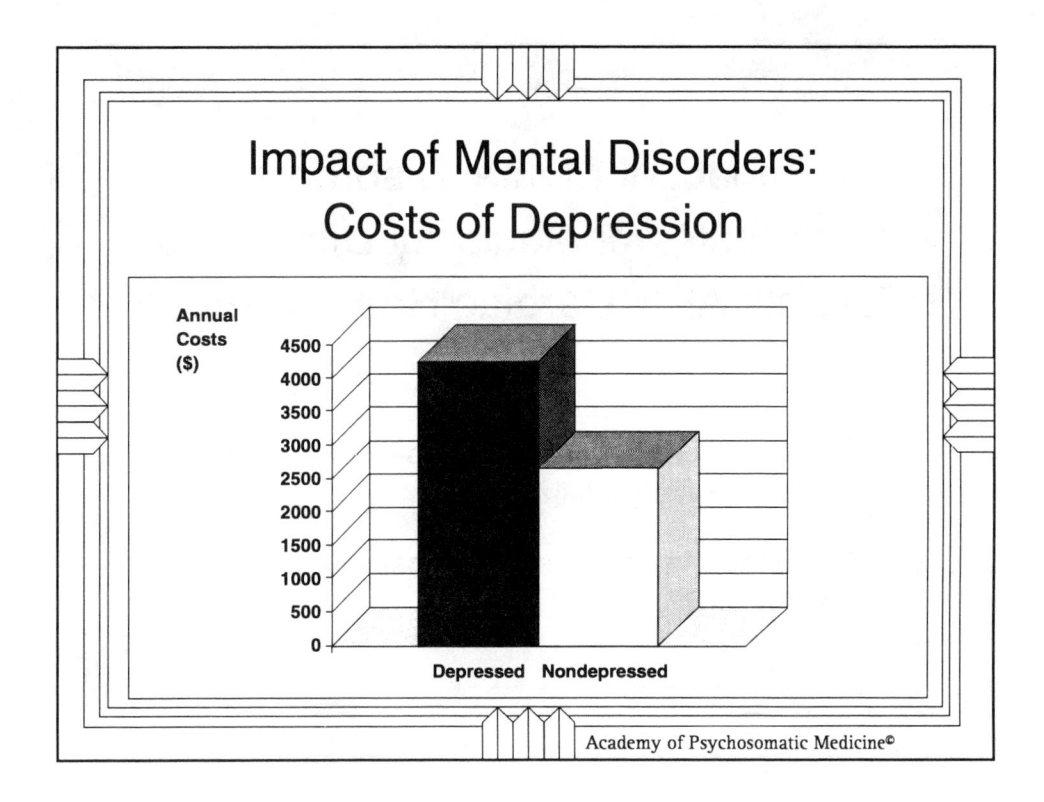

Impact of Mental Disorders: Costs of Depression

[Bar chart showing Annual Costs ($) for Depressed (~4250) vs Nondepressed (~2500) patients. Academy of Psychosomatic Medicine©]

SLIDE 16 Impact of Mental Disorders: Costs of Depression

High utilization rates associated with mental disorders have a direct effect on costs.

Using HMO accounting records, investigators at the Center for Health Studies in Seattle, Washington, compared the healthcare costs of some 6,000 primary care patients with recognized depression with the healthcare costs of an equal number of primary care patients without depression (Simon et al 1995b). Those with diagnosed depression had higher annual healthcare costs ($4,246) than did those without depression ($2,371). The pattern of increased costs held true across all categories including primary care visits, medical hospitalizations, labs, etc. This disparity existed before and after the initiation of treatment for depression. These findings suggest that recognition and primary care treatment alone without an integrated approach are inadequate to reduce utilization of medical services.

[In a similar study, overall healthcare costs associated with depression and anxiety were examined in 206 primary care patients of an HMO (Simon et al 1995a). Annual medical costs for patients with anxiety or depression was $2,390, compared to the annual medical costs of $1,397 for patients without anxiety or depression. Large cost differences were attributable to higher utilization of general medical services rather than to higher mental health costs.]

> **Impact of Mental Disorders: Costs in Psychologically Distressed Patients After Cardiac Hospitalization**
>
> - Significantly higher rates of subsequent cardiac events and rehospitalizations
> - Significantly higher costs of rehospitalizations ($9,504 vs $2,146)
>
> Academy of Psychosomatic Medicine©

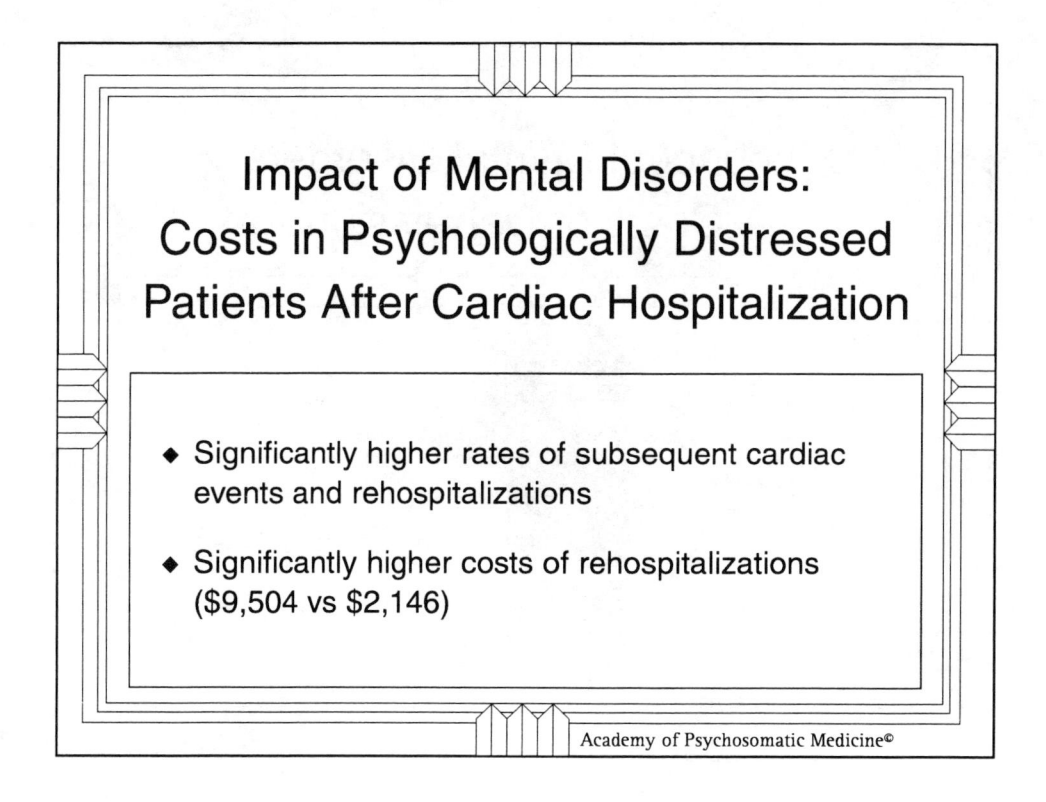

SLIDE 17   Impact of Mental Disorder: Costs in Psychologically Distressed Patients After Cardiac Hospitalization

The effect of psychologic distress on 6-month morbidity and rehospitalization costs was studied by Mayo Clinic researchers in 381 patients referred for cardiac rehabilitation after hospitalization for unstable angina, myocardial infarction, coronary angioplasty or coronary bypass procedure (Allison et al 1995). A Symptom Checklist-90-Revised score above the 90th percentile identified 41 patients as psychologically distressed. The researchers found that this subset of patients had significantly higher rates of cardiovascular rehospitalization and recurrent cardiac events than did the 340 nondistressed patients. Adjustment for other factors associated with risk of early rehospitalization and recurrent events did not reduce the strength or significance of the association between psychologic distress and rehospitalization and recurrent events.

Mean rehospitalization costs in the study were found to be $9,504 for distressed patients and $2,146 for nondistressed patients.

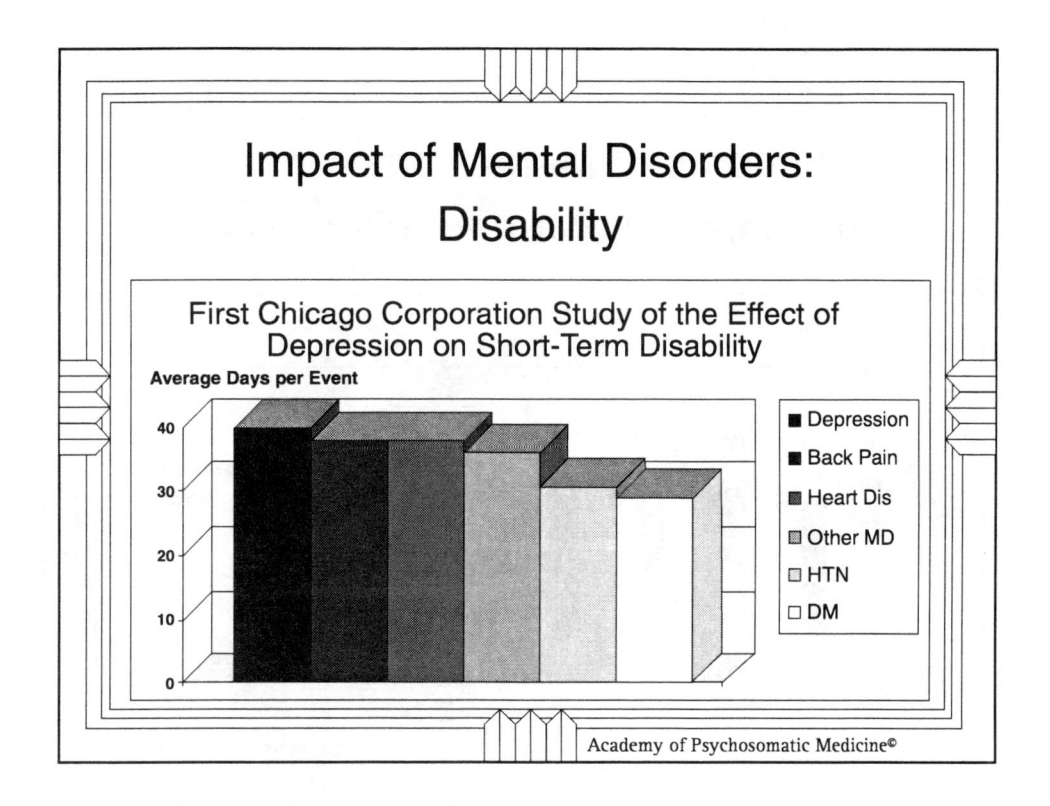

Impact of Mental Disorders: Disability

First Chicago Corporation Study of the Effect of Depression on Short-Term Disability

Average Days per Event

- Depression
- Back Pain
- Heart Dis
- Other MD
- HTN
- DM

Academy of Psychosomatic Medicine©

SLIDE 18 Impact of Mental Disorders: Disability

Mental disorders can be severely disabling, leading to costly losses in productivity.

In an attempt to quantify the direct costs to employers of employee depression, the First Chicago Corporation, a large Midwestern company employing 18,000 workers, undertook a review of treatment costs, absenteeism under the short-term disability program, and referrals to the Employee Assistance Program (Conti and Burton 1995). Employees with depression incurred more disability days and had a higher 2-month recidivism rate than did those with chronic physical disorders such as chronic back pain, heart disease, other mental disorders, hypertension and diabetes.

[In noting that mental disorders are commonly under-recognized or misdiagnosed, the authors concluded that the "current atmosphere of arbitrarily limiting behavioral healthcare benefits will encourage further misdiagnosis and inappropriate treatment with cost shifting to the medical-surgical ledger."]

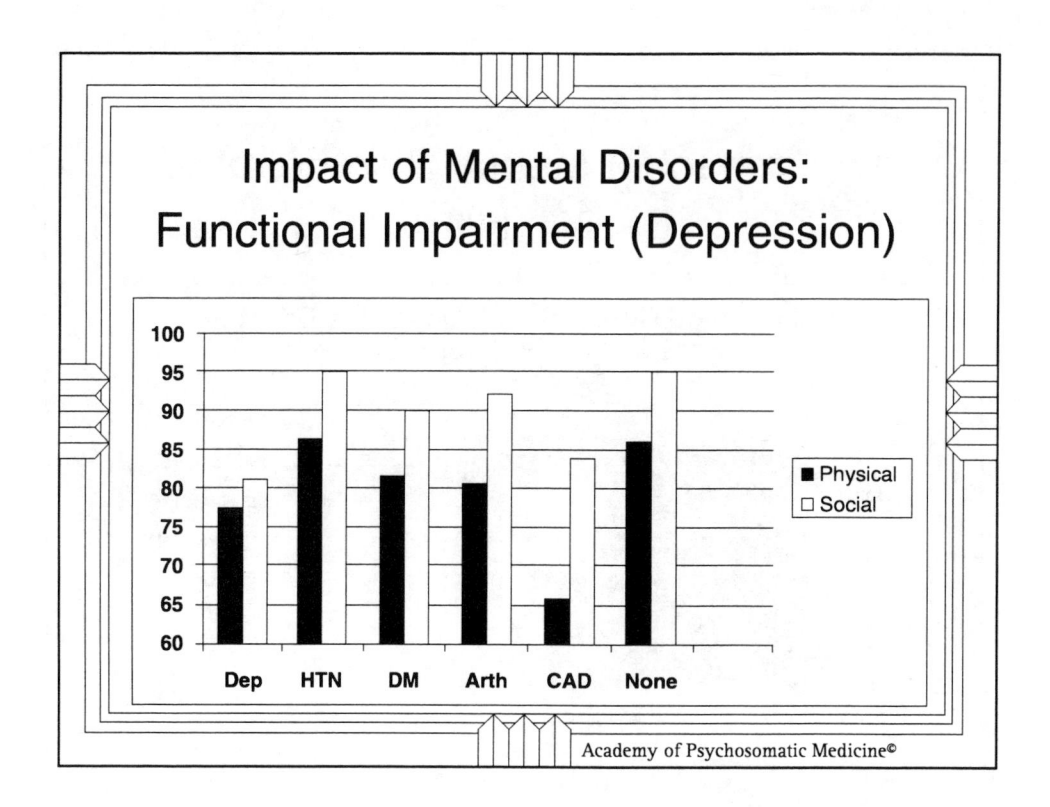

Impact of Mental Disorders: Functional Impairment (Depression)

[Bar graph showing physical and social functioning scores (Y-axis 60-100) for patients with Dep, HTN, DM, Arth, CAD, and None. Source: Academy of Psychosomatic Medicine©]

SLIDE 19   Impact of Mental Disorders: Functional Impairment

The impact of mental disorders on functioning is evident from the Medical Outcomes Study. As part of this study, the authors measured the physical, social and role functioning of patients with depressive symptoms and depressive disorders (Wells et al 1989). Data were obtained from 11,242 outpatients participating in three healthcare systems in three US cities. Higher scores on the Y-axis of the slide indicates better functioning. The bar graphs demonstrate selected findings concerning physical and social functioning of depressed patients (Dep) compared to patients with hypertension (HTN), diabetes (DM), arthritis (Arth), coronary artery disease (CAD), or no chronic conditions (None). Patients with depression were found to have worse physical, social, and role functioning, worse perceived current health, and greater bodily pain than did patients with no chronic conditions. Moreover, the functional impairment associated with depressive disorders was worse than seven other chronic conditions, including hypertension, diabetes and arthritis. Only patients with coronary artery disease had worse functioning.

[In a follow-up study, investigators found that functional impairment in depressed patients continued for at least two years and those limitations were similar to or worse than those attributed to chronic medical illnesses (Hays et al 1995).]

[Similar functional impairments were found to be true for patients with anxiety disorders or with somatoform disorders (Markowitz et al 1989; Spitzer et al 1995).]

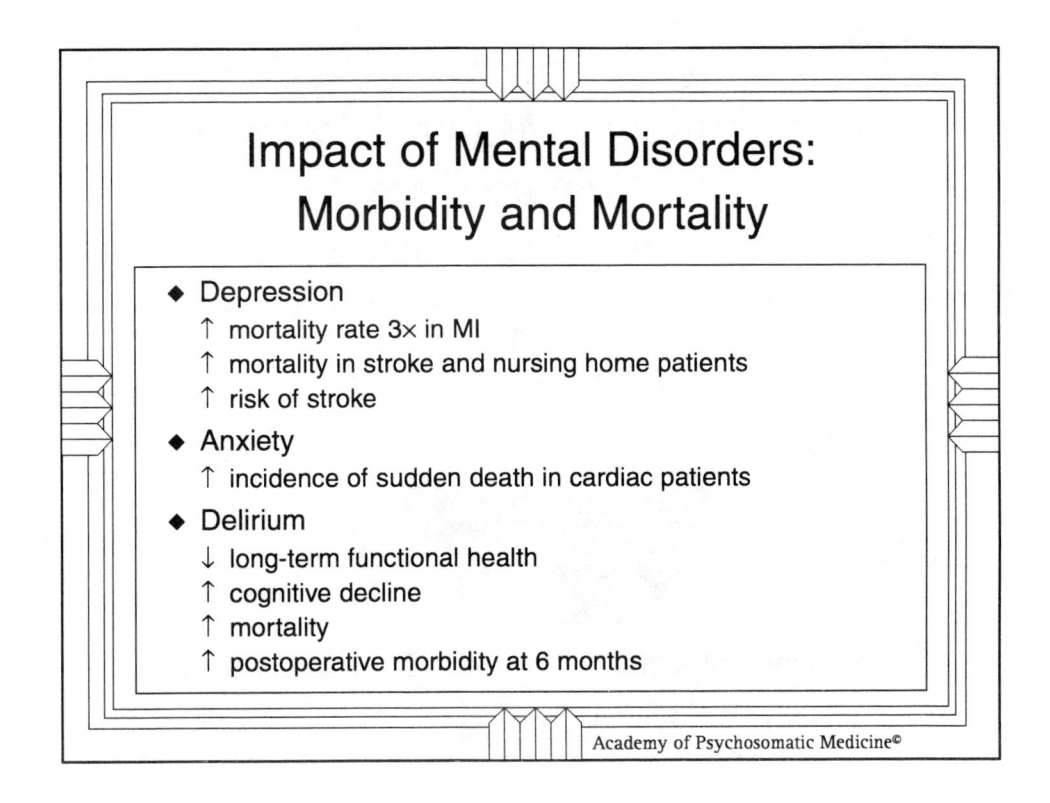

> **Impact of Mental Disorders:**
> **Morbidity and Mortality**
>
> - Depression
>   - ↑ mortality rate 3× in MI
>   - ↑ mortality in stroke and nursing home patients
>   - ↑ risk of stroke
> - Anxiety
>   - ↑ incidence of sudden death in cardiac patients
> - Delirium
>   - ↓ long-term functional health
>   - ↑ cognitive decline
>   - ↑ mortality
>   - ↑ postoperative morbidity at 6 months
>
> Academy of Psychosomatic Medicine©

SLIDE 20 Impact of Mental Disorders: Morbidity and Mortality

The Medical Outcomes Study also noted that depression and chronic medical conditions had unique and additive effects on clinical outcomes (Wells et al 1989). There are numerous other examples of the impact of mental disorders on medical morbidity and mortality. Frasure-Smith et al (1993), in a study of 222 post-MI patients, found major depression to be associated with a three-fold increase in 6-month mortality. Morris et al (1993) reported an increased 10-year mortality rate in socially isolated stroke patients (92%) compared to nondepressed stroke patients with strong social ties (38%). Rovner et al (1991) found that major depressive disorder in nursing home patients increased the one-year mortality by 60%. In a prospective study of 10,000 elderly hypertensives, Simonsick et al (1995) reported that subjects with depression had an incidence of stroke 2.7 times higher than non-depressed subjects. Kawachi et al (1994) report an association between anxiety and fatal coronary disease, especially with sudden death. Delirium in medical patients is associated with increased mortality, cognitive decline, poorer functional health (Frances et al 1992) and worse postoperative outcome (Rogers et al 1989).

The next three slides present data on the management of mental disorders in the general medical setting.

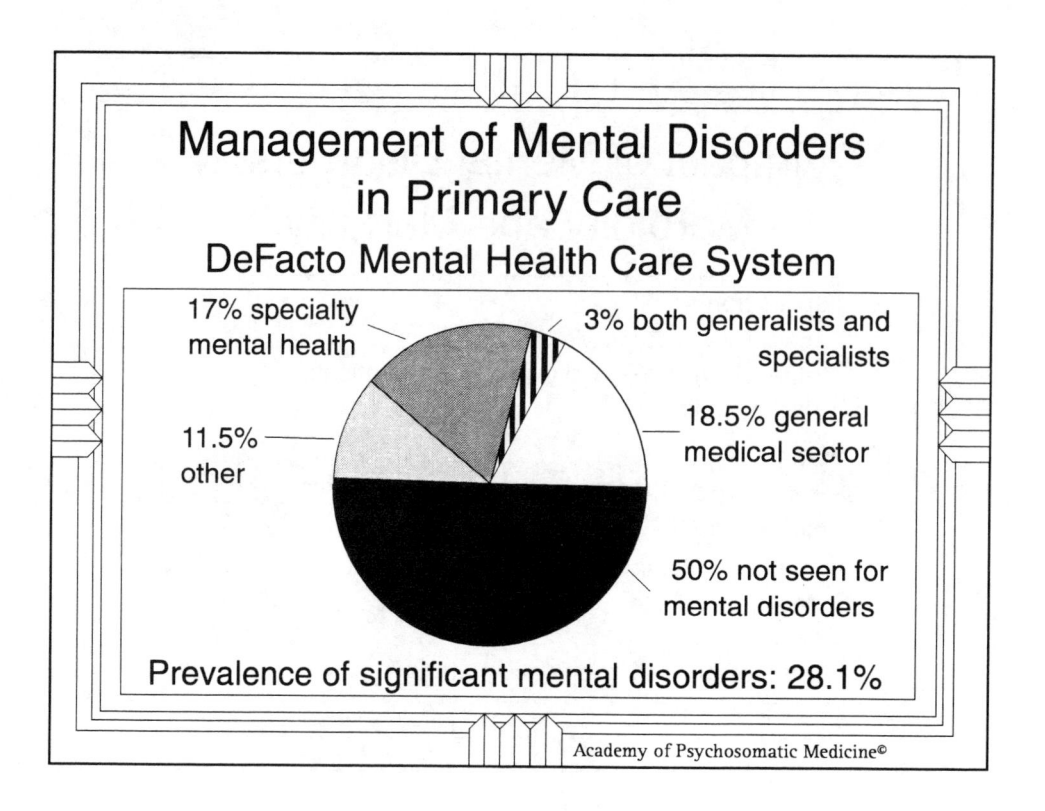

Management of Mental Disorders in Primary Care
DeFacto Mental Health Care System

- 17% specialty mental health
- 3% both generalists and specialists
- 18.5% general medical sector
- 11.5% other
- 50% not seen for mental disorders

Prevalence of significant mental disorders: 28.1%

Academy of Psychosomatic Medicine©

SLIDE 21 Management of Mental Disorders in Primary Care: The De Facto Mental Health Care System

Although 28% of the population have significant mental disorders, about half of these people never seek help (Regier et al 1993). Of those who do present for help, the majority are seen in the primary care sector (or the "de facto mental health system," Regier 1993). Approximately 18.5% of persons with mental or substance abuse disorders receive their only mental health care in the general medical sector, while 17% receive their only mental health care from mental health specialists (Miranda et al 1994; Narrow et al 1993, Regier et al 1993). About 11% of people with mental disorders receive their only mental health care in voluntary or other human service settings (religious, community, self-help programs, etc.). Considered from another perspective, among the group of individuals who do receive some type of help for their mental disorders, about 43.5% receive their only mental health care in the general medical sector and about 40% receive their care in the mental health sector (Narrow et al 1993).

Management of Mental Disorders in the General Medical Setting
Detection Rates

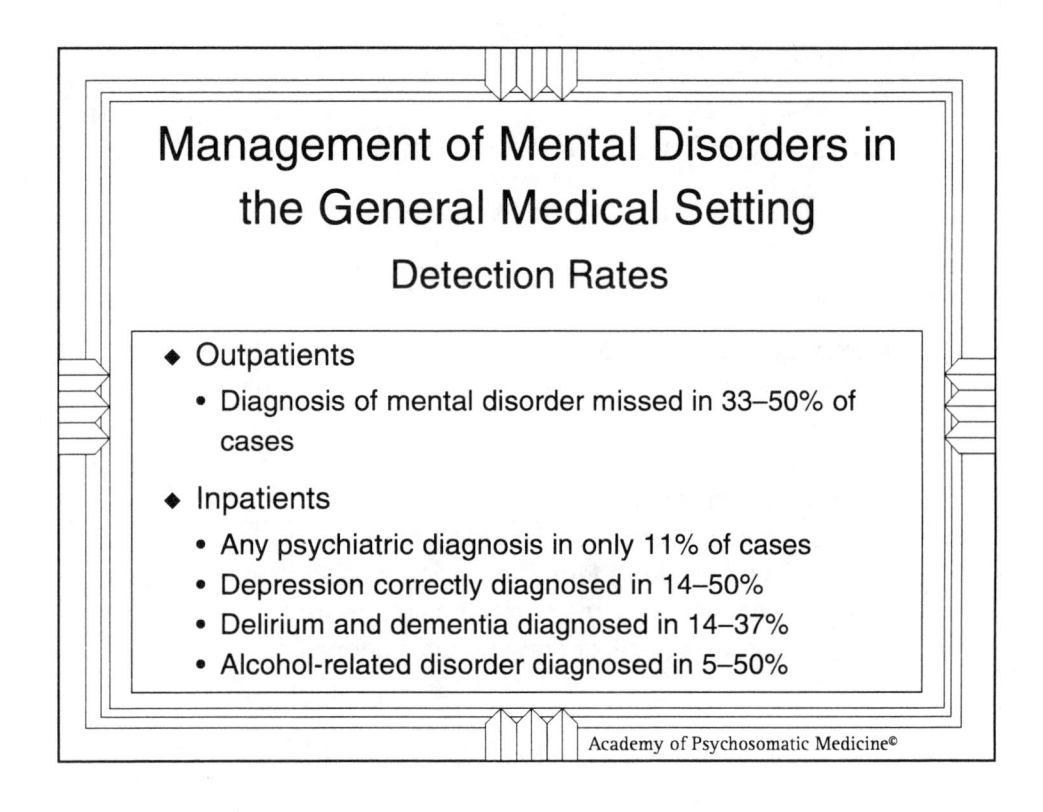

- ◆ Outpatients
  - Diagnosis of mental disorder missed in 33–50% of cases
- ◆ Inpatients
  - Any psychiatric diagnosis in only 11% of cases
  - Depression correctly diagnosed in 14–50%
  - Delirium and dementia diagnosed in 14–37%
  - Alcohol-related disorder diagnosed in 5–50%

Academy of Psychosomatic Medicine©

SLIDE 22   Management of Mental Disorders in Primary Care: Detection Rates

Despite the high prevalence of mental disorders in primary care, studies have established that the diagnoses of depression, anxiety and substance abuse/dependence are missed in between one-third to one-half of patients in this country (Rush et al 1993, Katon and Roy-Byrne 1989, Higgins 1994; Spitzer et al 1994, US Department of HHS 1990) and throughout the world (Sartorius et al 1993).

In hospitals, only 11% of patients with a mental disorder will have a formal diagnosis on discharge (Mayou et al 1988). Between 14% and 50% of patients with depression are correctly diagnosed (Moffic and Paykel 1975; Schubert et al 1992). Only 14–37% of patients with impairment due to delirium and dementia are diagnosed (Saravay et al 1991; Cavanaugh et al 1983; Francis et al 1990). Less than half (5–50%) of alcohol-related disorders are diagnosed (Moore et al 1989, Mayou et al 1991).

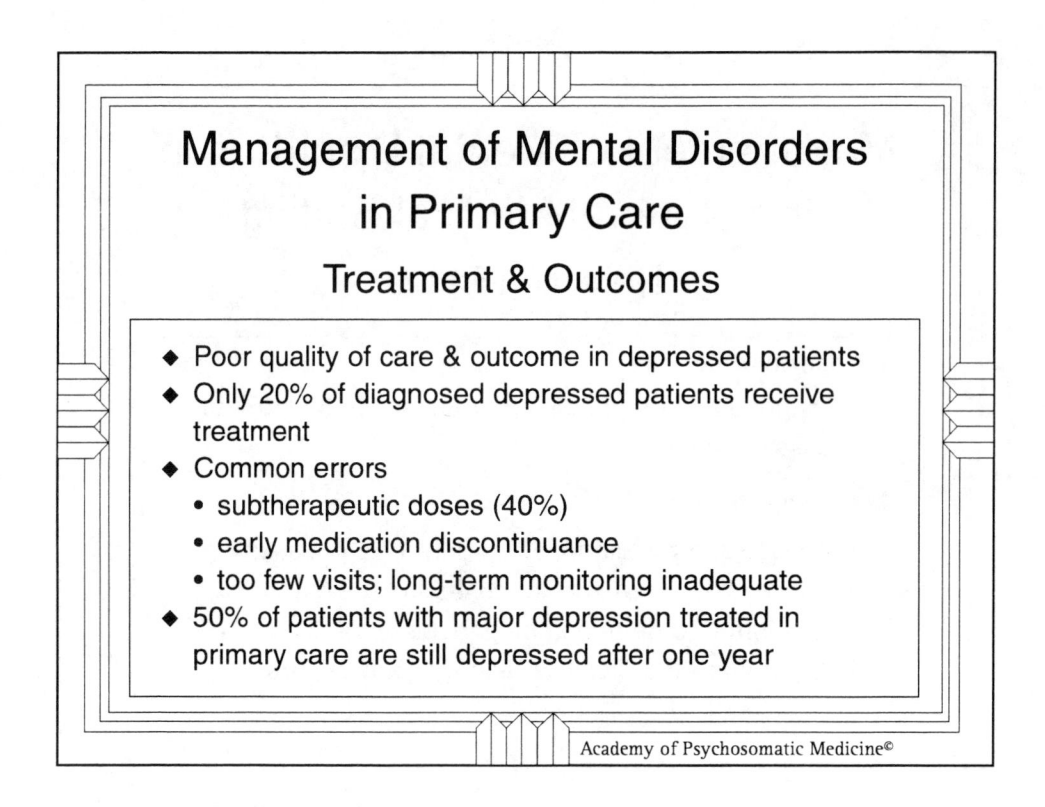

> **Management of Mental Disorders in Primary Care**
> **Treatment & Outcomes**
>
> - Poor quality of care & outcome in depressed patients
> - Only 20% of diagnosed depressed patients receive treatment
> - Common errors
>   - subtherapeutic doses (40%)
>   - early medication discontinuance
>   - too few visits; long-term monitoring inadequate
> - 50% of patients with major depression treated in primary care are still depressed after one year
>
> *Academy of Psychosomatic Medicine©*

SLIDE 23 Management of Mental Disorders in Primary Care: Treatment and Outcomes

In a review of three large health policy studies of the treatment of depression, Wells concluded that the quality of care given and the clinical outcome obtained in the general medical sector were inadequate (Wells 1994).

Antidepressants were prescribed only 20% of the time, and even then treatment was suboptimal. In 40% of the cases antidepressant dosages were subtherapeutic. Other common problems included inadequate medication instructions leading to early medication discontinuation by patients (50% in three months) (Lin et al 1995), too few visits (Wells 1994), and inadequate long-term monitoring (Simon et al 1993).

Perhaps as a consequence of these shortcomings, two prospective studies found that 50% of patients with major depression treated by primary care physicians in the "usual" manner of care were still depressed after one year (Schulberg et al, in press; Katon et al 1995).

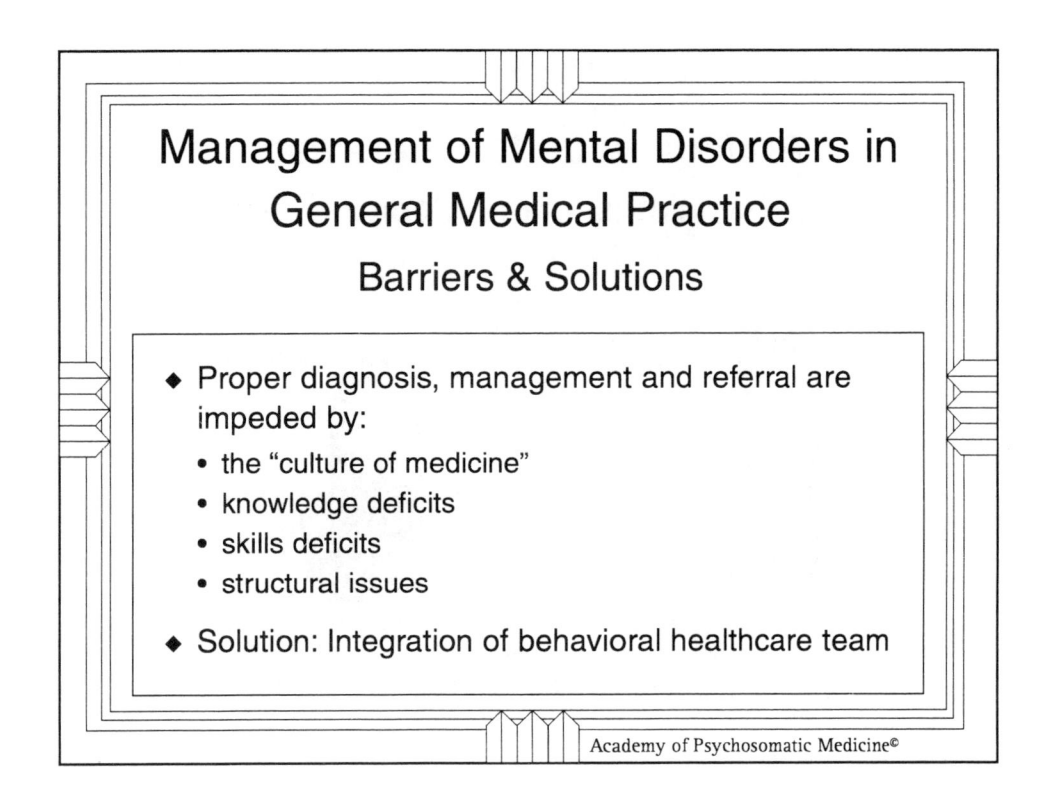

> **Management of Mental Disorders in General Medical Practice**
>
> **Barriers & Solutions**
>
> ◆ Proper diagnosis, management and referral are impeded by:
> - the "culture of medicine"
> - knowledge deficits
> - skills deficits
> - structural issues
>
> ◆ Solution: Integration of behavioral healthcare team
>
> Academy of Psychosomatic Medicine©

SLIDE 24 Management of Mental Disorders in Primary Care: Barriers and Solutions to Effective Care

Effective management of mental disorders within general medical practice may be impeded by several factors: (1) the "culture of medicine," in which the mind and body are viewed as separate entities; (2) limitations in physicians' knowledge and skills—that is, providers may have insufficient information or skill to manage mental disorders; and (3) structural issues, such as administrative hurdles, socio-economic obstacles, or "carve outs" that can act as disincentives to the recognition and treatment of mental disorders (Cole and Raju, in press).

Many of these barriers can be overcome, at least in part, by a combination of consultation and education provided by a behavioral healthcare team. This multidisciplinary team, composed of a psychiatrist, nurse, psychologist and social worker, should be integrated within general healthcare systems. The team should be coordinated by a psychiatrist with experience in treating mental disorders in the medically ill. The team together can provide care for patients; consult, support and educate general medical providers about mental disorders in the medically ill; and develop integrated programs and monitor outcomes.

The next four slides present data from intervention studies demonstrating the clinical and cost benefits of an integrated behavioral treatment approach.

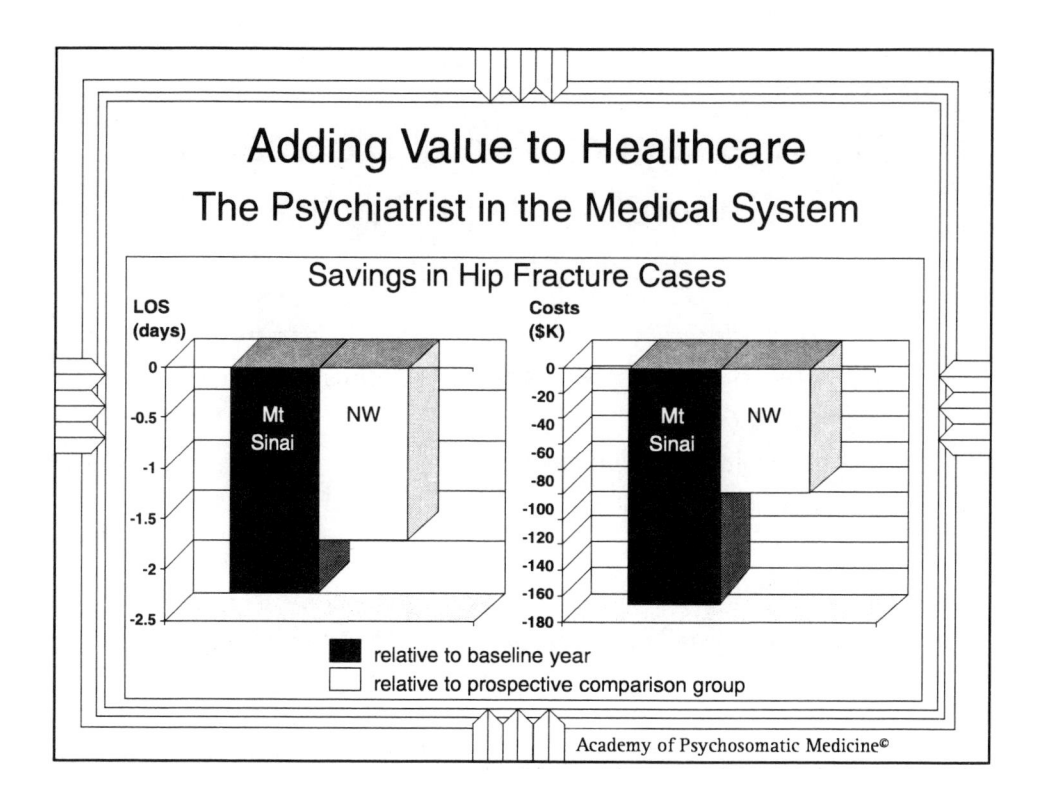

Adding Value to Healthcare
The Psychiatrist in the Medical System

Savings in Hip Fracture Cases

■ relative to baseline year
□ relative to prospective comparison group

Academy of Psychosomatic Medicine©

SLIDE 25 Adding Value to Healthcare:
The Psychiatrist in the Medical System
Savings in Hip Fracture Management

The value of psychiatric consultation in medical patients was dramatically demonstrated in a two-site study of patients with hip fractures at Mt. Sinai Medical Center in New York and Northwestern Memorial Hospital in Chicago (Strain et al 1991). All hip-fracture patients in the experimental groups received psychiatric consultations. Results showed that intervention significantly reduced the mean length of stay (LOS): at Mt. Sinai it dropped from 20.7 days during a baseline year, to 18.5 days during the experimental year—for a savings of 2.2 hospital days (the mean LOS for other orthopedic surgery patients at Mt. Sinai did not decrease between the baseline and subsequent study year); at Northwestern, mean LOS was 13.8 days in the study group, versus 15.5 days in a prospective comparison group—a difference of 1.7 days. At a hospital day rate of $647, the experiment resulted in Mt. Sinai saving nearly $167,000, and Northwestern over $97,000.

These findings were similar to an earlier psychiatric consultation study of hip fracture patients at Columbia-Presbyterian Hospital in New York (Levitan and Kornfeld 1981).

Adding Value to Healthcare: The Psychiatrist in the Medical System

Savings in Management of Alcoholism

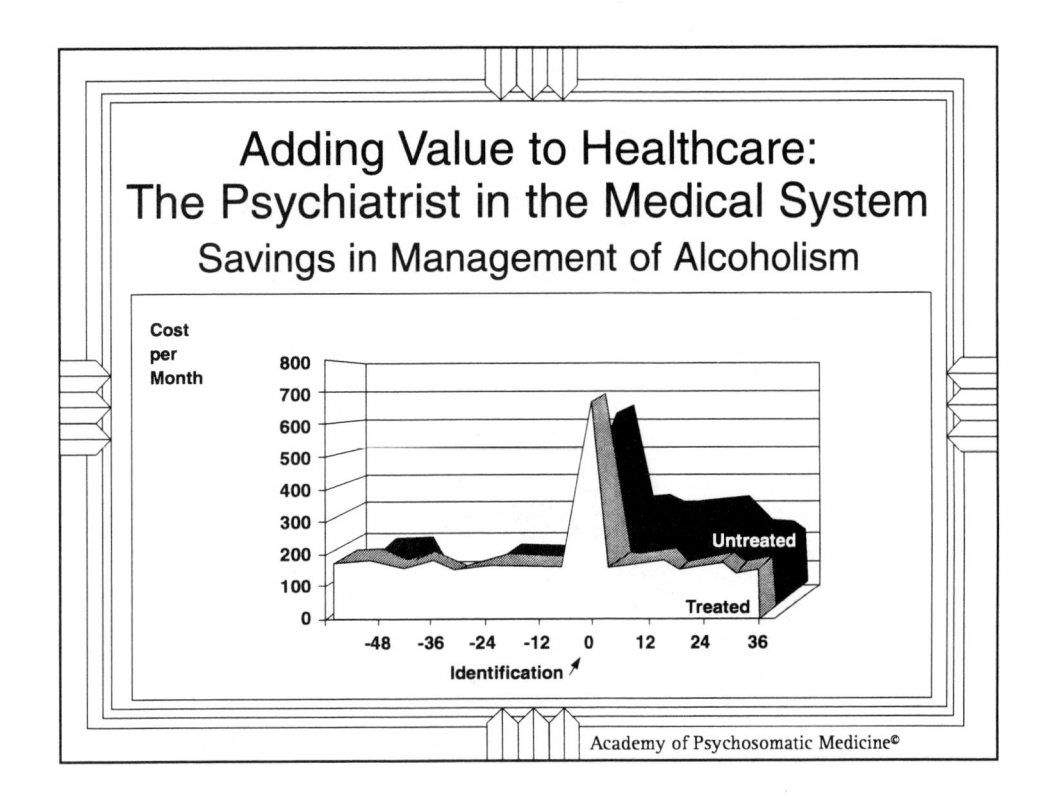

SLIDE 26 Adding Value to Healthcare:
The Psychiatrist in the Medical System

Savings in Alcoholism Management

Untreated alcoholism generates large healthcare costs, which can be offset by specialty treatment. Healthcare costs incurred by untreated patients are twice as high as those of people without alcohol problems. For those who do receive treatment, one-half the cost of this treatment is offset within one year by subsequent reductions in the use of general medical services, not only by the patient but also by the family of the patient. Two years after substance abuse treatment, one study documented a 40% reduction in the healthcare costs of participants (SAMHSA 1995).

Holder and Blose (1992) demonstrated savings in healthcare costs following alcoholism treatment. "In the longest longitudinal study of alcoholism treatment to date," this study reported total healthcare costs 4 years before and after treatment of 3068 alcoholics compared to 661 untreated alcoholics. After controlling for age, overall health status, and the costs of alcoholism treatment itself, the authors reported a 24% reduction in healthcare costs attributable to alcoholism treatment. For the treated patients, healthcare costs were lower than costs before treatment and also lower than costs of the untreated comparison group.

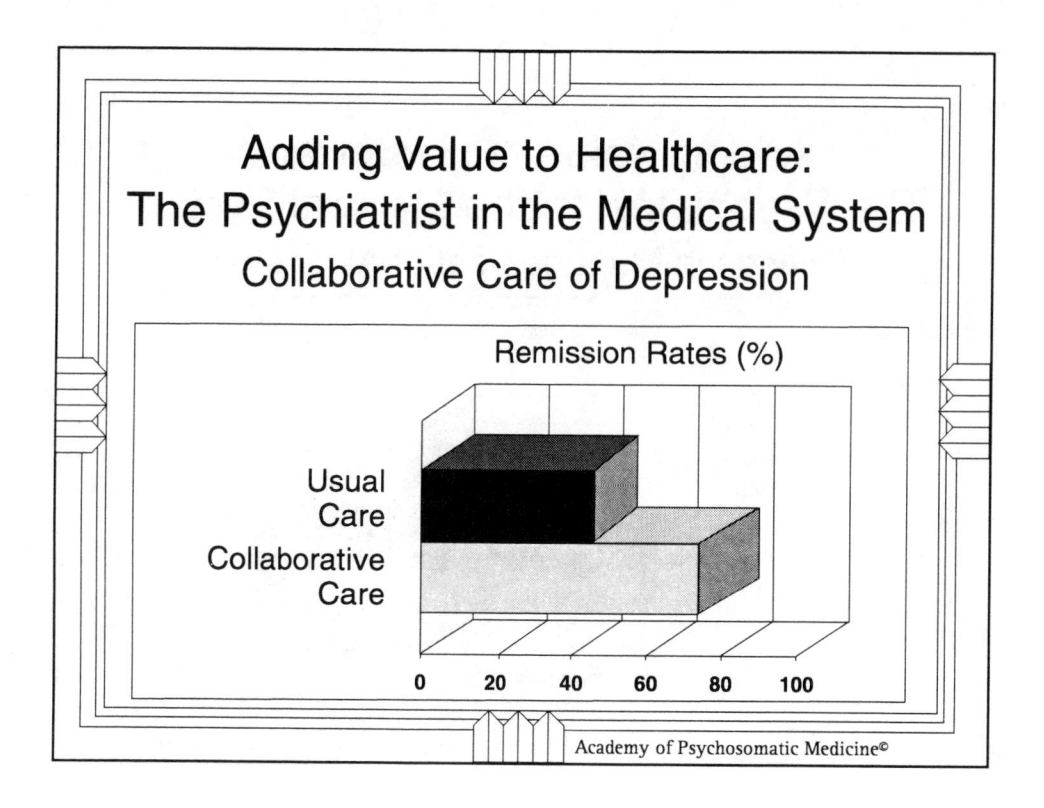

**Adding Value to Healthcare:
The Psychiatrist in the Medical System**
Collaborative Care of Depression

Remission Rates (%)

Usual Care
Collaborative Care

0 20 40 60 80 100

Academy of Psychosomatic Medicine©

SLIDE 27   Adding Value to Healthcare:
The Psychiatrist in the Medical System

Collaborative Care of Depression

Studies show that the suboptimal management of mental disorders in primary care can be improved when a psychiatrist is included in patient care.

In a one-year study, Katon and colleagues compared outcomes of the usual care of major depression with an integrated psychiatric intervention model. In this "collaborative" model, usual primary care treatment was supplemented by two visits with the consulting psychiatrist.

The investigators found that patients treated in the integrated model had significantly greater adherence to treatment and were more likely to rate the quality of care as good to excellent. In the intervention group, 74% of patients with major depression showed a 50% or more improvement in symptoms. In contrast, less than half the patients with major depression in the usual care group showed improvement (Katon et al 1995).

Based on their study's results, the authors suggested that the outcome of major depression in primary care settings can be improved by incorporating a collaborative role for a psychiatrist.

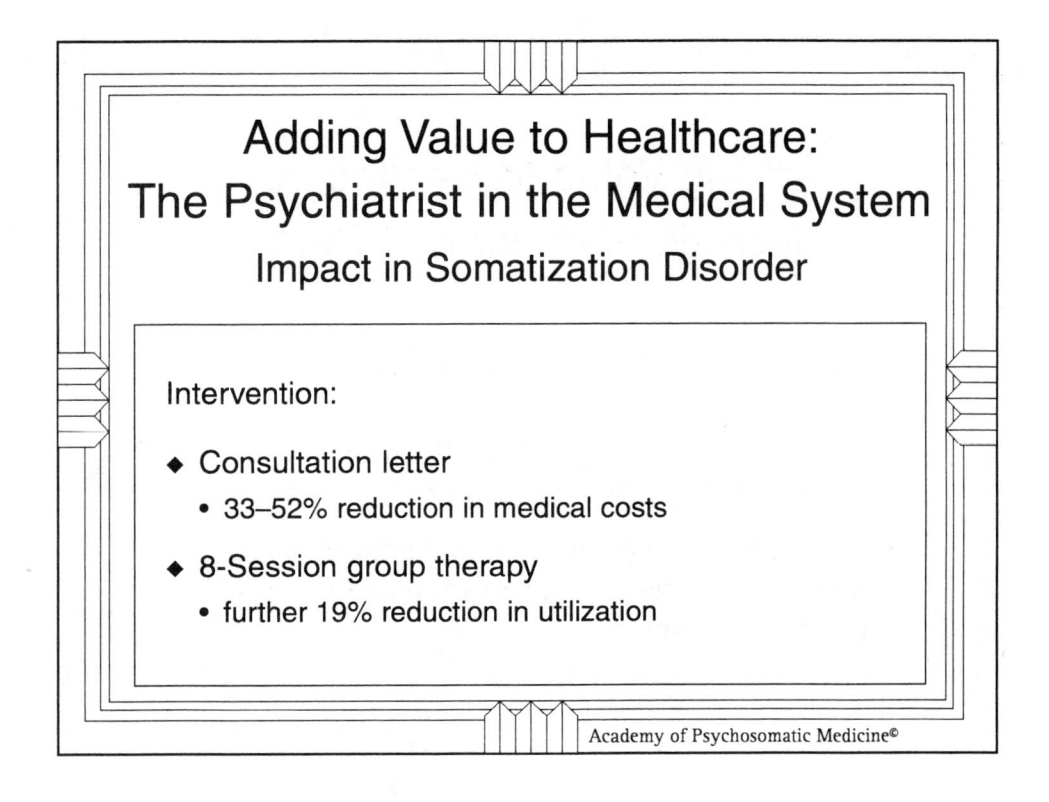

Adding Value to Healthcare: The Psychiatrist in the Medical System

Impact in Somatization Disorder

Intervention:

- ◆ Consultation letter
  - 33–52% reduction in medical costs
- ◆ 8-Session group therapy
  - further 19% reduction in utilization

Academy of Psychosomatic Medicine©

SLIDE 28 Adding Value to Healthcare: The Psychiatrist in the Medical System

Impact in Somatization Disorder

As mentioned earlier, the management of somatization disorder is particularly troublesome and costly in primary care, but it can be improved.

In a controlled, cross-over study, physicians treating half of 38 patients diagnosed as having somatization disorder were sent a psychiatric consultation letter providing explicit instructions on appropriate management. Physicians of the remaining patients received no advice about treatment. After nine months the control group was crossed over for intervention. Quarterly healthcare charges declined by 53% in the initial treatment group and by 49% in the control-crossover group (Smith et al 1986).

In a subsequent, enlarged replication study, the same University of Arkansas researchers were able to show that patients whose treatment included psychiatric consultation had improved physical and mental functioning and significantly greater physical capacity during the following year (Rost et al 1994). Overall costs decreased by 33% in this study (Smith et al 1995). Patients randomized to a 8-session group therapy program were able to achieve an additional 19% reduction in utilization (Kashner et al 1995).

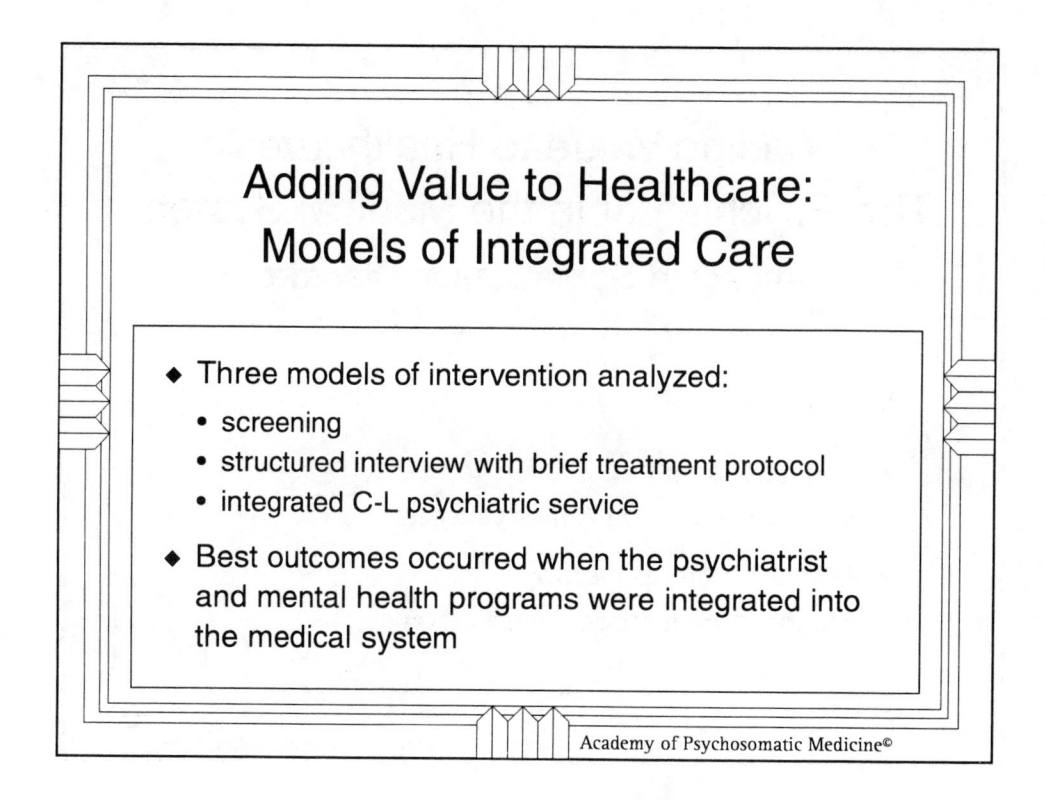

> **Adding Value to Healthcare: Models of Integrated Care**
>
> - Three models of intervention analyzed:
>   - screening
>   - structured interview with brief treatment protocol
>   - integrated C-L psychiatric service
> - Best outcomes occurred when the psychiatrist and mental health programs were integrated into the medical system
>
> Academy of Psychosomatic Medicine©

SLIDE 29 Adding Value to Healthcare: Models of Integrated Care

Katon and Gonzales (1994) reviewed the literature on the efficacy of psychiatric integration strategies for mental disorders in general medical settings. Prospective studies fell into three models: those that used only screening to identify patients with mental disorders; those that offered a brief treatment protocol after having identified patients by structured interview or screening; and those studies that used an integrated consultation-liaison psychiatric approach.

Katon and Gonzales found that consistently improved outcomes were seen only in the integrated model of care, such as we reviewed in the previous slides. Results were mixed and unimpressive in the other two models.

In interpreting these results, the authors suggested that the superior results seen with the integrated model might be due to the increased influence the psychiatrist has on both the provider and the patient.

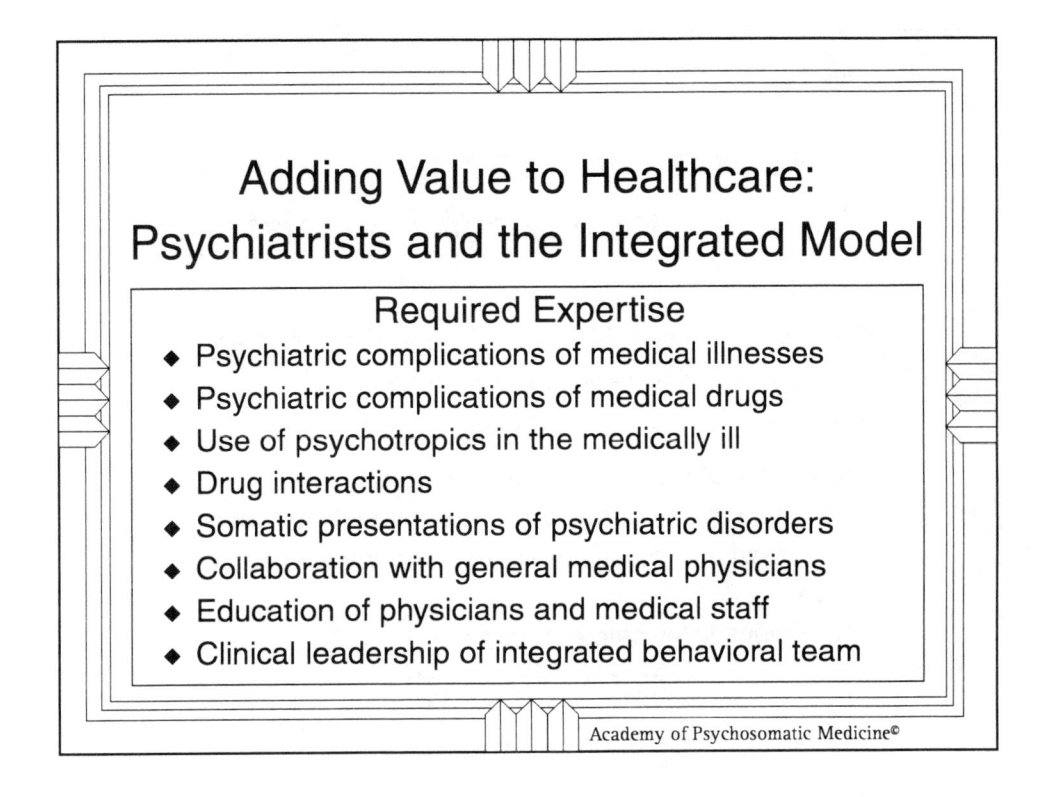

> # Adding Value to Healthcare:
> # Psychiatrists and the Integrated Model
>
> ## Required Expertise
> - Psychiatric complications of medical illnesses
> - Psychiatric complications of medical drugs
> - Use of psychotropics in the medically ill
> - Drug interactions
> - Somatic presentations of psychiatric disorders
> - Collaboration with general medical physicians
> - Education of physicians and medical staff
> - Clinical leadership of integrated behavioral team
>
> Academy of Psychosomatic Medicine©

SLIDE 30 Adding Value to Healthcare:
Mental Health Specialists and the Integrated Model

Required Expertise

Psychiatrists working in the integrated healthcare model will require highly developed skills to maximize the potential advantages of this management approach.

Clearly, they will need to be knowledgeable about the psychiatric complications of medical illnesses and of medical drug therapies. They must be experienced in the use of psychotropic agents to treat mental disorders in medically ill patients and they must be aware of potential drug interactions. They must be skilled in recognizing somatic presentations of psychiatric disorders.

Not least, psychiatrists in the integrated healthcare model must have the experience and skill for collaborating with and educating their general medical colleagues. Nurses, social workers, and psychologists should all be part of the multi-disciplinary behavioral intervention unit, all having some special skills to offer. Clinical leadership of the integrated behavioral team, however, needs to be provided by a psychiatric physician with the knowledge, skills, and experience to perform the complex tasks described above.

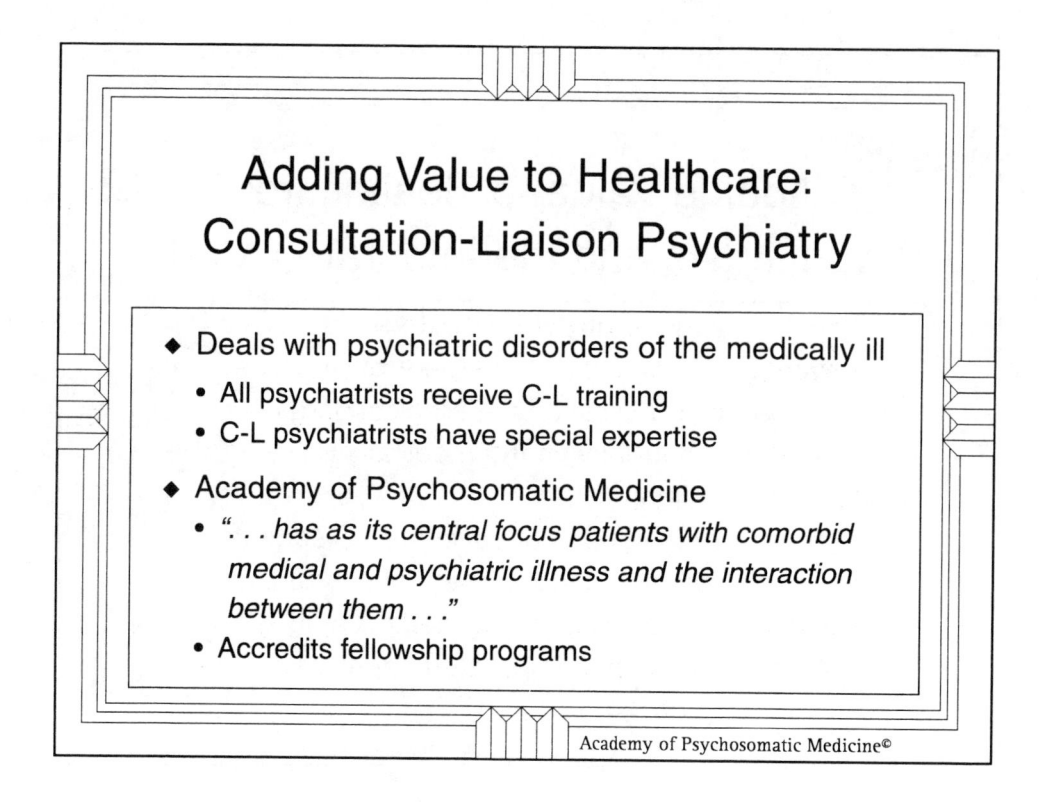

> **Adding Value to Healthcare: Consultation-Liaison Psychiatry**
>
> - Deals with psychiatric disorders of the medically ill
>   - All psychiatrists receive C-L training
>   - C-L psychiatrists have special expertise
> - Academy of Psychosomatic Medicine
>   - "... has as its central focus patients with comorbid medical and psychiatric illness and the interaction between them..."
>   - Accredits fellowship programs
>
> Academy of Psychosomatic Medicine©

SLIDE 31 Adding Value to Healthcare: Consultation-Liaison Psychiatry

Training in consultation-liaison psychiatry helps psychiatrists gain the knowledge and skill to provide the clinical interventions, education, and team leadership functions described previously. Consultation-liaison psychiatry is the subspecialty of psychiatry that deals with psychiatric disorders of the medically ill. "Consultation" refers to the process of evaluating and managing medical patients with psychiatric problems, while "liaison" refers to facilitating integrated care with a designated general medical provider or team.

All board-eligible psychiatrists who have been through accredited residencies receive several months of required training in consultation-liaison psychiatry. Consultation-liaison psychiatrists, however, devote the major proportion of their professional lives to the assessment and management of psychiatric problems in medical patients. For a program to receive accreditation for C-L specialty training, it must provide an additional year of training after general residency. C-L psychiatry has been approved by the American Psychiatric Association as a subspecialty warranting added qualifications of general psychiatry board certification.

The goals of C-L psychiatry are reflected in the mission statement of its national organization, the Academy of Psychosomatic Medicine: *"The Academy of Psychosomatic Medicine has as its central focus patients with comorbid medical and psychiatric illness and the interaction between them. The focus entails clinical work, research and teaching as well as leadership in the provision of consultation-liaison services."*

The Academy currently has reviewed and accredited 46 fellowship programs nationwide, and has established standards for psychiatry residency training in C-L psychiatry.

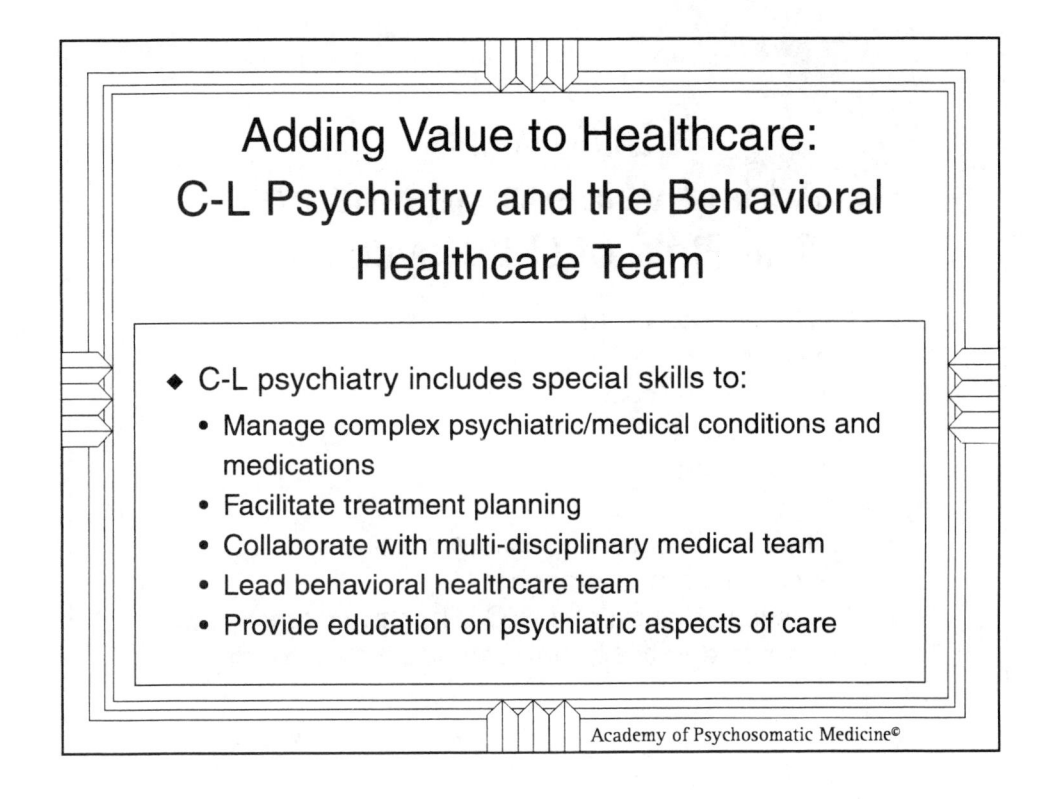

> **Adding Value to Healthcare: C-L Psychiatry and the Behavioral Healthcare Team**
>
> - C-L psychiatry includes special skills to:
>   - Manage complex psychiatric/medical conditions and medications
>   - Facilitate treatment planning
>   - Collaborate with multi-disciplinary medical team
>   - Lead behavioral healthcare team
>   - Provide education on psychiatric aspects of care
>
> Academy of Psychosomatic Medicine©

SLIDE 32   Adding Value to Healthcare: C-L Psychiatry and the Behavioral Healthcare Team

Psychiatrists with consultation-liaison experience and skill are uniquely equipped to manage the complex clinical problems that arise when mental disorders co-exist with medical conditions. These complexities include the detection of mental disturbances, the differential diagnosis of somatoform disorders and medical disorders producing psychiatric symptoms, the recognition of CNS drug effects as well as drug interactions between psychotropics and other medications.

Psychiatrists with consultation-liaison expertise are, therefore, well qualified to facilitate complex treatment planning and collaboration with a multi-disciplinary medical healthcare team for management of mental disorders in the medically ill; to provide clinical leadership of the behavioral healthcare team; and to offer education on the psychiatric aspects of medical care to general medical physicians and other providers.

> **SUMMARY**
> **Adding Value to Healthcare:**
> **The Role of C-L Psychiatry**
>
> - Psychiatric comorbidity
>   - common
>   - ↑ utilization and costs
> - Integrated model
>   - improves care
>   - ↓ costs
> - Optimal healthcare will include a behavioral healthcare team approach
> - The psychiatrist trained in C-L has the expertise to lead the integrated behavioral healthcare team
>
> *Academy of Psychosomatic Medicine©*

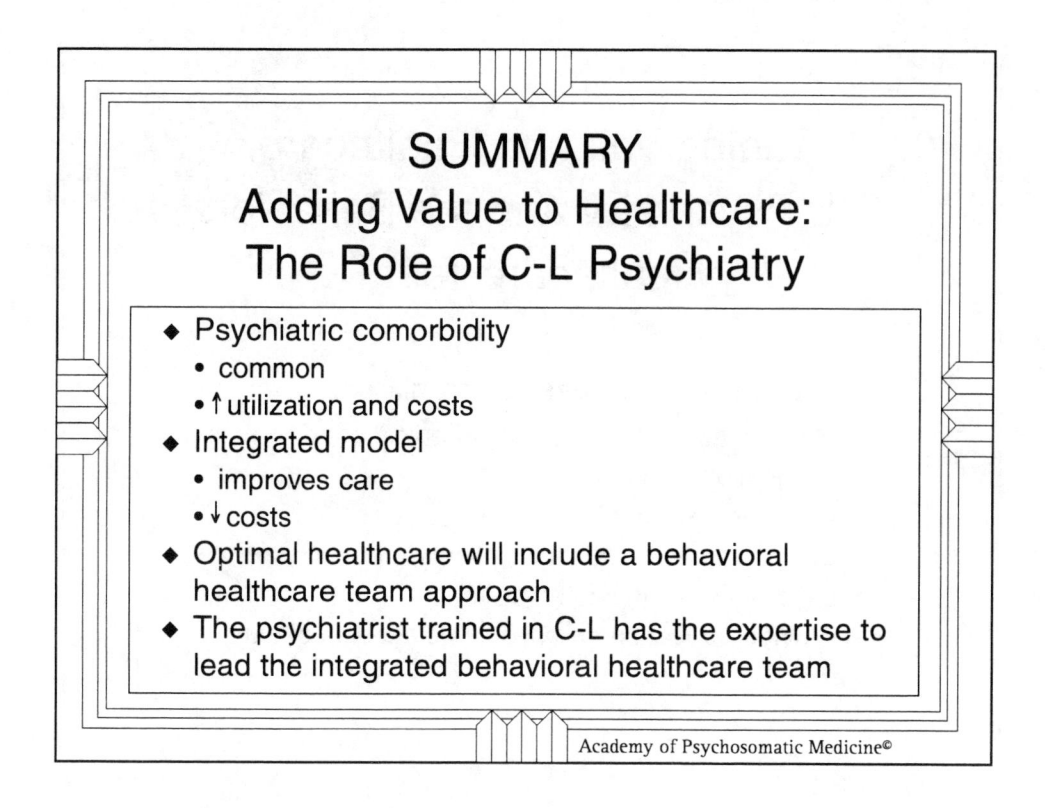

SLIDE 33   Summary: Adding Value to Healthcare
The Role of C-L Psychiatry

As this presentation has demonstrated, psychiatric comorbidity is common in general medical patients and leads to significant increases in healthcare utilization and costs. We have also seen that experimental models that integrate psychiatry and behavioral healthcare services within the general medical setting have led to better care and decreased costs. Given the improved outcomes with an integrated model, we believe that the optimal healthcare delivery system of the future necessarily will integrate a behavioral healthcare team into general medical practice. By training and experience, the psychiatrist with consultation-liaison expertise is uniquely qualified to provide clinical leadership of the integrated behavioral healthcare team.

References

Allison TG, Williams DE, Miller TD, et al: Medical and economic costs of psychologic distress in patients with coronary artery disease. *Mayo Clinic Proc* 70:734-742, 1995.

Ballenger JC: Unrecognized prevalence of panic disorder in primary care, internal medicine and cardiology. *American Journal of Cardiology* 60:39J-47J. 1987.

Borson S, McDonald GJ, Gayle T, et al: Improvement in mood, physical symptoms, and function with nortriptyline for depression in patients with chronic obstructive pulmonary disease. *Psychosomatics* 33(2):190-201, 1992.

Broadhead WE, Blazer DG, George LK, et al: Depression, disability days, and days lost from work in a prospective epidemiologic survey. *Journal of the American Medical Association* 264(19):2524-2528, 1990

Cavanaugh VS: The prevalence of emotional and cognitive dysfunction in a general medical population: using the MMSE, GHQ, and BDI. *General Hospital Psychiatry* 5:15-24, 1983.

Cohen-Cole SA, Kaufman K: Major depression in physical illness: Diagnosis, prevalence, and antidepressant treatment. (A ten year review: 1982-1992). *Depression* 1:181-204, 1993.

Cole S. Raju M, (in press): Overcoming barriers to integration of primary care and behavioral healthcare: focus on knowledge and skills. *Behavioral Healthcare Tomorrow.*

Conti DJ, Burton WN: The economic impact of depression in a workplace. *Journal of Occupational Medicine* 36:983-988, 1994

Coyne JC, Fechner-Bates S, Schwenk TL: Prevalence, nature, and comorbidity of depressive disorders in primary care. *General Hospital Psychiatry* 16:267-276, 1994.

Dalack GW, Roose SP: Perspectives on the relationship between cardiovascular disease and affective disorder. *Journal of Clinical Psychiatry* 51(7)Suppl.:4-7, 1990.

Francis J, Kapoor WN: Prognosis after hospital discharge of older medical patients with delirium. *Journal of the American Geriatric Society* 40:601-606, 1992.

Francis J, Martin D, Kapoor WN: A prospective study of delirium in hospitalized elderly. *Journal of the American Medical Association* 263(8):1097-1101, 1990.

Frasure-Smith N, Lesperance F, Talajic M: Depression following myocardial infarction: Impact on 6-months survival. *Journal of the American Medical Association* 270(15):1819-1825, 1993.

Fuller MG: More is less: Increasing access as a strategy for managing health care costs. *Psychiatric Services* 46:1015-1017, 1995.

Fuller MG, Jordan ML: The substance abuse consultation team: addressing the problem of hospitalized substance abusers. *General Hospital Psychiatry* 16:73-77, 1994.

Greenberg P, Stiglin LE, Finkelstein SN, et al: The economic burden of depression in 1990. *Journal of Clinical Psychiatry* 54:405-418, 1993.

Greenberg PE, Stiglin LR, Finklestein SN, et al: Depression: a neglected major illness. *Journal of Clinical Psychiatry* 54:419-424, 1993.

Hall CW, Wise MG: The clinical and financial burden of mood disorder: cost and outcome. *Psychosomatics* 36:S11-S18, 1995.

Hays RD, Wells KB, Sherbourne CD, et al: Functioning and well-being outcomes of patients with depression compared with chronic general medical illness. *Archives of General Psychiatry* 52:11-19, 1995.

Higgins ES: A review of unrecognized mental illness in primary care: prevalence, natural history, and efforts to change the course. *Archives of Family Medicine* 3:908-917, 1994.

Holder HD, Blose JO: Alcoholism treatment and total health care utilization and costs: a four-year longitudinal analysis of federal employees. *Journal of the American Medical Association* 256:1456-1460, 1986.

Holder HD, Blose JO: The reduction of healthcare costs associated with alcoholism treatment: a 14-year longitudinal study. *Journal of Studies on Alcoholism* 53:293-302, 1992.

Howland RH: General health, health care utilization and medical comorbidity in dysthymia. *International Journal of Psychiatry in Medicine* 23:211-238, 1993.

Johnson J, Weissman M, Klerman GL: Service utilization and social morbidity associated with depressive symptoms in the community. *Journal of the American Medical Association* 267:1478-1483, 1992.

Kashner TM, Rost K, Cohen B, et al: Enhancing the health of somatization disorder patients: effectiveness of short-term group therapy. *Psychosomatics* 36:462-470, 1995.

Katon W, VonKorff M, Lin E, et al: Collaborative management to achieve treatment guidelines: Impact on depression in primary care. *Journal of the American Medical Association* 273(13):1026-1031, 1995.

Katon W, Gonzales J: A review of randomized trials of psychiatric consulation-liaison studies in primary care. *Psychosomatics* 35:268-278, 1994.

Katon W, Roy-Byrne PP: Panic disorder in the medically ill. *Journal of Clinical Psychiatry* 50(8):299-302, 1989.

Katon W, Schulberg H: Epidemiology of depression in primary care. *General Hospital Psychiatry* 14:237-247, 1992.

Katon w, VonKorff M, Lin E, et al: Distressed high utilizers of medical care: DSM-III-R diagnoses and treatment needs. *General Hospital Psychiatry* 12:355-362, 1990.

Kawachi I, Sparrow D, Vokonas PS, et al: Symptoms of anxiety and risk of coronary disease: the normative aging study. *Circulation* 90:2225-2229, 1994.

Kessler LG, Burns BJ, Shapiro S, et al: Psychiatric diagnoses of medical service users: evidence from the Epidemiologic Catchment Area Program. *American Journal of Public Health* 77(1):18-24, 1987.

Levenson JL: Experimental study of psychiatric consultation for unrecognized psychopathology in general medical inpatients. *Psychiatric Medicine* 9:593-607, 1991.

Levenson JL: Psychosocial intervention in chronic medical illness: an overview of outcome research. *General Hospital Psychiatry* 14:43s-49s, 1992.

Levitan SJ, Kornfeld DS: Clinical and cost benefits of liaison psychiatry. *American Journal of Psychiatry* 138:790-793, 1981.

Lin E, VonKorff M, Katon w, et al: Primary care physician behavior and patient's adherence to antidepressant therapy. *Medical Care* 33:67-74, 1995.

Manderscheid RW, Ray DS, Narrow WE, et al: Congruence of service utilization estimates from the Epidemiologic Catchment Area Project and other sources. *Archives of General Psychiatry* 50:108-114, 1993.

Markowitz JS, Weissman MM, Ouellette R, et al: Quality of life in panic disorder. *Archives of General Psychiatry* 46:984-992, 1989.

Mayou R, Hawton K, Feldman E: What happens to medical patients with psychiatric disorders. *Journal of Psychosomatic Research* 32:541-549, 1988.

Mayou R, Hawton K, Feldman E, et al: Psychiatric problems among medical admissions. *International Journal of Psychiatry in Medicine* 21(1):71-84, 1991.

Miranda J, Munoz R: Intervention for minor depression in primary care patients. *Psychosomatic Medicine* 56:136-142, 1994.

Moffic HS, Paykel ES: Depression in medical inpatients. *British Journal of Psychiatry* 126:346-353, 1975.

Moore RD, Bone LR, Geller G, et al: Prevalence, detection and treatment of alcoholism in hospitalized patients. *Journal of the American Medical Association* 261(3):403-407, 1989.

Morris PLP, Robinson RG, Andrzejewski P, et al: Association of depression with 10-year poststroke mortality. *American Journal of Psychiatry* 150:124-129, 1993.

Mumford E, Schlesinger HJ, Glass GV, et al: A new look at evidence about reduced cost of medical utilization following mental health treatment. *The American Journal of Psychiatry* 141(10):1145-1158, 1984.

Narrow WE, Reiger DA, Rae DS, et al. Use of services by persons with mental and addictive disorders: findings from the National Institute of Mental Health Epidemiological Catchment Area program. *Archives of General Psychiatry* 50:95-107, 1993.

Ormel J, VonKorff M, Ustun TB, et al: Common mental disorders and disability across cultures: Results from the WHO collaborative study on psychological problems in general health care. *Journal of the American Medical Association* 272:1741-1748, 1994.

Pallack MS, Cummings NA, Dorken H, et al: Effect of mental health treatment on medical costs. *Foundation for Behavioral Health* 7-16, 1995.

Regier DA, Boyd JH, Burke JD, et al: One-month prevalence of mental disorders in the United States: based on five Epidemiologic Catchment Area sites. *Archives of General Psychiatry* 45:977-986, 1988.

Regier DA, Narrow WE, Rae DS, et al: The de facto US mental and addictive disorders service system: Epidemiologic Catchment Area propsective 1-year prevalence rates of disorders and services. *Archives of General Psychiatry* 50:85-94, 1993.

Rogers MP, Liang MH, Daltroy LH, et al: Delirium after elective orthopedic surgery: risk factors and natural history. *International Journal of Psychiatry in Medicine* 19(2):109-121, 1989.

Rost K, Kashner TM, Smith GR: Effectiveness of psychiatric intervention with somatization disorder patients: improved outcomes at reduced costs. *General Hospital Psychiatry* 16:381-387, 1994.

Rovner BW, German PS, Brant LJ, et al: Depression and mortality in nursing homes. *Journal of the American Medical Association* 265:993-996, 1991.

Rush AJ, Golden WE, Hall GE, et al: Depression in primary care: Clinical Practice Guidelines. Agency for Health Care Policy and Research. AHCPR publication No. 93-0550. US Department of Health and Human Services. Rockville, MD, 1993.

Saravay SM: Psychiatric interventions in the medically ill: outcome and effectiveness research. *Psychiatric Clinic of North America* 19:1-14, 1996.

Saravay SM, Lavin M: Psychiatric comorbidity and length of stay in the general hospital: a critical review of outcome studies. *Psychosomatics* 35:233-252, 1994.

Saravay SM, Steinberg MD, Weinschel B, et al: Psychological comorbidity and length of stay in the general hospital. *American Journal of Psychiatry* 148:324-329, 1994.

Saravay SM, Strain JJ: AMP task force on funding implications of consultation-liaison outcome studies. *Psychosomatics* 35:227-232, 1993.

Sartorius N, Ustun TB, Costa e Silva JA, et al: An international study of psychological problems in primary care: preliminary report form the WHO collaborative project on psychological problems in general health care. *Archives of General Psychiatry* 50:819-824, 1993.

Schneier FR, Heckelman RG, Garfinkel RC, et al: Functional impairment in social phobia. *Journal of Clinical Psychiatry* 55:322-331, 1994.

Schneier FR, Johnson J, Hornig CD, et al: Social phobia: comorbidity and morbidity in an epidemiologic sample. *Archives of General Psychiatry* 49:282-288,1992.

Schubert DSP, Burns R, Paras W, et al: Increase of medical hospital length of stay by depression in stroke and amputation patients: a pilot study. *Psychotherapy and Psychosomatics* 57:61-66, 1992.

Schubert DSP, Taylor C, Lee S, et al: Physical consequences of depression in the stroke patient. *General Hospital Psychiatry* 14:69-76, 1992.

Schulberg HC, Block MR, Madonia MJ, et al (in press). Treating major depression in primay care practice: eight-month clinical outcome. *Archives of General Psychiatry.*

Simon GE, Ormel J, VonKorff M, et al: Health care costs associated with depressive and anxiety disorders in primary care. *American Journal of Psychiatry* 152:353-357, 1995a.

Simon GE, VonKorff M, Barlow W: Health care costs of primay care patients with recognized depression. *Archives of General Psychiatry* 52:850-856, 1995b.

Simon GE, VonKorff M, Wagner EH, et al: Patterns of antidepressant use in community practice. *General Hospital Psychiatry* 15:399-408, 1993.

Simonsick EM, Wallace RB, Blazer DG, et al: Depressive symptomology and hypertension-associated morbidity in older adults. *Psychosomatic Medicine* 57:427-435, 1995.

Smith GR Jr.: The course of somatization and its effects on utilization of health care resources. *Psychosomatics* 35:263-267, 1994.

Smith GR Jr., Monson RA, Ray DC: Psychiatric consultation in somatization disorder: a randomized controlled study. *New England Journal of Medicine* 314:1407-1413, 1986.

Smith GR Jr., Monson RA, Ray DC: Patients with multiple unexplained symptoms: their characteristics, functional health, and health care utilization. *Archives of Internal Medicine* 146:69-72, 1986.

Smith GR Jr., Rost K, Kashner TM: A trial of the effect of a standardized consultation on health outcome and costs in somatizing patients. *Archives of General Psychiatry* 52:238-243, 1995.

Spitzer RL, Kroenke K, Linzer M, et al: Health related quality of life in primary care patients with mental disorders: results from the PRIME-MD 1000 study. *Journal of the American Medical Association* 274:1511–1517, 1995.

Spitzer RL, Williams JBW, Kroenke K, et al: Utility of a new procedure for diagnosing mental disorders in primary care: the PRIME-MD 1000 study. *Journal of the American Medical Association* 272:1749–1756, 1994.

Strain JJ, Hammer JS, Fulop G: APM Task Force on psychological intervention in the general hospital inpatient setting: a review of cost-offset studies. *Psychosomatics* 35:253–262, 1994.

Strain MD, Lyons JS, Hammer JS, et al: Cost offset from a psychiatric consultation-liaison intervention with elderly hip fracture patients. *American Journal of Psychiatry* 148,1044–1049, 1991.

Strain JJ, Pincus HA, Leslie HG, et al: The role of psychiatry in the training of primary care physicians. *General Hospital Psychiatry* 8:372–385, 1986.

Substance Abuse and Mental Health Services Administration (SAMHSA): *Cost of Addictive and Mental Disorders and Effectiveness of Treatment.* U.S. Department of Health and Human Services, Rockville, Maryland, 1995.

US Department of Commerce: *Statistical Abstract of the United States.* Bureau of the Census. Washington, D.C., 1994.

US Department of Health and Human Services (HHS): *Seventh Special Report to the U.S. Congress on Alcohol and Health.* Alcohol, Drug Abuse, and Mental Health Administration, Rockville, Maryland (1990).

Verbosy LA, Franco K, Zrull JP: The relationship between depression and length of stay in general hospital patients. *Journal of Clinical Psychiatry* 54:177–181, 1993.

Wells KB, Goldberg G, Brook R, et al: Management of patients on psychotropic drugs in primary care clinics. *Medical Care* 26:645–656, 1988.

Wells KB, Golding JM, Burman MA, et al: Psychiatric disorder in a sample of the general population with and without chronic medical conditions. *American Journal of Psychiatry* 145:976–981, 1988.

Wells KB: Depression in general medical settings: implications of three health policy studies for consultation–liaison psychiatry. *Psychosomatics* 35:279–296, 1994.

Wells KB: Cost containment and mental health outcomes: experiences from US studies. *British Journal of Psychiatry* Apr (27):43–51, 1995.

Wells KB, Stewart A, Hays R, et al: The functioning and well-being of depressed patients: results from the medical outcomes study. *Journal of the American Medical Association* 262(7):914–919, 1989.

Appendix 2

Levels of Systematic Collaboration Between Therapists and Other Health Professionals

William J. Doherty, Ph.D., Susan H. McDaniel, Ph.D., and Macaran A. Baird, Ph.D

The hierarchy of the five levels assumes that the greater the level of systemic collaboration, the more likely that the management of demanding cases will be adequate. Demanding cases generally challenge less collaborative settings beyond their ability to manage. The model does not prescribe the optimal model for all healthcare settings but does show the strengths and limitations of a variety of options.

The Levels of Systemic Collaboration model can be used by organizations to evaluate their current structures and procedures in light of their goals for collaboration and to set realistic steps for change. Their goals should reflect the developmental nature of the levels: moving from Level One distance to Level Two off-site linkages, for example; or moving from Level Two to Level Three on-site collaboration as the first step, with provision for the development of closer teams at Level Four. Level Five collaboration requires a significant amount of time with Level Four teamwork.

The model can be used for research, to assess outcomes and cost-effectiveness for different populations. Level Four utility might be best demonstrated on complex patients, for example. The model suggests that significant effort must be made to blend the cultures of medical and mental health professionals in order for high levels of collaboration to be feasible.

Copyright © 1996 by **Behavioral Healthcare *Tomorrow*.** All rights reserved. No part of this publication may be reproduced, stored in a retrieval system, or transmitted in any form or by any means, electronic, mechanical, photocopying, recording, or otherwise, without prior written permission of the copyright owner.

PRIMARY CARE MEETS MENTAL HEALTH

	Description	Where Practiced	Handles Adequately	Handles Inadequately
Level One Minimal Collaboration	Mental health and other healthcare professionals work in separate facilities, have separate systems, and rarely communicate about cases.	Most private practices and agencies.	Cases with routine medical or psychological problems that have little biopsychosocial interplay and few management difficulties.	Cases that are refractory to treatment or have significant biopsychosocial interplay.
Level Two Basic Collaboration from a Distance	Providers have separate systems at separate sites, but engage in periodic communication about shared patients, mostly by telephone and letter. Communication is driven by specific patient issues. Mental health professionals view each other as resources, but operate on their own, with little sharing of responsibility and little understanding of each other's cultures. There is little sharing of power and responsibility.	Settings with active referral linkages across facilities.	Cases with moderate biopsychosocial interplay, for example, a patient has diabetes and depression, and management of both problems proceeds reasonably well.	Cases that have significant biopsychosocial interplay, especially when the medical or mental health management is not satisfactory to one of the parties.
Level Three Basic Collaboration on Site	Mental health and other healthcare professionals have separate systems but share the same facility. They engage in regular communication about shared patients, mostly by phone or letter, but occasionally meet face to face because of the close proximity. They appreciate the importance of each other's roles, may have a sense of being part of a larger, though somewhat ill-defined team, but do not share a common language or an in-depth understanding of each other's worlds. As in Levels One and Two, medical physicians have considerably more power and influence over case management decisions than the other professionals, who may resent this.	HMO settings and rehabilitation centers where collaboration is facilitated by proximity, but there is no systemic approach to collaboration and misunderstandings are common. Also, medical clinics that employ therapists but engage primarily in referral-oriented collaboration rather than systemic mutual consultation and team building.	Cases with moderate biopsychosocial interplay that require occasional face-to-face interactions between providers to manage and coordinate complex treatment plans.	Cases with significant biopsychosocial interplay, especially those with ongoing and challenging management problems.

APPENDIX 2

	Description	Where Practiced	Handles Adequately	Handles Inadequately
Level Four Close Collaboration in a Partly Integrated System	Mental health and other healthcare professionals share the same sites and have some systems in common, such as scheduling or charting. There are regular face-to-face interactions about patients, mutual consultation, coordinated treatment plans for difficult cases, and a basic understanding and appreciation for each other's role and culture. There is a shared allegiance to a biopsychosocial/systems paradigm. However, the routines are still sometimes difficult, team-building meetings are held only occasionally, and there may be operational discrepancies such as co-pays for mental health but not for medical services. There are likely to be unresolved but manageable tensions over medical physicians' greater power and influence on the collaborative team.	Some HMOs, rehabilitation centers, and hospice centers that systematically build teams. Also some family practice training programs.	Cases with significant biopsychosocial interplay and management complications.	Complex cases with multiple providers and multiple large systems involvement, especially when there is the potential for tension and conflicting agendas among providers or triangling on the part of the patient or family.

	Description	Where Practiced	Handles Adequately	Handles Inadequately
Level Five Close Collaboration in a Fully Integrated System	Mental health and other healthcare professionals share the same sites, the same vision, and the same systems in a seamless web of biopsychosocial services. Providers and patients have the same expectations of a team offering prevention and treatment. All professionals are committed to a biopsychosocial systems paradigm and have developed an in-depth understanding of each other's roles and cultures. Regular collaborative team meetings are held to discuss patient issues and team issues. There are conscious efforts to balance power and influence among the professionals according to their roles and areas of expertise.	Some hospice centers and other special training and clinical settings.	The most difficult and complex biopsychosocial cases with challenging management problems.	Cases when the resources of the healthcare team are insufficient or when breakdowns occur in the collaboration with larger service systems.

Appendix 3

Symptom-Driven Diagnostic System—Primary Care (SDDS-PC)

SDDS-PC

The SDDS-PC (Symptom-Driven Diagnostic System—Primary Care) is a two stage diagnostic system with a longitudinal monitoring component developed to assist practitioners in detecting six key mental and addictive disorders, including:

- major depression
- panic disorder
- generalized anxiety
- obsessive-compulsive disorder
- drug and alcohol dependence/abuse
- suicidal ideation.

SDDS-PC is a computerized software tool which provides the practitioner with a systematized approach to evaluating potential for pathology based on symptom patterns, level of impairment, and appropriate medical rule outs. It facilitates recognition of common DSM-IV mental illnesses seen either alone or in conjunction with concomitant somatic disorders.

The SDDS-PC software is capable of providing the questionnaire in such formats as paper and pencil, direct entry computer screens, and computer assisted telephone interviews (CATI). Screen results are instantly scored by the computer with a summary of potential disorders, if any, in the form of diagnosis-specific modules. These modules can be administered by all practitioners. The completed module provides a one-page diagnostic summary with appropriate medical rule-outs, symptoms identified by the patient and practitioner, impairment scores, and DSM-IV criteria for the six major/minor mental and addictive disorders.

The SDDS-PC system is rapid and accurate, does not interfere with office dynamics and supports the practitioner in the ultimate diagnosis and formulation of a treatment plan. It is a comprehensive, scientifically based disease managment tool which will ultimately help the patient by early recognition, treatment and monitoring.

Copyrighted by Pharmacia & Upjohn—1995—All rights reserved. Furnished by Greenstone Healthcare Solutions.

SDDS-PC®
DSM-IV Patient Screening Form

Patient's Name: _____ Physician's Name/Number: _____ [# _____]
Number: _____ Information obtained by: _____ [# _____]
DOB: _____ Date of Administration: _____

In the LAST MONTH, have you been bothered by any of the following:

1. Unhappiness?
   - ☐ No
   - ☐ Yes

2. Trouble falling asleep?
   - ☐ No
   - ☐ Yes

3. Anxious/worried?
   - ☐ No
   - ☐ Yes

4. Others worried about your drinking?
   - ☐ No
   - ☐ Yes

5. Rapid pulse?
   - ☐ No
   - ☐ Yes

6. Fear of going crazy?
   - ☐ No
   - ☐ Yes

7. Feeling blue?
   - ☐ No
   - ☐ Yes

8. Wishing you were dead?
   - ☐ No
   - ☐ Yes

APPENDIX 3

SDDS-PC®
DSM-IV Patient Screening Form

Patient's Name: _____ Physician's Name/Number: _____ [# _____]
Number: _____ Information obtained by: _____ [# _____]
DOB: _____ Date of Administration: _____

9. Trembling or shaking?
   ☐ No
   ☐ Yes

10. Palpitations?
    ☐ No
    ☐ Yes

11. Tension?
    ☐ No
    ☐ Yes

12. High or hung over from drugs?
    ☐ No
    ☐ Yes

13. Drinking too much alcohol?
    ☐ No
    ☐ Yes

14. Sudden attacks of panic or fear?
    ☐ No
    ☐ Yes

15. Cleaning things over and over?
    ☐ No
    ☐ Yes

16. Worrying?
    ☐ No
    ☐ Yes

17. Checking or counting things over and over?
    ☐ No
    ☐ Yes

SDDS-PC®
DSM-IV Patient Screening Form

Patient's Name: _____   Physician's Name/Number: _____ [# _____]
Number: _____   Information obtained by: _____ [# _____]
DOB: _____   Date of Administration: _____

18. Feeling sad?
    ☐ No
    ☐ Yes

19. Your drug use causing problems with family or at work?
    ☐ No
    ☐ Yes

20. Feeling suicidal?
    ☐ No
    ☐ Yes

21. Thoughts or images that do not make sense?
    ☐ No
    ☐ Yes

22. Drinking alcohol in the morning?
    ☐ No
    ☐ Yes

23. Your family thinking you use drugs too much?
    ☐ No
    ☐ Yes

24. Trouble staying asleep?
    ☐ No
    ☐ Yes

25. Rapid heartbeat?
    ☐ No
    ☐ Yes

26. Depression
    ☐ No
    ☐ Yes

APPENDIX 3

| **SDDS-PC®** |
| **DSM-IV Patient Screening Form** |

Patient's Name: _____ Physician's Name/Number: _____ [#_____]
Number: _____ Information obtained by: _____ [#_____]
DOB: _____ Date of Administration: _____

27. Other than having a bodily illness, have there been any times in THE LAST MONTH that you felt so bad or ill that you missed days at work or missed school or were unable to do your housework?
    - [ ] No days missed
    - [ ] Missed 1 day
    - [ ] Missed 2, 3 or 4 days
    - [ ] Missed 5 or more days
    - [ ] Not Applicable

28. In the LAST MONTH, how well did you and your husband/wife/partner get along?
    - [ ] Very Well
    - [ ] Fairly Well
    - [ ] Not Well
    - [ ] Very Poorly
    - [ ] No Partner

29. What best describes your emotional health in the LAST MONTH?
    - [ ] Excellent
    - [ ] Good
    - [ ] Fair
    - [ ] Poor
    - [ ] Very Poor

Appendix 4

Prime-MD Patient Questionnaire

The PRIME-MD consists of two components. The first is a one-page Patient Questionnaire (PQ) that the patient completes prior to seeing the physician. It consists of 26 yes/no questions and a single question about overall health. The first 26 questions are divided into five broad diagnostic areas. The second PRIME-MD component is a Clinical Evaluation Guide (CEG) that the physician uses to gather additional information in diagnostic areas in which patients respond positively on the PQ.

This appendix contains the Patient Questionnaire. For a complementary copy of the Clinical Evaluation Guide, please write to: Pfizer Inc., 235 E. 42nd Street, Prime-MD 235-10-49, New York, NY 10017.

Prime-MD is a trademark of Pfizer Inc. Copyright Pfizer Inc. 1997. For a complementary copy of Prime-MD, please write to: Pfizer Inc., 235 E. 42nd Street, Prime-MD 235-10-49, New York, NY 10017.

PATIENT QUESTIONNAIRE

NAME: _____ SEX: ☐ Male ☐ Female   AGE: _____   TODAY'S DATE: _____

MARITAL STATUS
☐ Married
☐ Widowed
☐ Separated
☐ Divorced
☐ Never married

YOUR BACKGROUND
☐ Black (not Hispanic)
☐ Hispanic
☐ White (not Hispanic)
☐ Asian
☐ Other Describe: _____

HOW FAR YOU WENT IN SCHOOL
☐ 8th grade or less
☐ Some high school
☐ High school graduate or equivalency (GED)
☐ Some college or associate degree
☐ Completed college

INSTRUCTIONS: This questionnaire will help your doctor better understand problems that you may have. Your doctor may ask you more questions about some of these items. Please make sure to check a box for *every* item.

*During the **PAST MONTH**, have you **OFTEN** been bothered by . . .*						*During the **PAST MONTH** . . .*		
	Yes	No		Yes	No		Yes	No
1. stomach pain	☐	☐	12. constipation, loose bowels, or diarrhea	☐	☐	22. have you had an anxiety attack (suddenly feeling fear or panic)	☐	☐
2. back pain	☐	☐	13. nausea, gas, or indigestion	☐	☐			
3. pain in your arms, legs, or joints (knees, hips, etc)	☐	☐	14. feeling tired or having low energy	☐	☐	23. have you thought you should cut down on your drinking of alcohol	☐	☐
4. menstrual pain or problems	☐	☐	15. trouble sleeping	☐	☐			
			16. the thought that you have a serious undiagnosed disease	☐	☐	24. has anyone complained about your drinking	☐	☐
5. pain or problems during sexual intercourse	☐	☐						
6. headaches	☐	☐	17. your eating being out of control	☐	☐	25. have you felt guilty or upset about your drinking	☐	☐
7. chest pain	☐	☐	18. little interest or pleasure in doing things	☐	☐	26. was there ever a single day in which you had five or more drinks of beer, wine, or liquor	☐	☐
8. dizziness	☐	☐						
9. fainting spells	☐	☐	19. feeling down, depressed, or hopeless	☐	☐			
10. feeling your heart pound or race	☐	☐				Overall, would you say your health is: Excellent ☐ Very Good ☐ Good ☐ Fair ☐ Poor ☐		
11. shortness of breath	☐	☐	20. "nerves" or feeling anxious or on edge	☐	☐			
			21. worrying about a lot of different things	☐	☐			

Appendix 5

Quick Guide to Patient Problem Questionnaire (PPQ)

Quick Guide to Patient Problem Questionnaire

Purpose. The Patient Problem Questionnaire (PPQ) is designed to facilitate the recognition of the most common mental disorders in primary care patients.

Who Should Take the PPQ. Ideally, the PPQ should be used with all new patients, all patients who have not completed the questionnaire in the last year, and all patients suspected of having a mental disorder.

Making a Diagnosis. Since the questionnaire relies on patient self-report, definitive diagnoses must be verified by the clinician, taking into account how well the patient understood the questions in the questionnaire, as well as other relevant information from the patient, his or her family or other sources.

Interpreting the PPQ. To facilitate interpretation of patient responses, all clinically significant responses are found in the column furthest to the right. (The only exception is for suicidal ideation when diagnosing a depressive syndrome.) At the bottom of several of the pages, beginning with "FOR OFFICE CODING," in small type, are criteria for diagnostic judgments for summarizing the responses on that page. The names of the categories are abbreviated, e.g., Major Depressive Syndrome is Maj Dep Syn. The criteria for diagnostic judgments about Alcohol Abuse/Dependence are not presented because they are so simple, and to avoid possibly influencing patient answers to the alcohol questions.

Page 1

Somatoform Disorder if at least 3 of #1a–m bother the patient "a lot" and lack an adequate biological explanation.

Major Depressive Syndrome if answer to #2a or #b is "nearly every day" and 5+ of #2a–i are "nearly every day" (count #2i if present at all); Other Depressive Syndrome the same but only 2+ of the answers to #2a–i are "nearly every day."

Note: the diagnoses of Major Depressive *Disorder* and Other Depressive *Disorder* requires ruling out normal **bereavement (mild symptoms, duration less than 2 months),** a history of a **manic** episode (Bipolar Disorder) and a **physical disorder, medication or other drug** as the biological cause of the depressive symptoms.

© PPQ c/o Spitzer, Unit 74, 722 W. 168th Street, New York, NY, 10032 (212-960-5534).

> **Page 2**
>
> Panic Syndrome if #3a–d are 'Yes' and 4+ of #4a–k are 'Yes.'
>
> Other Anxiety Syndrome if #5a and answers to 3+ of #5b–g are "more than half the days."
>
> Note: The diagnoses of Panic *Disorder* and Other Anxiety *Disorder* require ruling out a **physical disorder, medication or other drug** as the biological cause of the anxiety symptoms.
>
> **Page 3**
>
> Bulimia Nervosa if #6a, b, and c and #8 are 'Yes'; Binge Eating Disorder the same but #8 is either 'NO' or left blank.
>
> Alcohol abuse/dependence if any of #10a–e are "Yes."

Additional Clinical Considerations. After making a provisional diagnosis with the PPQ, there are additional clinical considerations that may affect decisions about management and treatment.

Have current symptoms been triggered by psychosocial **stressor(s)***?*

What is the duration of the current disturbance and has the patient received any **treatment** *for it?*

To what extent are the patient's symptoms **impairing** *his or her usual work and activities?*

Is there a **history** *of similar episodes, and were they* **treated***?*

Is there a **family history** *of similar conditions?*

Patient Problem Questionnaire

This questionnaire is an important part of providing you with the best health care possible. Your answers will help in understanding problems that you may have. Please answer every question to the best of your ability unless you are requested to skip over a question.

TODAY'S DATE _____ NAME _____ AGE _____ SEX: ☐ Female ☐ Male

1. During the *last 4 weeks,* how much have you been bothered by any of the following problems?

	Not bothered at all	Bothered a little	Bothered a lot
a. Stomach pain	☐	☐	☐
b. Back pain	☐	☐	☐
c. Pain in your arms, legs, or joints (knees, hips, etc.)	☐	☐	☐
d. Menstrual cramps or other problems with your periods	☐	☐	☐
e. Pain or problems during sexual intercourse	☐	☐	☐
f. Headaches	☐	☐	☐
g. Chest pain	☐	☐	☐
h. Dizziness	☐	☐	☐
i. Fainting spells	☐	☐	☐
j. Feeling your heart pound or race	☐	☐	☐
k. Shortness of breath	☐	☐	☐
l. Constipation, loose bowels, or diarrhea	☐	☐	☐
m. Nausea, gas, or indigestion	☐	☐	☐

2. Over the *last 2 weeks,* how often have you been bothered by any of the following problems?

	Not at all	Several days	More than half the days	Nearly every day
a. Little interest or pleasure in doing things	☐	☐	☐	☐
b. Feeling down, depressed, or hopeless	☐	☐	☐	☐
c. Trouble falling or staying asleep, or sleeping too much	☐	☐	☐	☐
d. Feeling tired or having little energy	☐	☐	☐	☐
e. Poor appetite or overeating	☐	☐	☐	☐
f. Feeling bad about yourself—or that you are a failure or have let yourself or your family down	☐	☐	☐	☐
g. Trouble concentrating on things, such as reading the newspaper or watching television	☐	☐	☐	☐
h. Moving or speaking so slowly that other people could have noticed? Or the opposite—being so fidgety or restless that you have been moving around a lot more than usual	☐	☐	☐	☐
i. Thoughts that you would be better off dead or of hurting yourself in some way	☐	☐	☐	☐

FOR OFFICE CODING: Som Dis if at least 3 of #1a–m are "a lot" and lack an adequate biol explanation.
Maj Dep Syn if answer to #2a. or #b. are "nearly every day" and 5+ of #2a–#i are "nearly every day" (count #2i if present at all).
Other Dep Syn same but only 2, 3, or 4 of the answers to #2a–#i are "nearly every day."

3. **Questions about anxiety**   NO   YES

   a. In the *last 4 weeks,* have you had an anxiety attack—
      suddenly feeling fear or panic? . . . .   ☐   ☐

   | If you checked "NO," go to question #5. |

   b. Has this ever happened before? . . . .   ☐   ☐

   c. Do some of these attacks come *suddenly out of the blue—*
      that is, in situations where you don't expect to be nervous or
      uncomfortable? . . . .   ☐   ☐

   d. Do these attacks bother you a lot or are you worried about
      having another attack? . . . .   ☐   ☐

4. **Think about your last bad anxiety attack.**   NO   YES

   a. Were you short of breath? . . . .   ☐   ☐
   b. Did your heart race, pound, or skip? . . . .   ☐   ☐
   c. Did you have chest pain or pressure? . . . .   ☐   ☐
   d. Did you sweat? . . . .   ☐   ☐
   e. Did you feel as if you were choking? . . . .   ☐   ☐
   f. Did you have hot flashes or chills? . . . .   ☐   ☐
   g. Did you have nausea or an upset stomach, or the feeling
      that you were going to have diarrhea? . . . .   ☐   ☐
   h. Did you feel dizzy, unsteady, or faint? . . . .   ☐   ☐
   i. Did you have tingling or numbness in parts of your body? . .   ☐   ☐
   j. Did you tremble or shake? . . . .   ☐   ☐
   k. Were you afraid you were dying? . . . .   ☐   ☐

			Not at all	Several days	More than half the days

5. **Over the *last 4 weeks,* how often have you been bothered by any of the following problems?**

   a. Feeling nervous, anxious, on edge, or worrying a lot
      about different things . . . .   ☐   ☐   ☐

   | If you checked "Not at all," go to question #6. |

   b. Feeling restless so that it is hard to sit still . . . .   ☐   ☐   ☐
   c. Getting tired very easily . . . .   ☐   ☐   ☐
   d. Muscle tension, aches, or soreness . . . .   ☐   ☐   ☐
   e. Trouble falling asleep or staying asleep . . . .   ☐   ☐   ☐
   f. Trouble concentrating on things, such as reading a
      book or watching TV . . . .   ☐   ☐   ☐
   g. Becoming easily annoyed or irritable . . . .   ☐   ☐   ☐

FOR OFFICE CODING: Pan Syn if #3a–d are 'Y' and 4+ of #4a–k are 'Y.'
Other Anx Syn if #5a and answers to 3+ of #5b–g are "more than half the days."

6. **Questions about eating**   NO   YES

     a. Do you often feel that you can't control *what* or *how much* you eat? .... ☐ ☐

     b. Do you often eat, *within any 2-hour period,* what most people would regard as an unusually *large* amount of food? .... ☐ ☐

| If you checked "NO" to either #a or #b, go to question #9. |

     c. Has this been as often, on average, as twice a week for the last 3 months? .... ☐ ☐

7. **In the last 3 months have you *often* done any of the following in order to avoid gaining weight?**   NO   YES

     a. Made yourself vomit? .... ☐ ☐

     b. Took more than twice the recommended dose of laxatives? .... ☐ ☐

     c. Fasted—not eaten anything at all for at least 24 hours? .... ☐ ☐

     d. Exercised for more than an hour specifically to avoid gaining weight after binge eating? .... ☐ ☐

                                                                      NO   YES

8. If you checked 'YES' to any of these ways of avoiding gaining weight, were any as often, on average, as twice a week? ... ☐ ☐

                                                                      NO   YES

9. Do you ever drink alcohol (including beer or wine)? .... ☐ ☐

| If you checked "NO" go to question #11. |

10. **Have any of the following happened to you *more than once in the last 6 months?***   NO   YES

     a. You drank alcohol even though a doctor suggested that you stop drinking because of a problem with your health ...... ☐ ☐

     b. You drank alcohol, were high from the alcohol, or hung over while you were working, going to school, or taking care of children or other responsibilities .... ☐ ☐

     c. You missed or were late for work, school, or other activities because you were drinking or hung over .... ☐ ☐

     d. You had a problem getting along with other people while you were drinking .... ☐ ☐

     e. You drove a car after having several drinks or after drinking too much .... ☐ ☐

11. **If you checked off *any* problems on this questionnaire, how *difficult* have these problems made it for you to do your work, take care of things at home, or get along with other people?**

Not difficult at all	Somewhat difficult	Very difficult	Extremely difficult
☐	☐	☐	☐

FOR OFFICE CODING: Bul Ner if #6a, b, and c and #8 = 'Y'; Bin Eat Dis same but #8 either 'N' or left blank

Appendix 6

Teaching Medical Interviewing: The Lipkin Model

Mack Lipkin, Jr., Craig Kaplan, William Clark, and Dennis H. Novack

This appendix describes the evolution of a unique faculty development course and innovative educational model designed by Mack Lipkin, Jr. for teachers of medical interviewing. His approach integrates principles of learner-centered (or self-directed) learning with core human values, such as unconditional positive regard for others and attention to affect. We first describe some experiences that led Lipkin to the development of the course model. We then discuss the educational context and principles of the course and detail its structure, process, and problems. We end with some short examples of other applications of this approach in medical education.

Initial Experiences

Problem Solving and Groups

Lipkin's first relevant experience with a learner-directed approach to education was in a highly technical graduate course on invertebrate physiology. Although this subject might seem an unlikely candidate for non-traditional learning, the students quickly found otherwise. Every two weeks, rather than being asked to repeat established rote laboratory experiments, they were posed problems such as "Prove whether snail cellulose is endogenous or derived from a symbiotic bacterium in the snail gut." To solve this particular problem, Lipkin learned to create a bacterial culture medium, to pour cellulose-rich agar plates, to dissect a snail, and finally, to isolate cellulolytic bacteria from the snail's gut—all without benefit of a scripted laboratory manual! Other students undertook similarly challenging problems.

Each student presented results to the entire class. These presentations were notable for their enthusiasm, high energy, and triumphant creativity. Student learning was much more profound than expected. The creative discovery experience was exhilarating in comparison with accepted models in which laboratories consist of proving the accepted by replicating prescribed steps in rote fashion. He learned that students can be as creative as their teachers and that student standards were sometimes higher than their teachers'.

That physiology course introduced Lipkin to the powerful educational benefits to be found in discovering solutions to problems for oneself—an educational model now termed "problem based" (Schmidt et al., 1989). In this educational approach, learners

---

Reprinted from: Lipkin M Jr., Kaplan C, Clark W, Novack DH: Teaching medical interviewing: The Lipkin Model. *In:* The Medical Interview: Clinical Care, Education, and Research, Lipkin M Jr., Putnam SM, Lazare A (eds). Springer-Verlag, New York, 1995.

develop an intense interest in the subject and a sense of ownership of what is learned. The discovery process resulting from problem solving helps to demystify the subject. Learners feel empowered and independent of their teachers for solutions. Additionally, they learn to value one another as learning resources. Many preferred working in small groups rather than alone.

When Lipkin began to teach second-year medical students in Rochester, he wondered whether they too would prefer this type of educational model. That course, which focused on doctor/patient communication and psychosocial medicine, was previously taught in small groups following a tightly prescribed format. Instead, the author negotiated a separate task with his students during each three-week block. Not only did students solve problems, they chose which problems to solve. Lipkin arranged to have patients and related reading materials available. Students pursued their own approach to learning about such subjects as adult development, the human life cycle, the dying patient, breaking bad news, psychosis, and the team approach. Other instructors were skeptical, but the students enthusiastically undertook major learning projects.

The results were unexpectedly rewarding. Presentations demonstrated zest for learning. Not only did students learn from one another, but enduring respect and caring developed between them and between the students and the instructor.

An important lesson was that learners' personal feelings and affective responses can present serious impediments to learning medicine. A student who has lost a parent in adolescence found that he could not work with dying patients. Another student with a domineering father encountered authority problems during his patient interviews. Still another student, who craved love, having so little at home, became a compulsive giver, unable to set limits because she perceived them as inflicting on her patients or teachers the pain she had experienced. Sensitive and supportive discussion of personal issues led to personal and educational breakthroughs and to closeness and trust within the group. Failing to attend to the personal dimensions of learning would have inhibited both personal and professional growth.

One year following that group, Lipkin attended a group program run by Orenne Strode and Carl Rogers called Human Dimensions in Medical Education. This program adapted Rogerian group methods to medical education. It modeled a method of responding to feelings and emotions that was fast, efficient, and effective. Lipkin discovered that what he had learned about dealing with the affective domain from his own experience as student and teacher had been the subject of significant research (Rogers, 1983).

Accepting A New Challenge

Lipkin had the opportunity to apply these insights and educational experiences when he undertook to design a faculty development course for teachers of the medical interview in 1980. This course was designed to focus on the participants' interests and to allow exploration of feelings, based on problems in both clinical and educational practice. Participants would improve their knowledge and skills by designing their own curriculum, identifying relevant problems in their teaching and patient care activities, and using resources made available throughout the course, including faculty, patients, actors, and videotapes. When this process becomes blocked, which is common because most participants are not used to such a learning model, skilled facilitators are present to suggest possible approaches without taking over. An environment is created that enables participants to work on interactional skills, explore teaching dilemmas, and learn new teaching methods. In addition, by requiring self-selected groups of participants to complete projects of their own choosing during the course, he included a task orientation to provide a sense of time limitation, a degree of healthy, self-motivated performance, and a group focus. Finally, time is reserved for reflecting about the personal dimensions of the work and exploring the learners' responses to similar problems and barriers at their own institutions and in their own lives.

The first time Lipkin's course was offered, with the collaboration of W. Clark and D. Novack, the greatest challenge to overcome was the faculty belief that they had to be both the focus of student attention and the predominant source of learning. Not only did participants have to adapt to the new educational methods, so did the course faculty! Most teachers were conditioned to treat students as relatively passive recipients of knowledge and skills rather than as active participants in their own learning. They were tempted to do the work for the students rather than let students struggle to define their own problems and create their own learning situations. Nevertheless, the course was judged a success by most who attended it. Subsequently, course faculty have grown increasingly skilled at encouraging each learner to stretch and maximize their own knowledge, skills, and growth. (Details of the production of a course are contained in the Course Development Manual of the American Academy on Physician and Patient.)

Historical Context of the Educational Model

Until the turn of the century, physicians in training apprenticed with experienced clinicians. In return for providing care to patients, student-physicians received medical training. The apprentice depended on a single practitioner or small group of practitioners for the acquisition of medical knowledge and practical skills. A fractured form of apprenticeship persists in current medical education, particularly in the medical school clerkships and residency. Within these mini apprenticeships, the learner attempts to absorb relevant clinical education through exposure to more experienced teachers. Apprentice models are also used for learning basic clinical skills, including, at some levels, medical interviewing.

The persistence of the apprentice model relates to two educational strengths. First, learners enter an active and complex educational environment where they must decide which educational issues are most pertinent for personal development. In addition, the education takes place in the context of solving practical, real-world problems. On the negative side, apprenticeship creates a master-novice relationship, which places the learner in a dependent position with respect to defining learning needs and goals, regulating day-to-day activities, setting performance standards, and evaluating accomplishments. In this relationship, creativity and independent thinking may not be encouraged. There may be heavy reliance on teachers, whose motivation, skill, and commitment to teaching vary widely. Furthermore, the educational outcomes are dependent on the interactions between two people who, if poorly matched in personality, interests, learning styles, or cultural background, may diminish the educational value. A related problem is the lack of emphasis on group learning in the apprentice model. Even with several students assigned to a teacher, the important learning interactions are assumed to take place between each learner and the teacher, a parallel set of one-on-one relationships, rather than among the entire group. Evidence suggests that small groups generate learning as well or better than solo study (Cartwright and Zander, 1953).

In 1910, Flexner advocated sweeping changes in both the learning model and the settings for medical education. Flexner's era was marked by tremendous change and the closing of schools that did not insist on academic excellence or provide an adequate scientific or clinical education. Citing the thinking of Dewey (not published until 1916), Flexner emphasized that students in medicine should learn "a method of thinking [and] an attitude of mind" (Flexner, 1910) rather than simply memorize facts. Flexner stressed that the initiative should lie with the learner and that students should learn by doing. He believed that thinking and problem solving deserved emphasis and that learners should be actively involved with the process of their education.

The reforms Flexner suggested for the organization of the medical school were more widely accepted and understood than those he suggested for its learning model. The six decades following that reform period brought only limited implementation of his concepts of active student involvement. The teacher remained at the center of the educational process.

Although it improves in some ways over a pure apprenticeship model, the teacher-centered model also has limitations. Because the teacher directs most learning activities, students often attribute success or failure to their teacher's actions and qualities rather than their own. Passive students do not visualize themselves as independently defining and accomplishing learning. This leads to difficulties following completion of formal training when learners are forced to be independent or to stop learning.

In addition to being teacher centered, the currently dominant educational model fails to recognize that students and physicians have strong emotional reactions to patient care (Gorlin and Zucker, 1982) and learning (Reuben 1983; Smith et al., 1986), which can either retard or further their development. If the teacher does not acknowledge emotional reactions as an appropriate focus for learning and discussion, students may suppress feelings and miss opportunities to cope more effectively. Some of the cynicism that grows during medical training (Kopelman, 1983; Rezler, 1974) may arise from the failure to recognize and cope with the feelings inevitable throughout medical training.

Recognition of these educational dilemmas has spawned notable attempts at innovation and reform during the last two decades (Schmide et al., 1989). Advocates of problem-based learning (Barrows and Tamblyn, 1980; Neufeld and Barrows, 1974), in which students accept greater responsibility for independent problem solving and learning, have spread real-world clinical practice throughout all years of medical training. The Harvard New Pathway emphasizes small learning groups that focus on contextually derived problems. Other schools have developed innovative curricula and clarified faculty responsibilities. The report on the General Professional Education of the Physician (Physicians for the Twenty-first Century, 1984) stimulated further discussion and interest in identifying and resolving these problems. Manning et al. (1987) have noted that continuing medical educational efforts have sometimes emphasized self-directed learning.

We have applied Lipkin's model, which also provides attention to learner feelings, to faculty development. The model, described next, retains the strengths of the apprenticeship and teacher-centered models. It places more responsibility for learning in the hands of the learner and deemphasizes the teacher as the focus of attention and dependence.

A Teaching/Learning Model for Medical Faculty Development

Underlying Principles

Lipkin derived the model for his course from his experiences as learner and teacher and was delighted to find it fits principles from adult learning practices while going beyond that literature to combine didactic, skill learning, a task orientation, and personal awareness. In addition to accomplishing requisite learning, central goals include empowering learners, assisting them in maximizing their creativity and self-esteem as learners, and treating them with empathic understanding and positive regard. The following guiding principles help achieve these goals.

"Adults want to learn about topics which are relevant to their daily experience" (Cross, 1981). Learning must be individualized, because participants vary in prior experience, interests, and learning styles. "Adults learn best when they are able to determine their own learning goals and participate in evaluating their learning."

"Learning experiences must provide opportunities both to practice skills and knowledge and to reflect upon the effects of that experience." Freire and others (1986) refer to the cycle of action and reflection as praxis.

In our approach, teachers are facilitators of learning. They provide help and support to learners as they specify their goals, resources, and means of evaluation. This is a different role than that traditionally envisioned for teachers. Freire (1986) noted that facilitators of learning viewed themselves not as repositories of knowledge to be deposited in the learner (the "banking" theory of learning) but as partners in the learning enterprise. Knowles (1980) emphasized that facilitators viewed the past and present experience of their learners as the most important resource for learning. Brookfield (1987) discussed the differences between the roles of traditional teachers and facilitative teachers, writing that facilitators were teachers who promoted the development of "self directed, critically aware individuals capable of imagining and realizing alternative ways of thinking and living." Table 1 lists four major characteristics of facilitative teachers identified by Brookfield.

TABLE 1. CHARACTERISTICS OF FACILITATIVE TEACHERS

Show genuineness, acceptance, positive regard
Create trusting environment
Trust the abilities of the learner
Provide resources and negotiate goals

Rogers (1983) stated that the characteristics of good facilitators were those of genuineness, acceptance, and empathic understanding of the learner. The common theme of these descriptions is that facilitators trust the learner's ability to organize, accomplish, and evaluate their own learning activities. To encourage these activities, facilitators empower the learner and create an interpersonal environment in which learners feel comfortable sharing and reflecting on their experience and learning activities.

Process of the Course

The faculty development course provides an integrated environment for learners to practice interviewing and teaching skills, reflect on values and feelings towards interviewing and teaching, and develop specific skills to subsequently share with other course participants and bring back to their home settings. Courses are taught in two-and-a-half and five-day formats. Participants include senior and junior practitioners and faculty—physicians, nurses, psychologists, psychiatrists, social workers, and others.

Course goals are multiple and multidimensional, as shown in Table 2.

Four major activities constitute the bulk of time for participants during the course: didactic sessions, interview skills groups, personal awareness groups, and project groups. Didactic sessions are lectures, seminars, or workshops, presented by acknowledged experts. Topics have included an enormous variety such as the medical interview, evaluation of learners or curriculum, alcoholism, and somatization.

Interview skills groups comprise four or five learners and one faculty who work on interviewing and teaching skills during several two-hour sessions. Throughout the course, participants and group facilitators negotiate the goals and objectives for each session, so as to foster participants' responsibility for accomplishing tasks relevant to their own needs. Participants are encouraged to choose specific, relevant educational goals and activities. Facilitators take an active role, clarifying choices and broadening participants' perspectives on their choices and underlying values. When appropriate, they may challenge learners' choices to promote new insights about interviewing and

TABLE 2. DESIRED OUTCOMES OF THE COURSE

For medical education:

- Expand and support the network of skilled faculty committed to medical interview teaching.
- Expand the use of the Lipkin Model and of learner-centered methods in medical schools.

For participants:

- Improve interview and facilitation skills and knowledge.
- Improve knowledge of teaching methods, resources, evaluation.
- Improve small-group facilitation skills.
- Unleash creative potential of faculty and develop their trust in their own and others' abilities.
- Develop and deepen attitudes of respect, empathy, and unconditional positive regard.
- Impart core values of the model.
- Foster personal exploration, growth, and change.
- Empower learners.

teaching. Facilitators emphasize that ultimate responsibility for achieving satisfactory outcomes rests with the learner, and strongly suggest at the outset that learners will be successful in their endeavors.

The combination of personal responsibility, high expectation of success, and a discrete time period encourages the learner to make thoughtful choices and successfully accomplish learning activities. Faculty and group affirmation of the learner's ability to carry out significant learning and develop creative products facilitates their growth and promotes new teaching and learning behaviors which continue long after the course ends.

After taking time for needs assessment and goal setting, the group commences work on participants' chosen objectives. Specific content is impossible to predict and depends on the participants' experience and interests. Issues chosen for exploration vary dramatically. Interactive activities are the norm, such as interviewing an outpatient or hospital patient, with subsequent feedback from the group. Other common activities include role-play of interviews or teaching situations and interviews with standardized patients trained to play a consistent role and give feedback to the interviewer. Interviews may also be videotaped for review. Through this active process, participants develop and refine skills relevant to their perceived weaknesses and strengths in interviewing and teaching interviewing in a variety of settings. Facilitators are attuned to emotional issues and respond to them by demonstrating the importance of working with feelings and showing empathy, respect, and unconditional positive regard.

In addition, self-awareness sessions combining two skills groups spend one and a half to two hours per day together for the purpose of reflecting on the feelings that arise during the course and in the participants' outside activities. Such reflection improves their own patient care and teaching skills and makes them more sensitive to the feelings of those they teach.

Patient care and teaching are psychologically demanding and often arouse uncomfortable feelings. A natural tendency to deny or repress these feelings may hinder progress whenever interactions tap personal issues and, unconsciously or not, elicit behaviors that impede the work process. Insight into this mechanism and the ability to monitor and control one's feelings, where necessary, are part of becoming a competent professional interviewer and teacher. Exploration of learners' psychological reactions is an essential component of the model.

Group members are invited to reflect on the meaning of course experiences in relation to their sense of self, their family and other important relationships, and the work of patient care and teaching. Guidelines for creating an empathic, supportive, and respectful environment are that each person speaks for him or herself, that discussions are confidential, and that each participant speaks only as much as desired. Faculty encourage, but do not coerce, participants to explore feelings about patients, colleagues, and family in relation to the role of doctor, interviewer, and teacher. Each group evolves uniquely, and an individual session may resemble a discussion group, a psychotherapy group, or an encounter group (Yalom, 1985). A high degree of sophistication is needed to facilitate the self-awareness groups: facilitators are trained specifically and extensively for this task.

The fourth activity is project groups. Requiring individual learners or groups of learners to complete a learning project on a topic of their choice promotes consolidation of learning and augments learners' sense of creative accomplishment. The course requires participation in task groups because a project orientation focuses effort and gives control to the learners. Focusing on a task sets a time limit and produces objective results that a learner can identify. The results directly reward behaviors associated with the learning and channel group efforts toward a product rather than toward social successes or other such goals. A task group synergizes its learning efforts, generating an outcome greater than the expected sum of individual learners' input.

Project groups comprise individuals with similar interests. These groups explore relevant topics, of their choosing, as widely divergent as alcoholism, Balint groups, DNR orders, residency curriculum, somatization, networking, self-care, and uncertainty. On the final day, each task group reports to the entire course. These thoughtful and original presentations creatively wrestle with the issues, using a variety of media such as music, comedy, drama, video, a written report, a bibliography, a role-play or a questionnaire. Many groups have produced materials of lasting value, or ideas that spawned continuing efforts after the course such as a published paper, a finished teaching video, or a research project.

A fluid evaluation process is used throughout the course. Careful attention to details such as group composition and resource availability greatly enhance the process. During the introductory period, facilitators suggest that standards for success against which they can evaluate their progress. Learners and facilitators continue to discuss evaluation criteria during the process of negotiating goals and designating learning activities. Responsibility for gathering evidence of performance and applying standards rests with the learner, shifting the motivation for learning from external sources (teacher and professional standards) to internal (the learner's negotiated standards). One consistent finding in our evaluation is that over the course, learners' standards are raised and therefore their judgment of their own skill level falls.

Participant Resistance and Overcoming Initial Problems

At the beginning of the course, some participants find it difficult to adapt to a radically different curriculum and orientation. During the initial session, we acknowledge that the curriculum learners are about to embark upon may be different from those they have experienced previously. We suggest that the process may be difficult for some but that positive outcomes are likely if they remain flexible and engage in the process.

Participants naturally expect their facilitators to behave in the customary teacher-centered ways and may be reluctant or unable to state goals or propose activities, a role traditionally reserved for the teacher. Some report a feeling of betrayal—that the facilitator is not holding up his or her end of the bargain, while others suspect that the teacher actually has a hidden agenda that is not explicitly shared. Many participants feel threatened by and/or anxious about the sudden responsibility for active decision-making roles. Facilitators address this issue both cognitively, with nondefensive explanations, and emotionally, by noting the feelings and encouraging their discussion. Group members progressively assume more responsibility and control as they discover that facilitators respond to them as capable, motivated, and creative people and that the facilitators' agenda is to maximize learning.

As with many types of nondirective groups, the initial phase of group development, for both interview skills and personal awareness groups, includes a period of uncertainty (Rogers, 1983), which many find uncomfortable. Empathically and supportively acknowledging this as an expected part of the process and reemphasizing confidence in the learners' competence and eventual success usually enables them to get through this phase.

An angry phase is predictable in the course of any experiential group (Rogers, 1970; Yalom, 1985). As learners begin to share emotions, positive feelings are typically more easily expressed than negative ones. When negative feelings surface, they are often directed at the facilitator. The facilitator's nondirective behavior and the perceived lack of course structure commonly serve as the focus for this anger. The facilitator's primary role at this stage is to establish and reinforce the safety of the group by reacting nondefensively, conveying acceptance and empathic understanding to the learner. The acceptance of negative as well as positive feelings promotes honest and open exchange of feelings, usually moving the group toward cohesiveness. Further meaningful exchange and higher-order learning subsequently occur.

Frequently, the experiential nature of many of the curriculum components is questioned. Participants may question the relevance of sharing personal feelings and emotions in the context of a skills-based course.

Under pressure from participants to adopt a teacher-centered method, facilitators with their primary expertise as teacher-centered faculty may be uncomfortable. Indeed, at times, facilitators do become more directive, suggesting specific activities or giving brief talks to their groups. Although these are teacher-centered behaviors, facilitators agree to those behaviors with the goal of helping participants bridge their prior experience as passive students and our expectation of a more active role.

Other Examples of the Lipkin Model in Medical Education

An extraordinary variety of educational situations can be served by the approach described here. The method has been used by the authors in every level of medical education, from the first year through the advanced education of full professors and deans. Others (e.g., Gordon, 1991; Levinson and Roter, 1993) have used these methods as well.

A Third Year Elective Group

A group of medical students in the third year decided to meet each week with Lipkin to pursue issues of interest to them. They set the agenda either the week before or at the start of the meeting. Topics included adaptation to the wards, dealing with difficult patients, educating oneself while in a structured clerkship with limited time, caring for dying patients on the service, coping with difficult residents and faculty, and becoming a doctor.

It was a profound and moving experience for all. Attendance remained high all year, with students staying two or more hours each session. Five years later, when someone from the group developed leukemia, other group members came to his aid, helping his wife and children and supporting one another. (A student perspective on this has been published in Romano, 1976.)

This approach readily leads to profound personal discussion of the issues of great concern to learners, the humanistic elements often omitted from standard curricula. A more open format allows the learners to focus on and deepen the emotional component of the process. The group process formed was the key to this experience and became important in the development of caring, well-adjusted physicians. The daily experience of the learners became the focus of learning.

A Residency Elective in Psychosocial Aspects of Care

Lipkin was asked by a primary care residency director to train residents in psychosocial aspects of care. Several barriers, however, had to be overcome. Residents were skeptical about the effectiveness of such teaching. They doubted that psychological concepts could be adapted meaningfully to the medical setting. Furthermore, the material was potentially sensitive and threatening, and it was believed that it would be difficult to begin to recognize the magnitude of the feelings and travails of medical patients. Finally, the residents had enormously varied levels of knowledge, talents, and motivations, as well as varied defenses.

Lipkin decided that attempts to create a single homogenous course would exaggerate these difficulties rather than ameliorate them. Instead, he decided to get out of the role of telling residents they really "ought to want" to learn (Mager, 1968) what he thought was important and instead had residents assume responsibility for their learning. Faculty were to serve as facilitators for this learning.

Lipkin asked each resident beginning the elective to define goals and objectives for the month. Thus, he began with the learner's own needs and problems, formulated in a way acceptable to him or her. He encouraged that their work together be based on real experiences, using simulation for focused examination of problems uncovered.

Lipkin was concerned that residents might limit themselves to what they do well and avoid uncomfortable topics. But for the most part they went right for difficult issues, and when they didn't the problems arose in the course of contact with patients. They often began by seeing patients and discovered how much could be learned in a short time when observation was heightened and focused.

During the one-month block, residents typically made major progress in a variety of areas, such as improving their medical interviewing knowledge and skills, adapting to working with sick patients, interacting with difficult patient types such as borderline personalities, breaking bad news, understanding common psychiatric problems (including anxiety, depression, substance abuse, and somatization), and applying therapies such as supportive psychotherapy, relaxation, hypnosis, and behavior modification. This was much more than he ever would have designed into a rigid curriculum. Furthermore, the depth of curiosity, the enthusiasm shown for reading and studying, and the seriousness of grappling with the concepts was much greater than he had imagined possible. Residents felt personal ownership of the material, and they created a self-sustaining basis for continued growth and development.

Workshops at the Society of General Internal Medicine

Lipkin found that the problems encountered in teaching psychosocial issues to general internist faculty were similar to those of practitioners at national meetings. Many had negative views about the possibility of effective teaching in the area. Others felt the material was too "soft." To overcome these resistances, the objectives were reframed as expectations that learners bring. Brainstorming was used to engage learners with issues that they themselves identified. Thus, we began at the learner's level rather than at a defined starting place. Furthermore, we harnessed each learner's leadership instincts and competitiveness, challenging each to develop superior approaches. The resulting workshops led in brief spaces of time to dramatic engagement on the part of some learners. Others were disappointed by the lack of structure. For some, it was possible to achieve satisfaction by presenting a clear, albeit paradoxical, structure by defining what we would do and how long the different elements would take, without abandoning the core approach. Others were gratified by a presentation of useful learning tools such as an annotated bibliography or a core chapter.

Using Learning Contracts during Inpatient Attending Months

One of the authors (C. Kaplan) has used learning contracts during several different services by requesting that house staff and students complete learning contracts throughout the month. The major barrier to using learner-centered approaches, during inpatient months is the overwhelming patient care responsibility faced by the house staff team. They often resist taking the time to complete the learning contracts. The author has found that supportively acknowledging the difficulty and encouraging learners to specify realistic goals will enable them to succeed. Many team members acknowledge a sense of satisfaction at the end of the month in having accomplished come specific albeit limited goals, rather than simply having survived the service.

Aside from encouraging limited and realistic goal setting, which ensures a sense of success, a confident and persistent posture is helpful when trying to activate learners in the relatively chaotic setting of a busy inpatient ward team. Presently, Kaplan meets briefly with each team member individually halfway through the month to review progress on learning contracts and tries to refer to them frequently during the month, often choosing topics to discuss during attending and work rounds that were included on one or more team members' learning contracts. For medical students, the learning contracts become the basis for 10- to 15-minute educational presentations throughout the month. Students are informed that the learning contract will provide the basis for part of their clerkship evaluation. In this way, the learning contracts become a functional part of the teaching.

Summary

This chapter has presented a brief introduction to the evolution of Lipkin's model for faculty development. It has presented both the history of the method and some educational theory that followed these developments.

Outstanding questions are numerous. Does this method apply to certain learners or to particular learning situations? What constitutes adequate preparation for this teaching? Does it work only for certain facilitators? How does it apply in situations where an absolute standard must be met for societal reasons—does all the necessary material get covered and learned? These and many other questions are currently being examined.

Contributors

Foreword

Michael A. Freeman, M.D. is the Chairman of the **Behavioral Healthcare** *Tomorrow* national dialogue conference, the Editor-in-Chief of the **Behavioral Healthcare** *Tomorrow* journal, and the series editor of the Managed Behavioral Healthcare Library. He also serves as the CEO of the Partnership for Behavioral Healthcare and the President of the Institute for Behavioral Healthcare; organizations dedicated to improving American and Global mental health and addiction treatment benefits, management, services and outcomes. Dr. Freeman has previously served as a health services planner for the Medicaid program in the Health Care Finance Administration, and as the corporate medical director of two large managed behavioral healthcare companies—U.S. Behavioral Health and American Psych Management of California (now Value Behavioral Health). He currently serves as a consultant to self-insured employers, health plans, delivery systems and government agencies that are working to solve challenges related to behavioral healthcare benefits and services. Dr. Freeman is a faculty member at the Langley Porter Psychiatric Institute of the University of California, San Francisco Medical Center. He is a noted public speaker within the healthcare and employee benefits fields.

Introduction

Marcia Byrnes, RN, M.P.A. is the Director of Primary Care Initiatives, where her responsibilities include strategically advising the Partnership for Behavioral Healthcare/CentraLink on resources, tools, and services for the integration of behavioral healthcare and primary care. Ms. Byrnes has a strong background in medical and psychiatric nursing, behavioral healthcare service delivery, and managed care. She previously served as the administrative director for St. Mary's Hospital and Medical Center in San Francisco, California and as manager of the 18-state midwest region for United Behavioral Healthcare (formerly US Behavioral Health). Before joining the Partnership for Behavioral Healthcare/CentraLink, she worked as the Executive Director of Quality Care Consortium, a multigroup, provider-owned network in the San Francisco Bay Area.

Part I Introduction

Chapter 1 *From Fragmentation to Integration:*
A History of Comprehensive Patient Care

Don R. Lipsitt, M.D. is Clinical Professor of Psychiatry at Harvard Medical School and Chairman of the Department of Psychiatry at Mount Auburn Hospital in Cambridge, Massachusetts. Dr. Lipsitt is Editor-in-Chief of *General Hospital Psychiatry* and *Somatization Newsletter*. Dr. Lipsitt holds the elected positions of President and President-elect of the Massachusetts Psychiatric Society and the International College of Psychosomatic Medicine respectively. In 1962, Dr. Lipsitt founded the Integration Clinic at the Beth Israel Hospital in Boston.

Chapter 2 *Integration of Primary Care and Behavioral Health:*
The Driving Forces

David R. Selden, A.C.S.W., LICSW is the President and founder of Enterprise Health Solutions, an innovative consulting company specializing in managed behavioral healthcare. A clinical social worker, his more than 20 years of experience includes work in both mental health and substance abuse services as a provider, manager, and leader in outpatient, inpatient, and alternative delivery systems in private and public sector settings and in managed care organizations. For the past ten years, Mr. Selden has been involved in the development and management of managed care systems and the most recent four years has been spent evaluating and implementing CQI initiatives for HMO behavioral health programs across the country. In addition, Mr. Selden has been involved in the development of HEDIS, NCQA behavioral health standards, and was the lead author for the behavioral health section of the Digital Equipment Corporation 1995 HMO Behavioral Health Standards, recognized as a landmark effort in the field.

Chapter 3 The Roles of the Behavioral Health Professional in Integrated Systems

Keith Dixon, Ph.D. is a graduate of the University of Minnesota and received graduate training from The College of St. Thomas (St. Paul, Minnesota) and The Union Institute (Cincinnati, Ohio), where he earned a Ph.D. in psychology. Dr. Dixon's experience in the private sector began in the development and marketing of corporate employee assistance programs in the early 1980s, consultation to community mental health centers regarding private sector opportunities, and with the Vista Hill Foundation in hospital PPO contracting, IPA formation, and in the initial development of the Foundation's managed care operations in the mid-1980s. Dr. Dixon also was Corporate Vice-President for ASSURED Health Systems, Inc., a national for-profit EAP/managed mental healthcare company based in Boston subsequently acquired by American Biodyne/Merit Behavioral Care Corporation. Dr. Dixon assumed his current responsibilities for Vista Behavioral Health Plans (Vista) in January, 1991. In 1992, Dr. Dixon was appointed to a three-year term to an advisory committee of the California State Department of Corporations – the state's HMO regulator. Dr. Dixon is currently Chairman of the Managed Behavioral Healthcare Association. He has authored numerous papers on EAP and managed behavioral healthcare and is a frequent speaker on these topics.

Part II Barriers to Integration

Chapter 4 Overcoming Ecological Barriers to Integration

Carol L. Alter, M.D. is the Associate Medical Director of CCC Medical Group, Inc. and the Director of Psychosocial Services and Cancer Pain Management of the Temple University Cancer Center. She serves as Chairman of the Managed Care Committee of the Academy of Psychosomatic Medicine and has been extensively involved in the development of and payment mechanisms for programs aimed at delivering psychosocial services for medically ill patients.

Steven Cole, M.D. is Professor of Psychiatry, Albert Einstein College of Medicine (Hillside Hospital Division) and Medical Director, Management Group of Greater New York, Inc. He has devoted his clinical, research, and educational career to developing better methods of treating patients with both psychiatric and general medical conditions. Dr. Cole is a board certified geriatric psychiatrist and has specialized in the treatment of depressed patients with neurological conditions.

Mary Raju, RN, M.S.N. is the Editor of the Greater NY/NJ Metro edition *of The Nursing Spectrum.* She is former Project Director, MacArthur Foundation Depression Education Project for Primary Care. With over 15 years experience as a clinician and instructor in medical-surgical nursing, Ms. Raju holds a master's degree in nursing education and is currently enrolled in a family nurse practitioner program. She has worked in medical communications for the last 8 years, including 1 year as the producer of Executive Nurse Update, a syndicated nationwide cable program for executive nurses.

Chapter 5 How to Structure the Financing of an Integrated System/Medical Cost Offset Model

Stephen P. Melek, FSA, MAAA is a consulting actuary with the Denver office of Milliman & Robertson, Inc. He joined the firm in 1990 after 14 years of health insurance company experience. His areas of expertise include healthcare product development, management, and financial analysis, with a particular emphasis in behavioral healthcare. Mr. Melek is a graduate of the Illinois Institute of Technology, a Fellow of the Society of Actuaries, a Member of the American Academy of Actuaries, and a Master Fellow of the Life Office Management Association.

Part III   Successful Models of Integration

Chapter 6   *Building Partnerships of Lasting Value in Healthcare: The Blue Cross and Blue Shield/Raytheon Collaboration*

Nancy Langman-Dorwart, M.S., M.P.H. is Vice President of Clinical Integration, CareGroup in Boston, Massachusetts. She was formerly Director of Mental Health and Clinical Director for the Raytheon Account, Blue Cross and Blue Shield Massachusetts. Ms. Langman-Dorwart has 15 years of managed care experience at Harvard Community Health Plan, Private Healthcare Systems, and Neighborhood Health Plan. Prior to working in managed care, Ms. Langman-Dorwart was a clinician and consultant with a broad range of experience. She has published multiple articles and is a regular speaker at national and local forums.

Elizabeth Gatti, Psy.D. is a clinical psychologist specializing in behavioral medicine for the treatment of anxiety disorders and stress-related illness. She consults to Blue Cross and Blue Shield Massachusetts on issues of prevention, wellness, and behavioral health. She is an Advanced Clinical Fellow at Harvard Medical School and an adjunct faculty member at the Massachusetts School of Professional Psychology. She also practices behavioral medicine at the University of Massachusetts Medical School and maintains a private practice.

Diane Duval is Director of Corporate Benefits at Raytheon Company, an international high technology company headquartered in Lexingon, Massachusetts. Her areas of responsibility include strategic planning, design, implementation, and administration of health, welfare, retirement, and work/life benefit programs. Prior to joining Raytheon, Ms. Duval was the Corporate Benefits Manager for Lotus Development Corporation. Ms. Duval holds a B.S. in Medical Technology and a M.S. in Health Service Administration. She serves as Director on the Board of the Massachusetts Health Care Purchasers Group and was a member of the Governor's Task Force on the Health Care Industry in Massachusetts.

Chapter 7   *The Integration Experience in a Group Model HMO: Northern California Kaiser-Permanente*

Robin Dea, M.D. trained at the University of New Mexico, interned at Highland Hospital in Oakland, California, and completed residency at California Pacific Medical Center in San Francisco. She became Chief of the Department of Psychiatry at Kaiser-Permanente Medical Center in Redwood City in 1981. From 1987 to 1989 and from 1991 to the present, she has been the elected Chair of the Chiefs of Psychiatry for Northern California Kaiser-Permanente. Since 1991, she has been the leader of the Psychiatry Coordinating Committee, whose assigned task is to completely re-engineer the mental health and chemical dependency system for Kaiser's Northern California Region. She has spoken at national conferences on mental health re-engineering, primary care integration, and the role of outcomes measurement in the creation of practice guidelines.

Chapter 8   *Integrated Systems in the Workplace: The Delta/Cigna/MCC Depression Initiative*

David Whitehouse, M.D., M.B.A. is Senior Vice President/Corporate Medical Director for MCC Behavioral Care, Inc. Responsible for clinical standards, policies and programs, Dr. Whitehouse is a member of MCC's Senior Management Team. He joined MCC in 1995 from Charles River Hospital in Massachusetts where he served as CEO and Medical Director. Prior to that, he was Chief of Psychiatry at St. Mary's Hospital in Waterbury, Connecticut; and Medical Director at Northeast Kingdom Mental Health Services in St. Johnsbury, Vermont. Additionally, Dr. Whitehouse has been an Assistant Clinical Professor for the Departments of Psychiatry at both Yale University School of Medicine and Dartmouth Medical School. Dr. Whitehouse graduated from Dartmouth Medical School and received his M.B.A. from the University of Connecticut. Dr. Whitehouse completed his residency in psychiatry at Massachusetts General Hospital where he acted as chief resident during the last year.

Chapter 9 Depression and Its Management in Primary Care: The Harvard Pilgrim Health Care Experience

Steve Stelovich, M.D. is the Associate Medical Director for mental health for the Boston and North Region of Harvard Pilgrim Health Care. He has led quality assurance efforts for the Department of Mental Health in the Commonwealth of Massachusetts as its past Director of Quality Assurance and has devoted significant time to developing programs for residency education in psychiatry at Harvard Medical School. During the past three years, he has spent increasing amounts of time developing programs for the early identification and treatment of mental disorders in primary care settings.

Chapter 10 High Utilizers of Health Services: The Purchaser Perspective and Experience with the Personal Health Improvement Program (PHIP)

Paul B. Johnson, M.D. is the Corporate Medical Director of US WEST, Inc. where he has worked since 1988. Prior to that, he headed the Chest and Occupational and Environmental Health Sections of the Department of Internal Medicine at St. Paul-Ramsey Medical Center in St. Paul, Minnesota from 1972 to 1988. Dr. Johnson is a graduate of Dartmouth College, Dartmouth Medical School, and the University of Minnesota Medical School. He did his residency and fellowship training at the University of Southwestern Medical School in Dallas, Texas and is board-certified in Internal Medicine and Pulmonary Diseases.

Lawrence B. Staubach, M.D., M.B.A. is currently Medical Director and Professional & Scientific Relations Manager for Health Delivery Systems at the Procter & Gamble (P&G) Company. In this role, Dr. Staubach is the primary technical relations liaison regarding P&G Healthcare products and services between P&G and key managed care customers and national managed care professional and trade organizations. He is responsible for assuring alignment between managed care customer needs and P&G products and services though long term relationships with medical, pharmacy, and healthcare executives and industry leaders. Dr. Staubach serves as Medical Director for the Personal Health Improvement Program and has served in a variety of medical affairs and clinical development positions in the pharmaceutical, over-the-counter, and food and beverage industries.

Anna P. Millar, M.B.A. graduated from Harvard Business School with distinction in 1996. Prior to obtaining her degree, she worked in marketing for Procter & Gamble for three years developing strategic direction and advertising for several pharmaceutical products. Ms. Millar returned to Procter & Gamble upon graduation and is currently a Brand Manager in the Health Care Sector. Her responsibilities now include developing strategies and programs that extend beyond P&G's traditional product line, thus meeting the needs of their healthcare customers. One of these programs is the Personal Health Improvement Program.

Chapter 11 The Group Practice Model: Allina Health System

Michael Trangle, M.D. is the Executive Medical Director of the Behavioral Health Services, Allina Health System. He is a graduate of Cornell University, University of Minnesota Medical School, and University of Wisconsin Residency/Chief Resident Program. In addition to his administrative duties, Dr. Trangle currently treats adolescents and adult psychiatric outpatients. In the past he has helped start and run chemical dependency programs, adolescent crisis evaluation and stabilization programs, and eating disorder programs in various clinics and hospitals.

Chapter 12 The Quality Improvement Model of Behavioral Health Group Practices

Allen S. Daniels, Ed.D. is the Chief Executive Officer for Alliance Behavioral Care and the Executive Director for University Psychiatric Services both affiliated with the Department of Psychiatry at the

University of Cincinnati. He is also Senior Director, Behavioral Care for the Alliance Partners, a partnership of the Health Alliance of Greater Cincinnati & Alliance Physicians and Surgeons, Ltd. Dr. Daniels, an Associate Professor of Psychiatry at the University of Cincinnati, College of Medicine, is a clinical social worker with extensive experience in the operation of academic group practices and the development of managed care programs.

Part IV Working in Primary Care Settings: What You Need to Know

Chapter 13 *The Primary Care Perspective: Culture and Reality*

Michael D. Cirigliano, M.D. is an Assistant Professor of Medicine at the University of Pennsylvania School of Medicine. He currently practices general internal medicine and is also responsible for supervising medical residents in the outpatient setting.

Mary F. Morrison, M.D. is an Assistant Professor of Psychiatry and Internal Medicine at the University of Pennsylvania School of Medicine. She is Co-Director of Medical and Consultation Psychiatry and the recipient of a career development award from the National Institutes of Mental Health to study depressive disorders in women.

Chapter 14 *Depression in Primary Care: Assessment and Management*

Steven Cole, M.D. is Professor of Psychiatry, Albert Einstein College of Medicine (Hillside Hospital Division) and Medical Director, Management Group of Greater New York, Inc. He has devoted his clinical, research, and educational career to developing better methods of treating patients with both psychiatric and general medical conditions. Dr. Cole is a board certified geriatric psychiatrist and has specialized in the treatment of depressed patients with neurological conditions.

Mary Raju, RN, M.S.N. is the Editor of the Greater NY/NJ Metro edition *of The Nursing Spectrum.* She is former Project Director, MacArthur Foundation Depression Education Project for Primary Care. With over 15 years experience as a clinician and instructor in medical-surgical nursing, Ms. Raju holds a master's degree in nursing education and is currently enrolled in a family nurse practitioner program. She has worked in medical communications for the last 8 years, including 1 year as the producer of Executive Nurse Update, a syndicated nationwide cable program for executive nurses.

James Barrett, M.D. is Emeritus Research Professor of Community and Family Medicine and Psychiatry at Dartmouth Medical School. Trained in psychiatry and research methodology, he has followed a full time research career devoted to outcome studies, treatment evaluation, and epidemiology. For the past 17 years, as Principal Investigator on NIMH-funded research and training grants, his activities have focused on the interface between psychiatry and primary care with a long-term commitment to improving the recognition and management of depressive disorders in the primary care sector. Dr. Barrett played a major role in the development of the John D. and Catherine T. MacArthur Foundation Depression Project in Primary Care, and served as its Director from 1994-1996.

Chapter 15 *Anxiety Disorders in Primary Care*

Mack Lipkin, Jr., M.D. is Professor of Medicine and Director of the Division of Primary Care, New York University School of Medicine, Founding President of the American Academy on Physician and Patient, and was Past-President of the Society of General Internal Medicine from 1992-1993. Dr. Lipkin is Vice-Chairman and Vice-President of the Psychiatric Education in Primary Care Alliance. He has written or edited eleven books, authored hundreds of articles and chapters on the medical encounter, the doctor-patient relationship, and psychosocial and psychiatric issues in primary care, and talks, writes, researches, and consults on these issues internationally.

Chapter 16 *Clinical Presentation, Screening, and Treatment of Substance Abuse in the Primary Care Setting*

Thomas Horst, M.D., M.P.H. is Chief of Chemical Dependency Medical Services in the Behavioral Health

Division, and a practicing Family Physician at Group Health Cooperative of Puget Sound in Seattle, Washington. Board certified in Family Practice in 1982, Dr. Horst was certified in Addiction Medicine in 1994.

Chapter 17 Clinical Presentation, Screening, and Treatment of Somatization in Primary Care

Steven E. Locke, M.D. is the Chief of Behavioral Medicine at Harvard Pilgrim Health Care. He is also the Director of Psychiatric Informatics at Boston's Beth Israel-Deaconess Medical Center. Dr. Locke teaches at Harvard Medical School and Massachusetts Institute of Technology as an Associate Professor of Psychiatry. Dr. Locke received his undergraduate degree from Cornell University, his medical degree from Columbia University College of Physicians and Surgeons, his residency in psychiatry at McLean Hospital, and post-graduate fellowship in both consultation-liaison psychiatry and biobehavioral sciences research from Boston University School of Medicine. He served as Associate and Acting Director of the psychiatry consultation services at Boston's Beth Israel Hospital and was the founding director of the hospital's Stress Disorders Program. He also was the founding director of the primary care psychiatry service at the Beth Israel-Children's Hospital Medical Center in Lexington, Massachusetts. Dr. Locke has served on the editorial boards of *Psychotherapy and Psychosomatics, M.D. Computing, Biofeedback and Self-Regulation, Medical Psychotherapy, International Journal of Clinical and Experimental Hypnosis, Psychoanalytic Quarterly, American Journal of Health Promotion,* and *American Health* magazine. He is a Fellow of the American Psychiatric Association and author or editor of numerous books and journal articles.

Katharine M. Larsson, RN, M.S., CS is a behavioral medicine specialist. Ms. Larsson became interested in behavioral medicine during her years of medical and psychiatric nursing experience and has always wanted to bridge the gap between the two disciplines. She obtained her graduate degree in psychiatric mental health nursing from Boston College. Her graduate and postgraduate clinical training took place at The Cambridge Hospital in the outpatient Psychiatry and Behavioral Medicine Departments. Ms. Larsson currently works with Dr. Steven Locke at Harvard Pilgrim Health Care in their Behavioral Medicine Department and at The Cambridge Hospital as a biofeedback clinician.

Chapter 18 The Mind-Body Connection: Outcomes Research in the Real World

Marcie Parker, Ph.D., CFLE is Senior Qualitative Researcher and Manager of Senior Programs with Optum, a division of United HealthCare Corporation. She holds a Doctorate in Family Social Science from the University of Minnesota and is a Certified Family Life Educator and a Fellow in The Gerontological Society of America. Dr. Parker has served as Senior Research Associate with InterStudy, responsible for research and policy studies in health care, managed care, aging, long-term care, and case management. She is widely published in these areas as well as in rural and minority healthcare issues.

R. Edward Bergmark, Ph.D. has been President of Optum since June, 1990. Previously, he has held a number of positions with Control Data Corporation. He is a Licensed Psychologist and attended The University of St. Thomas for an M.A. in Counseling Psychology and The University of Minnesota for a Ph.D. in Counseling Psychology. Dr. Bergmark is widely published in managed care, case management, demand management, and employee assistance. He has also been keynote speaker at many national meetings, speaking on such topics as drug prevention in the workplace, balancing work and family, using technology to improve quality and efficiency, healthcare reform, managing the costs of mental health, confidentiality, and integrating medical and psychosocial healthcare for greater effectiveness of behavioral health interventions.

Mark Attridge, Ph.D. is Research Specialist with Optum. He consults on survey projects, measurement issues, statistical analysis, and database development for applied business problems in healthcare. His past positions include grant-funded academic research and teaching psychology and communication courses in various academic settings. Dr. Attridge's Doctorate is in social psychology. He has published several book chapters and empirical research papers and serves as a reviewer for several academic journals.

Part V The Future of Behavioral Health and Primary Care Integration

Chapter 19 Training for Interdisciplinary Practice: Trends in Clinical Psychology and Family Medicine

Thomas M. DiLorenzo, Ph.D. is an Associate Professor and Chair of the Department of Psychology at the University of Missouri in Columbia. Dr. DiLorenzo received a B.S. in Psychology and a B.A. in Economics from the University of Pittsburgh and a M.A. and Ph.D. in Clinical Psychology from West Virginia University. He completed his residency at the University of Mississippi Medical Center. Dr. DiLorenzo's main research interests are in the general area of health psychology and the interface of behavioral health and primary care.

Harold A. Williamson, M.D., M.S.P.H. is Professor and Associate Chair of the Department of Family and Community Medicine at the University of Missouri in Columbia. He received a B.A. in Biology from St. Olaf College and an M.D. from Case Western Reserve University. Dr. Williamson completed his residency at the University of Missouri in Columbia. His main research interests are in the areas of rural health, rural inpatient services, and physician staffing issues.

Chapter 20 Computerized Technology: Integrative Treatment Outcome Technology in Primary Care Practice

Len Sperry, M.D., Ph.D. is a Professor in the Departments of Psychiatry and Behavioral Medicine and in Preventive Medicine at the Medical College of Wisconsin. Board certified in both Psychiatry and Preventive Medicine, he has published dozens of professional books and hundreds of articles and chapters in these fields. He has taught primary care residents and has also been involved in health service delivery research involving primary care providers. In addition, Dr. Sperry has been involved in the development and clinical application of COMPASS-PC.

Peter L. Brill, M.D. the founder, CEO, and Chairman of Compass Information Services Inc., is a board certified psychiatrist with over 25 years experience in psychiatry and organizational counseling. At present, Dr. Brill is an Adjunct Associate Professor in the Department of Psychiatry at the University of Pennsylvania, and a Senior Fellow with the Medical College of Wisconsin. He has authored numerous papers, books, and articles, and has lectured and consulted at major corporations on issues such as corporate culture, work stress, employee assistance programs, mental health and substance abuse, case management, and adult development.

Chapter 21 The Future of Behavioral Health and Primary Care: How Are We Doing?

Grant E. Mitchell, M.D. is a co-owner of Prime Care Consultants, a consulting company dedicated to the integration of primary care and behavioral healthcare. He is also President and founder of Prime Care Psychiatric & Behavioral Health Services, a multidisciplinary group practice in White Plains, New York. Additionally, Dr. Mitchell serves as Director of Mental Health Services for The Mount Vernon Hospital. Dr. Mitchell received a B.A. from Vassar College, a M.D. from New York Medical College, and completed residency training and was Chief Resident Physician in psychiatry at The New York Medical College Consortium-Psychiatric Institute. Dr. Mitchell is the author and editor of numerous publications and speaks on issues related to the interface between primary care and behavioral health, chronic fatigue syndrome, and pain management.

Joel D. Haber, Ph.D. is a co-owner of Prime Care Consultants, a consulting company dedicated to the integration of primary care and behavioral healthcare. He is also founder and Clinical Director of Prime Care Psychiatric & Behavioral Health Services, a multidisciplinary group practice in White Plains, New

York. Additionally, he is developing a primary care/behavioral health alternative medicine program within a hospital setting. Previously, he directed two interdisciplinary pain centers in hospital/academic settings. He has published numerous articles on the relationship between psychological disorders seen in medical conditions. Dr. Haber received a B.A. from the State University of New York at Binghamton, and a M.S. and Ph.D. from the University of Georgia. Dr. Haber is the author and editor of numerous publications and speaks on issues related to primary care and behavioral healthcare integration, and pain and stress management.

Annotated Bibliography

Marcia Kaplan, M.D. is the Medical Director of Alliance Behavioral Care, a managed behavioral healthcare organization and of University Psychiatric Services, a multidisciplinary group practice affiliated with the University of Cincinnati Department of Psychiatry.

Index

Absence management, 99-103
  Managed Time Loss model, 22-23
Absenteeism, 20
  depression and, 141, 273
  somatization and, 182
Abuse, see Domestic violence
Access to behavioral healthcare, see also Referral
  carve-outs and, 37
  copayments and, 21-22, 239
  in group practices, 122, 123-124
  management of, 206
Accreditation, by NCQA, 30, 122-126, 207
ADHD
  costs of testing for, 28
  patient education, 81
Adherence, see Patient adherence
Adjustment disorder with anxious mood, 156-157, 161-162
Adjustment disorder with depressed mood, 141, 142, 143
Adolescents, substance abuse in, 168, 173
Affective disorders
  medical utilization and, 141
Agoraphobia, 155, 159
AHCPR Depression in Primary Care Guidelines, 43, 90
AIDS
  case management, 44
  substance abuse and, 167, 172
Alcohol abuse, see Substance abuse
Alcohol dependence, definition of, 168
Alcoholics Anonymous, 173, 202
Alcohol Use Disorders Inventory Test (AUDIT), 170
Alexithymia, 4, 181
Allina Health System, 115-119
  integration models
    former carve-outs, 118-119
    multispecialty group, 117-118
    site-based, 116-117
    works in progress, 118
  overall structure, 115-116
Alternative medicine, 185, 241
Americans with Disabilities Act
  medical costs and, 87

Angry patient, 134-135
Anhedonia, 141, 148
Antabuse (disulfiram), 174
Antidepressants
  for anxiety disorders
    generalized anxiety disorder, 161
    obsessive-compulsive disorder, 163
    panic disorder, 159
    post-traumatic stress disorder, 162
  for depression, 143-145, 151
    Harvard Pilgrim program, 96
  patient acceptance of SSRIs, 143-144, 239
  pharmacology of, 143-145
Anxiety disorders, 155-164
  with asthma, 269
  with coronary disease, 275
  diagnosis, 155-157, 158-159
    vs. medical disorders, 156, 158, 164
  excess medical costs with, 157-158, 159, 269
  functional impairment, 274
  primary care physician's role, 155, 157-158, 164
  specific disorders
    adjustment disorder with anxious mood, 156-157, 161-162
    generalized anxiety disorder, 156, 160-161
    obsessive-compulsive disorder, 157, 162-163
    panic disorder, 55, 63, 76-78, 112, 155, 159, 269
    post-traumatic stress disorder, 157, 162
    simple phobia, 157, 163-164
    social phobia, 157, 164
  treatment, 159-164
Asthma
  anxiety disorders with, 269
  disease management programs, 65-66, 208
  PHIP patient education program, 112
At-risk drinkers
  brief interventions, 172
  definition of, 168

Attention-deficit hyperactivity disorder, see ADHD
AUDIT (Alcohol Use Disorders Inventory Test), 170

Bad news, delivering to patient, 132-133
BATHE, 131, 242
Battered women, see Domestic violence
Beck Depression Inventory, 184
Behavioral healthcare, see also Integration of primary care and behavioral health
  interface with primary care, 17-19, 136-137
  as percent of healthcare budget, 13, 30, 261
Behavioral health disorders, see also Anxiety disorders; Depression; Somatization; Substance abuse
  prevalence, 13-16, 20, 237, 262-263
  undertreatment, 13
    with capitation, 22
    of depression, 16, 19, 20, 140
Behavioral health plans, see Carved-out behavioral health services
Behavioral health providers, 136-137; see also Psychiatric nurses; Psychiatrists; Psychologists; Social workers
  privileging for, 39-40, 41, 125
  in risk-sharing arrangements, 50-51, 52-54
  training of
    about medical illness, 22, 80, 242
    on BCBSMA integrated team, 63-64
    psychiatrists, for new roles, 28-29
    psychologists, 213-214, 216-218, 222-224, 226-227
Behavioral therapy, see Cognitive-behavioral therapy
Benefits, see Capitation; Financial structure of integrated systems; Reimbursement

INDEX

Benefits managers, survey of, 194–196
Bereaved patient, 135
Biases of physician, 132
Biomedical model, 129, 137, 180, 223
Biopsychosocial model, 9, 180
  economic forces and, 190
  medical training and, 223, 242
  in outcomes research, 193, 208
    Optum Care24 telephone service, 196–198
    public employee survey, 199
Blue Cross and Blue Shield/Raytheon collaboration, 59–74
  corporate partner (Raytheon), 59–60
  customer service, 69–70
  disease management, 64, 65–68
  employee transition, 61–63, 64, 70
  guiding principles, 59, 61
  healthcare company (BCBSMA), 60–61
  incentive performance standards, 64–65
  integrated care model, 63–64
  member services, 70–72
  prevention programs, 59, 60, 61, 64–65, 68–69, 70–72, 74
  results, first-year, 73–74
  strategy, 60, 61–62
  team building, 73–74
  technological support, 72–73
Body dysmorphic disorder, 180
Breast cancer
  BCBSMA/Raytheon initiatives, 67–68
Brief Symptom Inventory (BSI), 110, 184
Buprenorphine, for opioid dependence, 174
Burnout, of physicians, 133

CAGE questionnaire, 169–170
  in BCBSMA/Raytheon collaboration, 72
  built into routine forms, 171
Cancer
  breast, BCBSMA/Raytheon initiatives, 67–68
  comprehensive centers, 44–45
Capitation
  in carve-out models, 18, 37
    Allina Health System, 115, 116, 118–119
    Comprehensive Cancer Centers and, 44–45
    Harvard Pilgrim depression program and, 93, 96
  as incentive for inpatient treatment, 22
  in integrated systems, 24, 28
    ODS model, 23–24
  physicians' time limitations and, 29
Cardiovascular disease
  anxiety disorders with, 275
  disease management programs, 65, 67, 208
  excess costs in distressed patients, 272
  major depression after MI, 140, 275
  presurgery alternative healing program, 241
Carpal tunnel syndrome, 63
Cartesian dualism, 5–6, 10, 11, 35, 223
Carved-in behavioral health services, see Integration of primary care and behavioral health
Carved-out behavioral health services, 11, 16, 29–30
  in Allina Health System, 115, 116, 118–119
  inpatient case example, 38–41
  integration with, 18, 19, 30, 36–37
  medical cost offsets and, 30, 52, 87–88
  noncompliance with referrals, 90–91
  pre-authorization, 39, 41
Case finding, see also Screening
  in BCBSMA/Raytheon collaboration, 64
  in Kaiser-Permanente Northern California, 77–78, 84, 85
  medical cost offsets and, 55
  for somatizing patients, 184, 185, 187
Case management, see also Disease management
  of absences from work, 22–23, 99–103
  in BCBSMA/Raytheon collaboration, 63–64, 69–70
  in chronic illness, 44–45
Chemical dependency, see Substance abuse
Chronic depression (dysthymia), 139, 141, 142–143, 145
Chronic illness, see also Case management; Disease management
  prevalence of mental disorders with, 24, 263
  psychological distress and, 183, 186
  specialized services, 37, 44–45
Chronic pain, see Pain management
CIGNA, see Delta/CIGNA/MCC depression initiative
Claims submission, electronic, 72
Clinical protocols, 125, 241
Clinical psychologists, see Psychologists
Clinics, hospital-based, 3–4, 11, 184
Cocaine dependence, 173
Cognitive-behavioral therapy
  advantages for managed care, 213
  for anxiety disorders
    generalized anxiety disorder, 161
    obsessive-compulsive disorder, 163
    panic disorder, 159
    social phobia, 164
  for depression, 145, 241
  at Kaiser-Permanente, 80
  outcomes research, 194, 241
  by psychologists, 136
  for somatization, 186
Collaboration, see also Integration of primary care and behavioral health
  levels of, 242–243, 293–295
Commitment, involuntary, 150
Communication among providers, 40, 75–76, 77, 223
Communication skills, 131–133, 147–150
  with angry patient, 134–135
  with bereaved patient, 135
  with nonadherent patient, 135
  training in, 36, 242, 311–322
Community mental health movement, 9, 10
Comorbidities, psychological, see also High utilizers; Medical cost offsets
  in cardiac patients, 140, 272, 275
  in chronic illness, 24, 44–45, 263
  costs of inappropriate treatment, 45
  depression as, 139, 140
  integrated management of, 63–64
  in medical inpatients, 264, 277
    case example, 38–41
  prevalence, 13
  somatization with mental disorders, 181, 186
  in telephone consultation calls, 197–198
Compass-INT, 231

INDEX

Compass-OP, 231
Compass-PC, 230-231, 233, 235
Complementary medicine, 185, 241
Compliance, *see* Patient adherence
Comprehensive Cancer Centers, Inc., 44-45
Comprehensive care, *see* Integration of primary care and behavioral health
Computer systems
   in BCBSMA/Raytheon collaboration, 72-73
   for integrated healthcare, 23, 24, 190
   in Kaiser-Permanente Northern California, 77, 82-83
   for outcomes assessment, 229-234
   for telephone screening, 131, 240, 297
   for treatment planning, 231-232, 233-234
   for virtual team approach, 22
Confidentiality
   with chemical dependency, 83, 175
   employers and, 91, 102-103
   in integrated systems, 40, 223
      group practices, 123-124, 126
      Kaiser-Permanente, 82-83
   psychiatrists' attitudes, 136
Consultation, *see also* Referral
   with on-site behavioral health providers, 37, 42, 44, 124
      in Harvard Pilgrim Health Care, 185
      in hierarchy of collaboration, 243
      in Kaiser-Permanente, 80, 84
      for substance abuse treatment, 175
   with psychiatrists, 42
      consultation-liaison subspecialty, 9-10, 41, 255-288
      in Harvard Pilgrim depression program, 94, 96, 97
      inpatient case example, 38-41
      for somatization, 283
Consultation-liaison psychiatry, 9-10
   definition of, 286
   reimbursement issues, 41
   slide show with lecture notes, 255-288
Consumers
   as constituency for integration, 21-22
   ignorance about behavioral health, 19
   reliance on PCP, 18-19

Continuous Quality Improvement (CQI), 21, 23
Conversion disorder, 180
"Coordination of care" agreements, 36-37
Copayments, parity in, 21-22, 239
Cornell Medical Index, 184
Cost models
   for financing of integrated system, 47-48
   structural, 22-24
Costs, *see also* Medical cost offsets; Reimbursement
   of alcohol abuse, 16
   of behavioral healthcare
      carved-out, 37
      copayments, 21-22, 239
      fraction of healthcare budget, 13, 30, 261
      inpatient treatment, 22
      by PCPs, 24
   of healthcare
      aging population and, 16-17
      employer stake in, 21, 87-88
      inflation of, 16
      prevention and, 65
   of mental disorders, 35, 43, 45, 63
      after cardiac hospitalization, 272
      anxiety disorders, 157-158, 159, 269
      depression, 15, 93, 139, 141, 268, 271
      somatization, 106, 182, 184, 267
   of psychological testing, 28
   of quality improvement programs, 123
Counseling, *see* Psychotherapy; Supportive counseling
Counselors, nondoctoral-level
   for telephone consultation, 196, 206
   training of, 217
CQI (Continuous Quality Improvement), 21, 23
Credentialing, for managed care companies, 125
Cultural factors
   in depression treatment, 140
   in doctor-patient relationship, 132
   in somatization, 183
Customer service
   in BCBSMA/Raytheon collaboration, 69-70

Deductibles, parity in, 21-22
Delirium, in medical patients, 275, 277

Delta/CIGNA/MCC depression initiative, 87-92
   comprehensive plan, 89-91
   goals, 87-89
   issues to be resolved, 91-92
Demand-side management, *see* Utilization management
Dementia, missed diagnosis of, 277
Depression
   bereavement causing, 135
   in cardiac patients, 140, 275
   with chemical dependency, 174
   clinical guidelines (AHCPR), 43, 90
   consumer ignorance about, 19
   Delta/CIGNA/MCC initiative, 87-92
   economics of, 15, 93, 139, 141, 268, 271
   fatigue presenting as, 129
   functional impairment, 274
   Harvard Pilgrim Health Care program, 93-98
   morbidity and mortality, 140, 275
   patient education about, 81, 111
   physical causes of, 139
   practice guidelines, Kaiser-Permanente, 76-77
   prevalence, 15, 93, 139
   primary care physicians and
      AHCPR guidelines, 43, 90
      communication with patient, 147-151
      consultation with psychiatrist, 282
      diagnosis, 139-140, 141-142
      follow-up, 145
      management strategies, 142-143
      outcomes, 278
      pharmacotherapy, 143-145, 151
      physician reluctance, 230
      referral to specialist, 145, 147, 150, 151
      supportive office counseling, 145, 147
      training programs, 36, 139
   psychotherapy for, 145, 147, 241
   screening
      in BCBSMA/Raytheon collaboration, 70, 72
      Beck Depression Inventory, 184
      in Delta/CIGNA/MCC initiative, 90, 91
      in Harvard Pilgrim program, 94-95, 97

Depression, screening (*cont.*)
  National Depression Screening Day, 16, 239
  simplified test, 94, 95
  secondary to panic disorder, 159
  types of, 139, 141–142
  undertreatment of, 16, 19, 20, 140
Depressive disorder not otherwise specified (NOS), 141
Diabetes
  disease management programs, 66–67, 208
  PHIP patient education, 112
Diagnosis, *see* Screening
Difficult bosses, research on, 200
Difficult patients, *see also* High utilizers
  angry, 134–135
  computer profiling and, 231
  somatizing, 189
Disability
  depression and, 273
  employer management of, 22–23, 99–102, 103, 238
  in primary care setting, 134
Disease management, *see also* Case management
  in BCBSMA/Raytheon collaboration, 64, 65–68
  Delta/CIGNA/MCC depression initiative as, 89
  in Kaiser-Permanente Northern California, 84
  programs developed by Optum, 207–208
Disease model, vs. psychosocial factors, 104–105
Disulfiram (Antabuse), 174
Doctor-patient relationship, 132, 244; *see also* Communication skills
Domestic violence
  primary care physician and, 133–134
  telephone consultation, 202–203
Drug abuse, *see* Substance abuse
Drug dependence, definitions of, 167, 168, 172
DSM IV PC, 43, 129–130, 131
  subsyndromal conditions and, 238
Dualism, 5–6, 10, 11, 35, 223
Dysthymia (chronic depression), 139, 141, 142–143, 145

Early Start Program, 20, 55, 78
Ecology, of healthcare systems, 35, 36–37
Economics, *see* Costs

Education, *see* Medical education; Patient education; Training
Elderly patients
  depression in, 140
  medical cost offsets for, 24, 88
Electronic claims submission, 72
Employee assistance programs
  alcohol treatment in, 16
  as carve-outs, 30
  of Raytheon, 63
Employers
  absence management by, 22–23, 99–103
  carve-outs and, 129–31
  cost-consciousness of, 21
  difficult bosses, research on, 200
  risk management survey, 194–196
Engel, George, 9, 180
Evidence-based medicine, 213, 220
Exercise programs, 72, 186

False negatives and positives, 169
Families
  in BCBSMA/Raytheon collaboration, 62, 64
  employer services for, 195, 196
  medical claims study, 199–200
Family medicine training, *see also* Primary care physicians
  current models, 219–220
  financing for, 223–224, 242
  historical perspectives, 9, 215–216
  integrated with behavioral health, 10, 213, 218, 219–220
  managed care and, 220, 221
  potential changes, 220–221
  residency curriculum, 219, 228
Family therapy, by social workers, 136
Fatigue, depression presenting as, 129
Fax on demand, of medical policies, 73
Fee-for-service, vs. integrated care, 11
Fee structures, 41, 48, 51, 239
Financial structure of integrated systems, 47–55; *see also* Reimbursement
  continual improvement process, 47, 51
  cost model development, 47–48
  fee structures, 41, 48, 51, 239
  medical cost offsets, 51–55
    aggregate approach, 52–53, 55
    specific approach, 53–55

  provider incentives, 48–49
  risk pools, 49–51
Flexner Report, 8, 215, 314
Fragmentation, *see* Carved-out behavioral health services; Integration of primary care and behavioral health
FRAMES, 172

Gatekeeper systems
  consultants' role in, 40
  fragmentation of services in, 18, 24, 123
  psychosocial medicine in, 9, 11
General Health Questionnaire, 184
Generalized anxiety disorder (GAD), 156, 160–161
Government healthcare policies, 45
Group model HMO, *see* Kaiser-Permanente Northern California
Group practice
  Allina Health System, 115–119
  defining characteristics, 121
  quality improvement model, 121–126
    access and referral, 123–124
    clinical records, 126
    credentialing, 125
    prevention services, 125–126
    quality programs, 122–123, 126
    rights and responsibilities, 124
    utilization management, 124
Group therapy
  for panic disorder, 159
  for post-traumatic stress disorder, 162
  by social workers, 136
  for somatization disorder, 283
Guidelines
  for depression in primary care, 43, 90
  Kaiser-Permanente, 76–77, 84

Hamilton Anxiety Scale, 184
Harvard Pilgrim Health Care
  depression program, 93–98
  Personal Health Improvement Program, 104–112, 186
  somatization, team approach, 185–186
Health assessment surveys
  in BCBSMA/Raytheon collaboration, 71–72
  Health Status Questionnaire 2.0, 110
  with routine physical exams, 238, 240

INDEX

Health Care Financing Administration, 220-221, 223-224
Health psychology, 214, 216, 217, 218
Health Wire, 72-73
HEDIS (Health Employer Data Information Set), 30, 207
High utilizers, 3-4; *see also* Somatization
  in capitation systems, 18
  depression in, 139, 141
  employer/purchaser perspective, 99-104
  medical cost offsets and, 88
  patient education for, 104-112, 186
  percent of services used by, 265
  prevalence of psychiatric disorders in, 266
  prevention and, 125
  referral out, by PCP, 19
  somatization in, 4, 106, 182
  undiagnosed behavioral health conditions in, 13-15, 184
HIV, *see* AIDS
HMOs, *see also* Harvard Pilgrim Health Care; Kaiser-Permanente Northern California
  carve-outs acquired by, 30
  medical education and, 223
  Minnesota licensure requirements, 115
  withhold arrangements with, 49
Hospitalization, *see* Inpatient behavioral healthcare
Hospital privileges, 39-40, 41, 125
Hospital risk pools, 49, 50
Hysteria, *see* Somatization

Incentives
  financial structuring of, 47, 48-49, 239
  performance standards, BCBSMA/Raytheon, 64-65
Indirect costs, *see* Medical cost offsets
Inflation of healthcare costs, 16
Inpatient behavioral healthcare
  involuntary, of suicidal patient, 150
  overuse, in fragmented systems, 22
  for substance abuse, 174
Insomnia, 129
Insurance companies, *see also* Reimbursement
  in Allina Health System, 115, 116

integrated care and, 239
medical records and, 223
Requests for Proposals and, 45
Integration Clinic, 3-4, 11, 184
Integration of primary care and behavioral health, *see also* Carved-out behavioral health services; Financial structure of integrated systems
  barriers to, 31, 186-187, 229-230
  ecological, 35, 36-37
  computer systems for, 23, 24, 190, 229-234
  consultation-liaison psychiatry in, 284-285
  definition of, 4-5
  driving forces for
    costs, 16-17
    dysfunction in current system, 17-22
    prevalence of behavioral health disorders, 13-16
  historical aspects
    integrated training, 7-10
    Integration Clinic, 3-4, 11, 184
    integration of disciplines, 7-10
    integration of healthcare systems, 10-12
  levels of collaboration, 242-243, 293-295
  mechanisms for, 37-38
    inpatient example, 38-41
    outpatient example, 41-44
  mind-body connection and, 5-7, 9-10, 35
  models of
    Allina Health System, 115-119
    BCBSMA/Raytheon collaboration, 59-74
    Delta/CIGNA/MCC depression initiative, 87-92
    Harvard Pilgrim depression program, 93-98
    Kaiser-Permanente Northern California, 75-85
    Personal Health Improvement Program, 104-112, 186
    quality improvement group model, 121-126
    US West, for high utilizers, 102-104
  outcomes research and, 193, 194, 208
  problems and solutions, 237-242
    appropriate management, 239
    recognition of mental disorders, 237-238

screening issues, 239-240
training issues, 242
treatment issues, 240-242
professional roles and, 27-31
somatization and, 184-185, 189-190
structural models for, 22-24, 30
for substance abuse treatment, 171-172, 175
training for
  in medical education, 10, 213, 218, 219-220, 221, 242
  in psychology curriculum, 213, 218, 222-223, 226-227
Interdisciplinary education, 213, 221-224
Internet, *see also* Web sites
  as screening tool, 240
Internists, *see also* Primary care physicians
  in multidisciplinary teams, 185, 186, 187
  training of, 10, 216, 221, 242
Interviewing, *see also* Communication skills
  Lipkin model, 311-322
Investors, integration and, 22

Kaiser-Permanente Northern California, 75-85
  basic structure of system, 75
  Early Start Program, 20, 55, 78
  pre-1993 system, 75-76
  primary care integration, 76-85
    behavioral health education, 80-81
    case finding, 77-78, 84, 85
    data systems, 77, 82-83
    on-site integration, 80, 84
    Psychiatry Model of Care for, 76-77, 85
    redesigning primary care, 83-85
    specialized programs, 78-79

Lawsuits, 134-135
Legitimation, of patient emotions, 149, 151
Lifestart program, 70
Limit setting, 189
Lipkin model, 311-322
  educational model, 311-315
  faculty development model, 315-319
  other uses of, 319-322
Low back pain, chronic, 63, 134

Major depression, 141, 142, 143-147

INDEX

Managed care, *see also* Integration of primary care and behavioral health
　BCBSMA reorganization for, 60
　behavioral group practices under, 122
　clinical psychology training and, 217, 218, 224
　contracts for, 45
　cost control results, 16, 261
　cost models and, 47
　credentialing for, 125
　family medicine training and, 220, 221
　as opportunity for integration, 9, 10–11
　short-term behavioral therapies for, 213, 217
　specialists' roles under, 27–29
　time limitations under, 130
Managed Time Loss model, 22–23
MCC, *see* Delta/CIGNA/MCC depression initiative
Medical cost offsets, 87–88; *see also* Comorbidities, psychological
　in BCBSMA/Raytheon collaboration, 64
　carve-out market and, 30, 52, 87–88
　documentation of, 123, 189–190, 194
　evidence for, 19–20, 24, 88, 194
　　in adjustment disorder, 233–234
　　in alcoholism treatment, 16, 51, 281
　　in hip fracture management, 280
　　with telephone consultation, 199–200, 203–207
　financial structures for, 51–55
　in Kaiser-Permanente, 77, 79
　from prevention services, 125
Medical education, *see also* Training, of primary care physicians
　curricula, 215, 219, 220, 221, 222
　historical perspectives, 7–9
　proposed changes, 242
　emotions in, 312, 314, 317, 319–320
Medical illness, *see* Chronic illness; Comorbidities, psychological; Medical cost offsets
Medical records, *see also* Confidentiality
　for behavioral group practices, 126

electronic, 190, 242
　as legal documentation, 135
　sharing, in integrated systems, 40
Medical tests, unnecessary
　with anxiety disorders, 55, 157–158
　with somatization, 179, 182
Medications, *see also* Antidepressants
　for chemical dependency, 174
　depression caused by, 139
　on-line prescription records, 82
　psychotropic, prescribed by PCPs, 20, 27–28
Meditrax, 72–73
Mental health services, *see* Behavioral healthcare
Mental illness, *see* Behavioral health disorders
Methadone, for opioid dependence, 174
Michigan Alcoholism Screening Test, 169
Mind-body connection, 5–7, 9–10, 35, 180; *see also* Somatization
　patient education about, 81, 105, 106–107, 111
Minor depression, 141, 142, 143
Multidisciplinary teams, *see* Team approaches

Naltrexone (Revia), 174
NCQA (National Committee for Quality Assurance), 30, 122–126, 207
Nurse practitioners
　counseling services by, 137
　in primary care, 83, 179
Nurses
　counseling services by, 137
　interdisciplinary education for, 222
　on Kaiser-Permanente team, 83
　in telephone consultation services, 70–71, 196, 204–207
Nursing home patients, depression in, 140
Nutrition information
　in BCBSMA/Raytheon collaboration, 71

Obsessive-compulsive disorder, 157, 162–163
ODS (Organized Delivery Systems) model, 23–24
Opioid dependence, pharmacotherapy of, 174

Optum research programs, *see* Outcomes research
OSC (Organized Systems of Care) model, 23
Outcome for Windows, 230, 231–232, 233, 235
Outcome Questionnaire-10, 232, 235
Outcome Questionnaire-45, 230, 232, 235
Outcomes assessment
　computerized systems for, 229–234
　for depression treatment, 145, 146
　for somatization treatment, 189–190
Outcomes research, 193–194; *see also* Medical cost offsets, evidence for
　annotated bibliography on, 248–250
　on behavioral health treatment, 16, 194
　depression in primary care, 278
　on cognitive-behavioral therapy, 194, 241
　on disease management program, 208
　on Personal Health Improvement Program, 111–112
　on telephone consultation services, 200–203
　　deferred healthcare visits, 203–204
　　diversions by NurseLine, 204–206
　　family effects, 199–200
　　medical cost offsets, 199–200, 203–207
Oversupply of physicians, 220–221
Overutilization, *see* High utilizers

Pain disorder, 180
Pain management
　alternative treatments, 241
　in BCBSMA/Raytheon collaboration, 63, 64
　Kaiser-Permanente pain clinic, 78–79
　in Personal Health Improvement Program, 186
　in primary care setting, 134
Panic disorder, 155, 159
　case finding, 55, 63, 77–78
　excess medical costs with, 269
　PHIP patient education for, 112

practice guidelines (Kaiser-
    Permanente), 76-78
Patient adherence, *see also* Stigma
    of behavioral disorders
  with antidepressant therapy, 151
  with behavioral health referrals,
    20, 90-91, 155, 189
  with cancer therapy, 67
  computerized prediction of, 231
  expectations of patient
    and, 149
  in somatization disorders, 182
Patient education, *see also*
    Personal Health Improvement
    Program
  about depression, 81, 111
  in disease management pro-
    grams, 65-68, 207, 208
  Kaiser-Permanente programs,
    80-81, 84
  for partnership with pro-
    viders, 244
  proposed national data
    bank, 241
Patient Problem Questionnaire
    (PPQ), 240, 305-309
Patients' rights and responsibili-
    ties, 124
PCCs (primary care clinicians), 179
PCPs, *see* Primary care physicians
Pediatrics training, 216, 221, 242
Performance standards, *see*
    Incentives; Quality assurance
Permanente Medical Group, *see*
    Kaiser-Permanente Northern
    California
Personal Health Improvement
    Program (PHIP),
    104-112, 186
  background, 104-106
  future uses of, 112
  health assessment tools, 110
  implementation, 107, 108
  marketing, 107, 109-110
  outcomes research, 111-112
  program elements, 106-107
  quality assurance, 110
  target population, 106
Pew Health Professions
    Commission, 221
PHIP, *see* Personal Health
    Improvement Program
Phobias, 157, 163-164
  agoraphobia, 155, 159
Physical therapists
  interdisciplinary education
    for, 222
  in Kaiser-Permanente team, 83
Physician assistants, 29, 179
Point-of-service technology, 72

Politics of healthcare policy, 45
Post-traumatic stress disorder
    (PTSD), 157, 162
PPQ (Patient Problem
    Questionnaire), 240, 305-309
Practice guidelines, Kaiser-
    Permanente, 76-77, 84
Pre-authorization, 39, 41
Pregnancy
  high-risk, case management, 70
  substance abuse in
    alcohol screening, 170, 173
    Early Start Program, 20,
      55, 78
    prevalence, 20
Prejudices of physician, 132
Presurgery relaxation programs,
    55, 241
Prevention programs, *see also*
    Disease management; Patient
    education
  in BCBSMA/Raytheon collabo-
    ration, 59, 60, 61, 64-65,
    68-69, 70-72, 74
  in group practices, 125-126
  in OSC structural model, 23
  outcomes research on,
    111-112, 193
  for prenatal substance abuse,
    20, 55, 78
Primary care physicians (PCPs),
    see also Consultation;
    Integration of primary care
    and behavioral health;
    Referral; Training, of primary
    care physicians
  anxiety disorders and, 155,
    157-158, 164
  avoidance of behavioral issues,
    29, 35-36, 230, 239
  behavioral disorders presenting,
    133-135
    differentiating from medical
      illness, 129-132
    missed diagnosis, 20, 130,
      237-238, 277
  behavioral healthcare by, 27,
    35, 139, 240-242,
    276-279
    appropriate conditions, 93
    billing issues, 43, 130
    case example, 41-44
    efficacy of, 24
  burnout of, 133
  chronic illness providers desig-
    nated as, 40
  culture of, 129, 132
  depression and (*see* Depression,
    PCPs and)
  disease management by, 207

  doctor-patient relationship,
    132-133, 244
  interface with behavioral
    health, 17-19, 136-137
  outcomes assessment, comput-
    erized, 229-234
  psychotropic medications and,
    20, 27-28
  risk pools and, 49-51
  somatization and, 179-180,
    182, 187-189
  substance abuse and, 167,
    173-176
  time limitations, 29, 43, 130
PRIME-MD, 43, 130, 131, 303-304
  anxiety disorders and, 158
  lack of physician accep-
    tance, 240
  somatization and, 184
Privileging, for behavioral health
    providers, 39-40, 41, 125
Problem drinker, definition
    of, 168
PROS (Psychosocial Review of
    Systems), 130
Protocols, clinical, 125, 241
Providers, *see* Behavioral health
    providers; Primary care
    physicians
Psychiatric disorders, *see*
    Behavioral health disorders
Psychiatric nurses
  inpatient consultation by, 39
  on multidisciplinary teams, 185
  role in managed care, 10, 27, 29
Psychiatrists
  consultation-liaison sub-
    specialty, 9-10
  definition of, 286
  reimbursement issues, 41
  slide show with lecture notes,
    255-288
  consultation with, 42
    for depression, 282
    in Harvard Pilgrim depres-
      sion program, 94, 96, 97
    inpatient case example,
      38-41
  historical roles, 7, 9-10
  on multidisciplinary teams, 185
  referral to, 136
    for depression, 147, 150, 151
    in Kaiser-Permanente system,
      75, 84
    patient resistance, 3
  role in managed care, 10,
    27-29
Psychological Factors Affecting
    a Medical Condition
    (DSM-IV), 183

INDEX

Psychological testing
  by clinical psychologists, 136
  cost-effectiveness of, 28
Psychologists
  medication and, 28, 39
  on multidisciplinary teams, 185
  referral to, 136
  role in managed care, 10, 27–28
  training of
    current models, 216–217
    historical perspectives, 213–214
    integrated with primary care medicine, 213, 218, 222–223, 226–227
    managed care and, 217, 218, 224
    potential changes, 217–218
Psychosis
  referral to behavioral health provider, 147, 151
  screening for, 184
Psychosocial medicine, see Biopsychosocial model
Psychosocial Review of Systems (PROS), 130
Psychosocial support services
  in chronic illness, 37, 44–45
Psychosomatic medicine, see also Somatization
  Academy of Psychosomatic Medicine, 255, 286
  future of, 190
  historical perspectives, 6–7, 9–10
Psychotherapy, see also Cognitive-behavioral therapy
  for depression, 145, 147
  future of, 28
  managed care and, 218
  by nondoctoral-level clinicians, 217
  outcomes research, 194
  by psychologists, 136
Public policy, 45
Purchasers, see Employers

Quality assurance
  annotated bibliography on, 251
  NCQA standards, 30, 122–126, 207
  quality improvement programs, 122–123, 126
  Total Quality Management, 21, 220, 221
Questionnaires, see also Health assessment surveys; Screening instruments
  for outcome assessment, 231, 232

Raytheon, see Blue Cross and Blue Shield/Raytheon Collaboration
Records, see Confidentiality; Medical records
Reductionism, 10, 35
Referral, see also Access to behavioral healthcare; Consultation
  to PCP by telephone line, 196, 197, 200, 201, 203–206
  by PCP to behavioral health provider, 19, 37
  for anxiety disorders, 164
  barriers to, 186–187, 230
  for depression, 145, 147, 150, 151
  noncompliance with, 20, 90–91, 155, 189
  for somatization, 186–188
  standards for, 123–124
  by PCP to substance abuse program, 174, 175
Reflection, of patient emotions, 149, 151
Reimbursement, see also Capitation; Financial structure of integrated systems
  copayments for behavioral healthcare, 21–22, 239
  in fragmented systems, 18
    inpatient case example, 38–41
    outpatient case example, 43
  for psychosocial services, in chronic illness, 44–45
Relaxation methods
  for anxiety disorders, 159, 161, 162, 163, 164
  at complementary care center, 241
  presurgery, 55, 241
  for somatization, 186
Requests for Proposals, 45
Research, see also Outcomes research
  breast cancer, psychological study, 68
Resistance to treatment, see Patient adherence; Stigma of behavioral disorders
Revia (naltrexone), 174
Rewards, as provider incentives, 48–49, 50
Risk pools, 49–51
Risk sharing, 41, 49–51
  for behavioral health providers, 18, 50–51
  medical cost offsets and, 52–55

Scientist-practitioner model, 213–214

SCL-90R (Symptom Checklist 90 Revised), 110, 184
Screening
  for alcohol abuse, 168–172
    in BCBSMA/Raytheon collaboration, 72
    in pregnancy, 170, 173
  for anxiety disorders, 158, 159
  biopsychosocial, 130, 197
  for depression
    in BCBSMA/Raytheon collaboration, 70, 72
    Beck Depression Inventory, 184
    in Delta/CIGNA/MCC initiative, 90, 91
    in Harvard Pilgrim program, 94–95, 97
    National Depression Screening Day, 16
    simplified test, 94, 95
  for drug abuse, 168–169, 171–172
  for psychiatric disorders, 43, 130, 131–132, 184
  OQ-10 questionnaire, 232
  in PHIP, 110
  routine, 238
  for somatization, 184
Screening instruments, see also PPQ; PRIME-MD; SCL-90R; SDDS-PC
  accuracy of, 169
  as behavioral lab tests, 230
  computer-assisted, by telephone, 131, 240, 297
  improvements needed, 239–240
SDDS-PC, 43, 131, 297–301
  anxiety disorders and, 158
  in Delta/CIGNA/MCC initiative, 90
  lack of physician acceptance, 240
  somatization and, 184
Secondary gain, 131, 134
Sensitivity, of screening test, 169
Shareholders, integration and, 22
Short-term therapy, see Cognitive-behavioral therapy; Supportive counseling
Simple phobias, 157, 163–164
Social phobias, 157, 164
Social workers
  interdisciplinary training for, 222
  on multidisciplinary teams, 185
  referral to, 136
  role in managed care, 10, 27–28, 29

Somatization, 179-190; see also
Psychosomatic medicine
common complaints, 182, 237
comorbidity with mental disorders, 181, 186
cultural factors, 183
definitions of, 106, 179, 180
detection of, 183-184
DSM-IV disorders, 179, 180-181, 183
economic impact, 106, 182, 184, 267
functional impairment, 274
future directions, 190
at Integration Clinic, 3-4
vs. medical illness, 183
multidisciplinary team approach, 184-186
outcomes assessment, 189-190
Personal Health Improvement Program and, 106-107, 109, 111, 186
predisposing factors, 181
prevalence, 106, 182
psychiatric consultation, 283
referral to behavioral health providers, 186-188
treatment issues, 179-180, 182, 188, 189
Somatization disorder *(DSM-IV)*, 179, 180-181, 183
Somatoform disorders *(DSM-IV)*, 179, 180-181, 183
Specialty risk pools, 49, 50
Specificity, of screening test, 169
Stigma of behavioral disorders, 3, 18-19, 129, 239
with depression, 140, 141, 148, 151
Delta/CIGNA/MCC initiative and, 89, 91
medical cost offsets and, 87
reduced by routine screening, 238
with somatization, 186
Stress management
Personal Health Improvement Program as, 111-112, 186
for physicians, 133
in primary care setting, 29, 30, 42
workplace screening and, 238
Subcapitation, 47, 48
Substance abuse, 167-176
affective disorders and, 141
definitions of terms, 167-168
employer programs, 195, 196
excess medical costs with, 16, 19-20, 270

physician attitudes, 167
in pregnancy
Early Start Program, 20, 55, 78
effect of early intervention, 173
prevalence, 20
screening instruments, 170, 173
prevalence, 167, 168, 270
in pregnancy, 20
screening
alcohol in pregnancy, 78, 170, 173
in BCBSMA/Raytheon collaboration, 72
indications for, 168-169
instruments for, 169-171, 173
system supports for, 171-172
treatment
brief interventions, 172-174
by carve-outs, 30, 38-39
follow-up, 173, 174-175
integrated care, 171-172, 175
in Kaiser-Permanente, 76-77, 78, 80, 83, 84
medical cost offsets, 16, 51, 281
pharmacotherapy, 174
primary care physician's role, 167, 173-176
referral to specialized programs, 174
telephone consultation, 197, 198, 201-202
Subsyndromal anxiety and depression, 186, 187, 238
Subsyndromal somatization, 179
Suicidal ideation
with chemical dependency, 174
psychiatric evaluation for, 147, 151
questioning patient about, 148, 150
Suicide, 133, 140
with panic disorder, 155, 159
Support groups
for anxiety disorders, 162
for breast cancer patients, 68
Supportive counseling
for adjustment disorder with anxious mood, 161-162
for depression, 145, 147
for post-traumatic stress disorder, 162
by psychologist, 136
Surveying questions, 148
Symptom Checklist 90 Revised (SCL-90R), 110, 184

Team approaches, 10, 37, 126; see also Integration of primary care and behavioral health
in BCBSMA/Raytheon collaboration, 63-64, 73-74
education for, 222
in Kaiser-Permanente primary care, 83-85
for management of somatization, 184-186
virtual, by computer, 22
Technology, see also Computer systems; Web sites
for BCBSMA/Raytheon collaboration, 72-73
Telephone consultation services
in BCBSMA/Raytheon collaboration, 70-71
employer ratings of, 195-196
NurseLine, 204-207
Optum Care24 biopsychosocial model, 196-199
Telephone screening, computer-assisted, 131, 240, 297
Testing, see Medical tests, unnecessary; Psychological testing; Screening
Time limitations, 29, 43, 130
Total Quality Management (TQM), 21, 220, 221
Training, of behavioral health providers
about medical problems, 22, 80, 242
on BCBSMA integrated team, 63-64
psychiatrists, new roles, 28-29
psychologists
current models, 216-217
historical perspectives, 213-214
integrated with primary care, 213, 218, 222-223, 226-227
managed care and, 217, 218, 224
potential changes, 217-218
Training, of primary care physicians
about behavioral disorders, 36, 42-43, 238, 242
depression management, 139
historical efforts, 9, 10
need for, 19, 20, 22, 35, 44
somatization, 187-188
family medicine training
current models, 219-220
financing for, 223-224, 242
historical perspectives, 9, 215-216

Training, of primary care physicians, family medicine training (*cont.*)
    integrated with behavioral health, 10, 213, 218, 219–220
    managed care and, 220, 221
    potential changes, 220–221
    residency curriculum, 219, 228
  proposed changes, 221
  in successful models of integration
    BCBSMA/Raytheon collaboration, 63–64
    Harvard Pilgrim depression program, 95–96
    Kaiser-Permanente, 80
Trans-disciplinary, definition of, 222
Treatment algorithms, 125, 241
Treatment outcome, *see* Outcomes assessment; Outcomes research
Treatment planning, computerized, 231–232, 233–234
Triage, *see* Access to behavioral healthcare
TWEAK questionnaire, 173

Undertreatment of behavioral health disorders, 13
  with capitation, 22
  depression, 16, 19, 20, 140
Uni-disciplinary education, 219, 221
United HealthCare Corporation, 193
US West, high utilizers and, 99–104
Utilization management
  in integrated systems, 124
  with telephone consultation, 206–207
Utilization rates, *see also* High utilizers; Risk sharing
  annotated bibliography on, 247–248
  copayments and, 21–22, 239
  in cost models, 47
  incentives and, 48, 49
  medical cost offsets and, 53, 87–88
  reduction in integrated system, 84

Violence, *see* Domestic violence

Washington Business Group on Health, 21, 23
Ways to Wellness, 104–105, 106, 110, 111
Web sites, *see also* Internet
  for health plans, 21, 72
Wellness programs, *see* Patient education; Personal Health Improvement Program; Prevention programs
Winnicott, Donald, 6–7, 9, 10
Withhold arrangements, of HMOs, 49
Workers' compensation
  case management for, 22–23, 30, 99–100, 103
  primary care physician and, 134
Workplace screening programs, 238
Work-related cost offsets, 87–88
Work-related problems, *see also* Absence management; Absenteeism
  telephone consultation for, 202
Worried well, 180

Zung Self-rating Depression Scale, 70, 184